Clinical Biochemistry

AN ILLUSTRATED COLOUR TEXT

Commissioning Editor: Timothy Horne
Development Editor: Hannah Kenner
Project Manager: Christine Johnston
Design Direction: Erik Bigland
Illustration Manager: Gillian Richards

Clinical Biochemistry

AN ILLUSTRATED COLOUR TEXT

Allan Gaw MD PhD FRCPath FFPM
Director
Glasgow Clinical Research Facility
Glasgow, UK

Michael J. Murphy FRCP Edin FRCPath
Clinical Senior Lecturer
Division of Pathology and Neuroscience
University of Dundee
Dundee, UK

Robert A. Cowan BSc PhD
Formerly Lecturer in Pathological Biochemistry
Department of Pathological Biochemistry
University of Glasgow
Glasgow, UK

Denis St. J. O'Reilly MSc MD FRCP FRCPath
Consultant Clinical Biochemist
Department of Clinical Biochemistry
University of Glasgow
Glasgow, UK

Michael J. Stewart PhD FRCPath
Director, Forensic Pathology Service
Department of Health
Pretoria
South Africa

James Shepherd PhD FRCP FRCPath FMedSci FRSE
Formerly Professor of Vascular Biochemistry
Glasgow Royal Infirmary
Glasgow, UK

Illustrated by Cactus Design and Illustration, Robert Britton and the authors

FOURTH EDITION

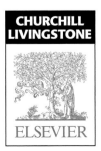

CHURCHILL
LIVINGSTONE

ELSEVIER

EDINBURGH   LONDON   NEW YORK   OXFORD   PHILADELPHIA   ST LOUIS   SYDNEY   TORONTO   2008

CHURCHILL
LIVINGSTONE
ELSEVIER

First edition 1995
Second edition 1999
Third edition 2004
Fourth edition 2008

ISBN 978-0-443-06932-1

British Library Cataloguing in Publication Data
A catalogue record for this book is available from the British Library

Library of Congress Cataloging in Publication Data
A catalog record for this book is available from the Library of Congress

---

Note
Knowledge and best practice in this field are constantly changing.
As new research and experience broaden our knowledge, changes
in practice, treatment and drug therapy may become necessary
or appropriate. Readers are advised to check the most current
information provided (i) on procedures featured or (ii) by the
manufacturer of each product to be administered, to verify the
recommended dose or formula, the method and duration of
administration, and contraindications. It is the responsibility of the
practitioner, relying on their own experience and knowledge of
the patient, to make diagnoses, to determine dosages and the best
treatment for each individual patient, and to take all appropriate
safety precautions. To the fullest extent of the law, neither the
Publisher nor the Authors assume any liability for any injury and/
or damage to persons or property arising out or related to any use
of the material contained in this book.

The Publisher

ELSEVIER your source for books,
journals and multimedia
in the health sciences

www.elsevierhealth.com

Working together to grow
libraries in developing countries

www.elsevier.com | www.bookaid.org | www.sabre.org

ELSEVIER   **BOOK AID**
International   **Sabre Foundation**

The
publisher's
policy is to use
**paper manufactured
from sustainable forests**

Printed in China

Preface to the fourth edition

It is heartening that more than a decade after the first edition of this book appeared it is still very widely read and deemed to be a useful addition to academic bookshelves throughout the world. With translations into French, Italian, Spanish, Portuguese, Chinese, Japanese and Greek we have not merely amassed a colourful collection of trophies on our own bookshelves – rather we now find ourselves speaking to an even wider audience than we originally envisaged.

We have taken this opportunity to update many sections of the book, for once again we find ourselves at the centre of a moving field. The sections on renal disease, potassium and hypertension have been completely rewritten, and virtually no double-page spread has escaped the authors' pen. We have also updated a number of photographic illustrations. Guiding us in these revisions we have had helpful comments from academic and clinical colleagues and students around the world. If there was a better way to say or illustrate it we have tried to find it and we have focused on clarity, but not, we hope, at the expense of brevity.

With each new edition this book continues to evolve. It has had to adapt to new practices both in clinical medicine and in education. It is, of course, only by changing that we can hope that our book remains fit for its original purpose – introducing Clinical Biochemistry to students across the health professions. We hope that the edition we now present is superior to its predecessors and will serve its users, both students and teachers, well.

Allan Gaw
Michael J. Murphy
Robert A. Cowan
Denis St. J. O'Reilly
Michael J. Stewart
James Shepherd

Preface to the first edition

Medical education is changing, so the educational tools we use must change too. This book was designed and written for those studying Clinical Biochemistry for the first time. We have placed the greatest emphasis on the foundations of the subject while covering all those topics found in a medical undergraduate course on Clinical Biochemistry. The format is not that of a traditional textbook. By arranging the subject in double-page learning units we offer the student a practical and efficient way to assimilate the necessary facts, while presenting opportunities for problem solving and self-testing with case histories. Clinical notes present channels for lateral thinking about each learning unit, and boxes summarizing the key points may be used by the student to facilitate rapid revision of the text.

The book is divided into four main sections. Introducing Clinical biochemistry outlines the background to our subject. In Core biochemistry we cover the routine analyses that would form the basic repertoire of most hospital laboratories. The Endocrinology section covers thyroid, adrenal, pituitary and gonadal function testing, and in Specialized investigations we discuss less commonly requested, but important analyses.

This book relies on illustrations and diagrams to make many of its points and these should be viewed as integral to the text. The reader is assumed to have a basic knowledge of anatomy, physiology and biochemistry and to be primarily interested in the subject of Clinical Biochemistry from a user's point of view rather than that of a provider. To this end we have not covered analytical aspects except in a few instances where these have direct relevance to the interpretation of biochemical tests. What we have tried to do is present Clinical Biochemistry as a subject intimately connected to Clinical Medicine, placing emphasis on the appropriate use of biochemical tests and their correct interpretation in a clinical setting.

Glasgow
1995

Allan Gaw, Robert A. Cowan
Denis St. J. O'Reilly
Michael J. Stewart and
James Shepherd

Acknowledgements

The following have helped in many different ways in the preparation of the first, second, third and fourth editions of this book: in providing illustrations, in discussions, and in suggesting improvements to the manuscript.

Bryan Adamson
Bill Bartlett
Sally Beard
Graham Beastall
Iain Boyle
Sharon Boyle
John Card
Sam Chakraverty
Brain Cook
Ellie Dow
Frances Dryburgh
Andy Duncan
Gordon Fell
Roy Fisher
Alan Foulis

Callum Fraser
Moira Gaw
Dairena Gaffney
Brian Gordon
Christina Gray
Helen Gray
David Halls
John Hinnie
Fiona Jenkinson
Jennie Johnston
Witsanu Kumthornthip
Kim Lim
Grace Lindsay
Greig Louden
Tom MacDonald
Jean McAllister
Neil McConnell
Derek McLean
Ellen Malcolm
Hazel Miller
Heather Murray
Brian Neilly

John Paterson
Nigel Rabie
Margaret Rudge
Naveed Sattar
Rajeev Srivastava
Heather Stevenson
Ian Stewart
Judith Strachan
Mike Wallace
Janet Warren
Philip Welsby
Peter H. Wise
Helen Wright

Special mention must be made of our editorial and design team at Elsevier without whose encouragement and wise counsel this book would not have been written.

Contents

Introducing Clinical Biochemistry

The clinical biochemistry laboratory

Clinical biochemistry, chemical pathology and clinical chemistry are all names for the subject of this book, that branch of laboratory medicine in which chemical and biochemical methods are applied to the study of disease (Fig. 1). While in theory this embraces all non-morphological studies, in practice it is usually, though not exclusively, confined to studies on blood and urine because of the relative ease in obtaining such specimens. Analyses are made on other body fluids, however, such as gastric aspirate and cerebrospinal fluid. Clinical biochemical tests comprise over one-third of all hospital laboratory investigations.

The use of biochemical tests

Biochemical investigations are involved, to varying degrees, in every branch of clinical medicine. The results of biochemical tests may be of use in diagnosis and in the monitoring of treatment. Biochemical tests may also be of value in screening for disease or in assessing the prognosis once a diagnosis has been made (Fig. 2). The biochemistry laboratory is often involved in research into the biochemical basis of disease and in clinical trials of new drugs.

Core biochemistry

Biochemical facilities are provided in every hospital, although not necessarily to the same extent. All biochemistry laboratories provide the 'core analyses', commonly requested tests that are of value in many patients, on a frequent basis (Table 1). The clinician will often request specific groupings of tests, and clinical biochemistry assumes a cryptic language of its own as request forms arrive at laboratory reception for 'U & Es' (urea and electrolytes), 'LFTs' (liver function tests) or 'blood gases'.

Specialized tests

There are a variety of specialties within clinical biochemistry (Table 1). Not every laboratory is equipped to carry out all possible biochemistry requests. Large departments may act as reference centres where less commonly asked for tests are performed. For some tests that are needed in the diagnosis of rare diseases, there may be just one or two laboratories in the country offering the service.

Urgent samples

All clinical biochemistry laboratories provide facilities for urgent tests, and can expedite the analysis of some

Table 1 **The clinical biochemistry repertoire**
Core biochemical tests
■ Sodium, potassium, chloride and bicarbonate
■ Urea and creatinine
■ Calcium and phosphate
■ Total protein and albumin
■ Bilirubin and alkaline phosphatase
■ Alanine aminotransferase (ALT) and aspartate aminotransferase (AST)
■ Thyroxine (T_4) and Thyroid Stimulating Hormone (TSH)
■ γ-glutamyl transpeptidase (γGT)
■ Creatine kinase (CK)
■ H^+, PCO_2 and PO_2 (blood gases)
■ Glucose
■ Amylase
Specialized tests
■ Hormones
■ Specific proteins
■ Trace elements
■ Vitamins
■ Drugs
■ Lipids and lipoproteins
■ DNA analyses

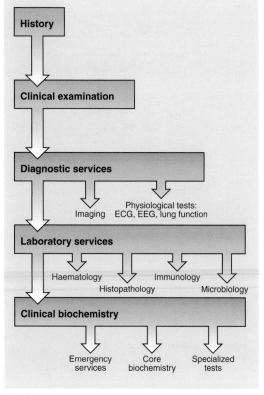

Fig. 1 **The place of clinical biochemistry in medicine.**

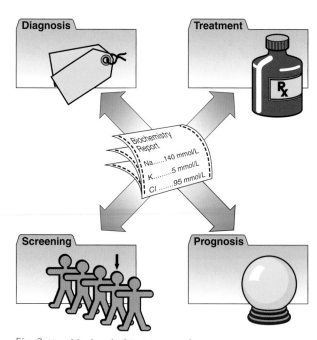

Fig. 2 **How biochemical tests are used.**

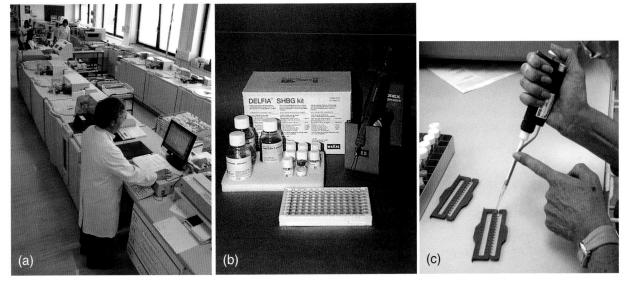

Fig. 3 **Analysing the samples: (a)** the automated analyser, **(b)** 'kit' analyser and **(c)** manual methods.

samples more quickly than others. Laboratories also offer an 'out of hours' service, in those cases where analyses are required during the night or at weekends. The rationale for performing such tests is based on whether the test result is likely to influence the immediate treatment of the patient.

Some larger hospitals have laboratory facilities away from the main laboratory, such as in the theatre suite or adjacent to the diabetic clinic (see pp. 8–9).

Automation and computerization

Most laboratories are now computerized, and the use of bar-coding of specimens and automated methods of analysis allows a high degree of productivity and improves the quality of service. Links to computer terminals on wards and GP surgeries allow direct access to results by the requesting clinician.

Test repertoire

There are over 400 different tests that may be carried out in clinical biochemistry laboratories. They vary from the very simple, such as the measurement of sodium, to the highly complex, such as DNA analysis, screening for drugs, or differentiation of lipoprotein variants. Many high volume tests are done on large automated machines. Less frequently performed tests may be conveniently carried out by using commercially prepared reagents packaged in 'kit' form. Some analyses are carried out manually (Fig. 3). Assays that are performed infrequently may be sent to another laboratory where the test is carried out regularly. This has both cost and reliability benefits.

Dynamic tests require several specimens, timed in relation to a biochemical stimulus, such as a glucose load in the glucose tolerance test for the diagnosis of diabetes mellitus. Some tests provide a clearcut answer to a question; others are only a part of the diagnostic jigsaw.

This book describes how the results of biochemistry analyses are interpreted, rather than how the analyses are performed in the laboratory. An important function of many departments is research and development. Advances in analytical methodology and in our understanding of disease continue to change the test repertoire of the biochemistry department as the value of new tests is appreciated.

Laboratory personnel

As well as performing the analyses, the clinical biochemistry laboratory also provides a consultative service. The laboratory has on its staff both medical and scientific personnel, who are familiar with the clinical significance and the analytical performance of the test procedures, and they will readily give advice on the interpretation of the results. Do not be hesitant to take advantage of this advice, especially where a case is not straightforward.

Clinical note

The clinical biochemistry laboratory plays only a part in the overall assessment and management of the patient. For some patients, biochemical analyses may have little or no part in their diagnosis or the management of their illness. For others, many tests may be needed before a diagnosis is made, and repeated analyses may be required to monitor treatment over a long period.

The clinical biochemistry laboratory

■ Biochemical tests are used in diagnosis, monitoring treatment, screening and for prognosis.

■ Core biochemical tests are carried out in every biochemistry laboratory. Specialized tests may be referred to larger departments. All hospitals provide for urgent tests in the 'emergency laboratory'.

■ Laboratory personnel will readily give advice, based on their knowledge and experience, on the use of the biochemistry laboratory, on the appropriate selection of tests, and about the interpretation of results.

The use of the laboratory

Every biochemistry analysis should attempt to answer a question that the clinician has posed about the patient. Obtaining the correct answers can often seem to be fraught with difficulty.

Specimen collection

In order to carry out biochemical analyses, it is necessary that the laboratory be provided with both the correct specimen for the requested test, and also information that will ensure that the right test is carried out and the result returned to the requesting clinician with the minimum of delay. As much detail as possible should be included on the request form to help both laboratory staff and the clinician in the interpretation of results. This information can be very valuable when assessing a patient's progress over a period, or reassessing a diagnosis. Patient identification must be correct, and the request form should include some indication of the suspected pathology. The requested analyses should be clearly indicated. Request forms differ in design. Clinical biochemistry forms in Europe are conventionally coloured green.

A variety of specimens are used in biochemical analysis and these are shown in Table 1.

Blood specimens

If blood is collected into a plain tube and allowed to clot, after centrifugation a *serum* specimen is obtained (Fig. 1). For many biochemical analyses this will be the specimen recommended. In other cases, especially when the analyte in question is unstable and speed is necessary to obtain a specimen that can be frozen quickly, the blood is collected into a tube containing an anticoagulant such as heparin. When centrifuged, the supernatant is called *plasma*, which is almost identical to the cell-free fraction of blood but contains the anticoagulant as well.

Urine specimens

Urine specimen containers may include a preservative to inhibit bacterial growth, or acid to stabilize certain metabolites. They need to be large enough to hold a full 24-hour collection. Random urine samples are collected into small 'universal' containers.

Other specimen types

For some tests, specific body fluids or tissue may be required. There will be specific protocols for the handling

> Table 1 **Specimens used for biochemical analyses**
>
> - Venous blood, serum or plasma
> - Arterial blood
> - Capillary blood
> - Urine
> - Faeces
> - Cerebrospinal fluid (CSF)
> - Sputum and saliva
> - Tissue and cells
> - Aspirates, e.g.
>   pleural fluid
>   ascites
>   joint (synovial) fluid
>   intestinal (duodenal)
>   pancreatic pseudocysts
> - Calculi (stones)

and transport of these samples to the laboratory. Consult the local lab for advice.

Dangerous specimens

All specimens from patients with dangerous infections should be labelled with a yellow 'dangerous specimen' sticker. A similar label should be attached to the request form. Of most concern to the laboratory staff are hepatitis B and HIV.

Sampling errors

There are a number of potential errors that may contribute to the success or failure of the laboratory in providing the correct answers to the clinician's questions. Some of these problems arise when a clinician first obtains specimens from the patient.

- *Blood sampling technique.* Difficulty in obtaining a blood specimen may lead to haemolysis with consequent release of potassium and other red cell constituents.
- *Prolonged stasis during venepuncture.* Plasma water diffuses into the interstitial space and the serum or plasma sample obtained will be concentrated. Proteins and protein-bound components of plasma, such as calcium or thyroxine, will be falsely elevated.
- *Insufficient specimen.* It may prove to be impossible for the laboratory to measure everything requested on a small volume.
- *Errors in timing.* The biggest source of error in the measurement of any analyte in a 24-hour urine specimen is in the collection of an accurately timed volume of urine.
- *Incorrect specimen container.* For many analyses the blood must be collected into a container with anticoagulant and/or preservative. For example, samples for glucose should be collected into a special container containing fluoride, which inhibits glycolysis; otherwise the time taken to deliver the sample to the laboratory can affect the result. If a sample is collected into the wrong container, it should never be decanted into another type of tube. For example, blood that has been exposed, even briefly, to EDTA (an anticoagulant

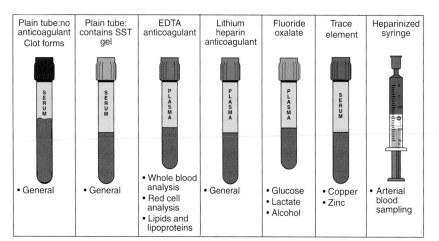

Plain tube: no anticoagulant Clot forms	Plain tube: contains SST gel	EDTA anticoagulant	Lithium heparin anticoagulant	Fluoride oxalate	Trace element	Heparinized syringe
SERUM	SERUM	PLASMA	PLASMA	PLASMA	SERUM	
• General	• General	• Whole blood analysis • Red cell analysis • Lipids and lipoproteins	• General	• Glucose • Lactate • Alcohol	• Copper • Zinc	• Arterial blood sampling

Fig. 1 **Blood specimen tubes for specific biochemical tests.** The colour-coded tubes are the vacutainers in use in the authors' hospital and laboratory.

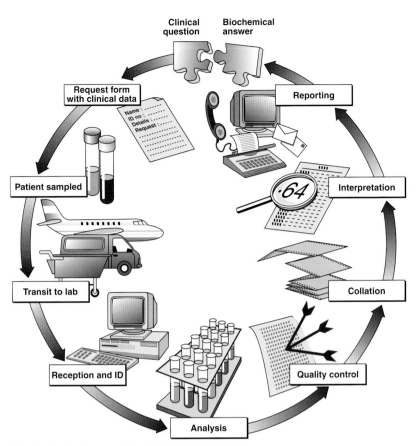

Fig. 2 **Circuit diagram of the clinical biochemistry process.**

Labels in figure: Clinical question · Biochemical answer · Request form with clinical data · Reporting · Patient sampled · Interpretation · Transit to lab · Collation · Reception and ID · Quality control · Analysis

Analysing the specimen

Once the form and specimen arrive at the laboratory reception, they are matched with a unique identifying number or bar-code. The average lab receives many thousands of requests and samples each day and it is important that all are clearly identified and never mixed up. Samples proceed through the laboratory as shown in Figure 2. All analytical procedures are quality controlled and the laboratory strives for reliability.

Once the results are available they are collated and a report is issued. Cumulative reports allow the clinician to see at a glance how the most recent result(s) compare with those tests performed previously, providing an aid to the monitoring of treatment (see p. 12).

Unnecessary testing

There can be no definite rules about the appropriateness, or otherwise, of laboratory testing because of the huge variety of clinical circumstances that may arise. Clinicians should always bear in mind that in requesting a biochemical test they should be asking a question of the laboratory. If not, both the clinician and the laboratory may be performing unnecessary work, with little benefit to the patient.

used in sample containers for lipids) will have a markedly reduced calcium concentration, approaching zero.

- *Inappropriate sampling site.* Blood samples should not be taken 'downstream' from an intravenous drip. It is not unheard of for the laboratory to receive a blood glucose request on a specimen taken from the same arm into which 5% glucose is being infused. Usually the results are biochemically incredible but it is just possible that they may be acted upon with disastrous consequences for the patient.
- *Incorrect specimen storage.* A blood sample stored overnight before being sent to the laboratory will

show falsely high potassium, phosphate and red cell enzymes, such as lactate dehydrogenase, because of leakage into the extracellular fluid from the cells.

Timing

Many biochemical tests are repeated at intervals. How often depends on how quickly significant changes are liable to occur, and there is little point in requesting repeat tests if a numerical change will not have an influence on treatment. The main reason for asking for an analysis to be performed on an urgent basis is that immediate treatment depends on the result.

Clinical note

Clinical biochemistry is but one branch of laboratory medicine. Specimens may be required for haematology, microbiology, virology, immunology and histopathology, and all require similar attention to detail in filling out request forms and obtaining the appropriate samples for analysis.

Case history 1

A blood specimen was taken from a 65-year-old women to check her serum potassium concentration as she had been on thiazide diuretics for some time. The GP left the specimen in his car and dropped it off at the laboratory on the way to the surgery the next morning.

Immediately after analysing the sample, the biochemist was on the phone to the GP. Why?

Comment on page 162

The use of the laboratory

- Each biochemistry test request should be thought of as a question about the patient; each biochemical result as an answer.
- Request forms and specimens must be correctly labelled to ensure that results can be communicated quickly to the clinician.
- Many biochemical tests are performed on serum, the supernatant obtained from centrifugation of clotted blood collected into a plain container. Others require plasma, the supernatant obtained when blood is prevented from clotting by an anticoagulant.
- A variety of sampling errors may invalidate results.

The interpretation of results

It can take considerable effort, and expense, to produce what may seem to be just numbers on pieces of paper. Understanding what these numbers mean is of crucial importance if the correct diagnosis is to be made, or if the patient's treatment is to be changed.

How biochemical results are expressed

Most biochemical analyses are quantitative, although simple qualitative or semi-quantitative tests, such as those for the presence of glucose in urine, are commonly encountered methods used for point of care testing. Many tests measure the amount of the analyte in a small volume of blood, plasma, serum, urine or some other fluid or tissue. Results are reported as concentrations, usually in terms of the number of moles in one litre (mol/L) (Table 1).

The concept of concentration is illustrated in Figure 1. The concentration of any analyte in a body compartment is a ratio: the amount of the substance dissolved in a known volume. Changes in concentration can occur for two reasons:

- The amount of the analyte can increase or decrease.
- The volume of fluid in which the analyte is dissolved can similarly change.

Enzymes are not usually expressed in moles but as enzyme activity in 'units'. Enzyme assays are carried out in such a way that the activity measured is directly proportional to the amount of enzyme present. Some hormone measurements are expressed as 'units' by comparison to standard reference preparations of known biological potency. Large molecules such as proteins are reported in mass units (grams or milligrams) per litre. Blood gas results (PCO_2 or PO_2) are expressed in kilopascals (kPa), the unit in which partial pressures are measured.

Variation in results

Biochemical measurements vary for two reasons. These are described as 'analytical variation' and 'biological variation'. Analytical variation is a function of analytical performance; biological variation is related to the actual changes that take place in patients' body fluids over a period of time.

Laboratory analytical performance

A number of terms describe biochemical results. These include:

- precision and accuracy
- sensitivity and specificity
- quality assurance
- reference ranges.

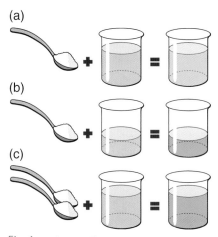

Fig. 1 **Understanding concentrations.**
Concentration is always dependent on two factors: the amount of solute and the amount of solvent. The concentration of the sugar solution in the beaker can be increased from 1 spoon/beaker **(a)** to 2 spoons/beaker by either decreasing the volume of solvent **(b)** or increasing the amount of solute **(c)**.

Precision and accuracy

Precision is the reproducibility of an analytical method. Accuracy defines how close the measured value is to the actual value. A good analogy is that of the shooting target. Figure 2 shows the scatter of results which might be obtained by someone with little skill, compared with that of someone with good precision where the results are closely grouped together. Even when the results are all close, they may not hit the centre of the target. Accuracy is therefore poor, as if the 'sights' are off. It is the objective in every biochemical method to provide good precision and accuracy. Automation of analyses has improved precision in most cases.

Analytical sensitivity and specificity

The analytical sensitivity of an assay is a measure of how little of the analyte the method can detect. Analytical specificity of an assay relates to how good the assay is at discriminating between the requested analyte and potentially interfering substances. These terms describing the analytical properties of tests should not be confused with 'test' specificity and sensitivity, as applied to the usefulness of various analyses (see below).

Quality assurance

Laboratory staff monitor performance of assays using quality control samples to give reassurance that the method is performing satisfactorily with the patients' specimens. Internal quality control samples are analysed regularly. The expected values are known and the actual results obtained are compared with previous values to monitor performance. In external quality assurance programmes, identical samples are distributed to laboratories; results are then compared.

Table 1 **Molar units**		
Mole	**Abbreviation**	**Definition**
Millimole	mmol	$\times 10^{-3}$ of a mole
Micromole	μmol	$\times 10^{-6}$
Nanomole	nmol	$\times 10^{-9}$
Picomole	pmol	$\times 10^{-12}$
Femtomole	fmol	$\times 10^{-15}$

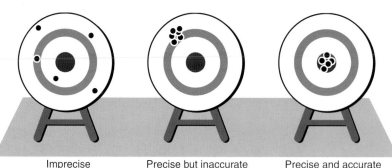

Imprecise · Precise but inaccurate · Precise and accurate

Fig. 2 **Precision and accuracy.**

Reference intervals

Analytical variation is generally less than that from biological variation. Biochemical test results are usually compared to a reference interval chosen arbitrarily to include 95% of the values found in healthy volunteers (Fig. 3). This means that by definition, 5% of any population will have a result outside the reference interval. In practice there are no rigid limits demarcating the diseased population from the healthy; however, the further a result is from the limits of the reference interval, the more likely it is to indicate pathology. In some situations it is useful to define 'action limits', at which appropriate intervention should be made in response to a biochemical result. An example of this is plasma cholesterol.

There is often a degree of overlap between the disease state and the 'normal value' (Fig. 3). An abnormal result in a patient who is subsequently found not to have the disease is called a 'false positive'. A 'normal result' in a patient who has the disease is a 'false negative'.

Specificity and sensitivity of tests

The specificity of a test measures how commonly negative results occur in people who do not have a disease. Sensitivity is a measure of the incidence of positive results in patients who are known to have a condition. As noted above, the use of the terms specificity and sensitivity in this context should not be confused with the same terms used to describe analytical performance. An ideal diagnostic test would be 100% sensitive, showing positive results in all diseased subjects, and 100% specific, with negative results in all persons free of the disease. Figure 3 shows the effect of changing the 'diagnostic cut-off value' on test specificity and sensitivity.

Biological factors affecting the interpretation of results

The discrimination between normal and abnormal results is affected by various physiological factors that must be considered when interpreting any given result. These include:

- *Sex.* Reference intervals for some analytes such as serum creatinine are different for men and women.
- *Age.* There may be different reference intervals for neonates, children, adults and the elderly.

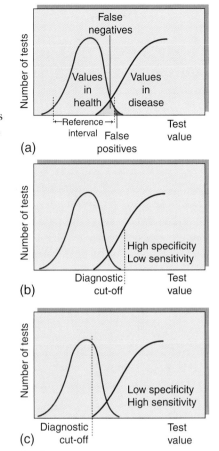

Fig. 3 **(a) Overlap of biochemical results in health and disease. (b) and (c) The effect of changing the diagnostic cut-off on test specificity and sensitivity**.

- *Diet.* The sample may be inappropriate if taken when the patient is fasting or after a meal.
- *Timing.* There may be variations during the day and night.
- *Stress and anxiety.* These may affect the analyte of interest.
- *Posture of the patient.* Redistribution of fluid may affect the result.
- *Effects of exercise.* Strenuous exercise can release enzymes from tissues.
- *Medical history.* Infection and/or tissue injury can affect biochemical values independently of the disease process being investigated.

- *Pregnancy.* This alters some reference intervals.
- *Menstrual cycle.* Hormone measurements will vary throughout the menstrual cycle.
- *Drug history.* Drugs may have specific effects on the plasma concentration of some analytes.

Other factors

When the numbers have been printed on the report form, they still have to be interpreted in the light of a host of variables. The clinician can refer to the patient or to the clinical notes, whereas the biochemist has only the information on the request form to consult.

The clinician may well ask the following questions on receiving a biochemistry report:

- 'Does the result fit with the history and clinical examination of the patient?'
- 'If the result is not what I expected, can I explain the discrepancy?'
- 'How can the result change my diagnosis or the way I am managing the patient?'
- 'What should I do next?'

What is done in response to a biochemistry report rests with the clinical judgement of the doctor. There is a maxim that doctors should always 'treat the patient, rather than the laboratory report'. The rest of this book deals with the biochemical investigation of patients and the interpretation of the results obtained.

Clinical note

It is important to realize that an abnormal result does not always indicate that a disease is present, nor a normal result that it is not. Beware of over-reacting to the slightly abnormal result in the otherwise healthy individual.

The interpretation of results

- Biochemistry results are often reported as concentrations. Concentrations change if the amount of the analyte changes or if the volume of solvent changes.
- Variability of results is caused by both analytical factors and biological factors.
- The reference range supplied with the test result is only a guide to the probability of the results being statistically 'normal' or 'abnormal'.
- Different reference intervals may apply depending on the age or sex of the patient.
- Sequential changes observed in cumulative reports when placed in clinical context are as important as the absolute value of the result.
- If a result does not accord with that expected for the patient, the finding should be discussed with the laboratory reporting office and a repeat test arranged.

Point of care testing

The methods for measuring some biological compounds in blood and urine have become so robust and simple to use that measurements can be made away from the laboratory – by the patient's bedside, in the ward sideroom, at the GP's surgery, in the home or even in the shopping centre! Convenience and the desire to know results quickly, as well as expectation of commercial profit by the manufacturers of the tests, have been the major stimuli for these developments. Experience has shown that motivated individuals, e.g. diabetics, frequently perform the tests as well as highly qualified professionals.

The immediate availability of results at the point of care can enable the appropriate treatment to be instituted quickly and patients' fears can be allayed. However, it is important to ensure that the limitations of any test and the significance of the results are appreciated by the tester to avoid inappropriate intervention or unnecessary anxiety.

Outside the laboratory

Table 1 shows what can be measured in a blood sample outside the normal laboratory setting. The most common blood test outside the laboratory is the determination of glucose concentration, in a finger stab sample, at home or in the clinic. Diabetic patients who need to monitor their blood glucose on a regular basis can do so at home or at work using one of many commercially available pocket-sized instruments.

Figure 1 shows a portable bench analyser. These analysers may be used to monitor various analytes in blood and urine and are often used in outpatient clinics.

Table 2 lists urine constituents that can be measured away from the laboratory. Many are conveniently measured, semi-quantitatively, using test strips which are dipped briefly into a fresh urine sample. Any excess urine is removed, and the result assessed after a specified time by comparing a colour change with a code on the side of the test strip container. The information obtained from such tests is of variable value to the tester, whether patient or clinician.

The tests commonly performed away from the laboratory can be categorized as follows:
A. *Tests performed in medical or nursing settings.* They clearly give valuable information and allow the practitioner to reassure the patient or family or initiate further investigations or treatment.
B. *Tests performed in the home, or non-clinical setting.* They can give valuable information when properly and appropriately used.
C. *Alcohol tests.* These are sometimes used to assess fitness to drive. In clinical practice alcohol measurements need to be carefully interpreted. In the Accident and Emergency setting, extreme caution must be taken before one can fully ascribe confusion in a patient with head injury to the effects of alcohol, a common complicating feature in such patients.

Table 1 **Common tests on blood performed away from the laboratory**	
Analyte	**Used when investigating**
Blood gases	Acid–base status
Glucose	Diabetes mellitus
Urea	Renal disease
Creatinine	Renal disease
Bilirubin	Neonatal jaundice
Therapeutic drugs	Compliance or toxicity
Salicylate	Detection of poisoning
Paracetamol	Detection of poisoning
Cholesterol	Coronary heart disease risk
Alcohol	Fitness to drive/confusion, coma

Table 2 **Tests on urine performed away from the laboratory**	
Analyte	**Used when investigating**
Ketones	Diabetic ketoacidosis
Protein	Renal disease
Red cells/haemoglobin	Renal disease
Bilirubin	Liver disease and jaundice
Urobilinogen	Jaundice/haemolysis
pH	Renal tubular acidosis
Glucose	Diabetes mellitus
HCG	Pregnancy test

Methodology

It is a feature of many sideroom tests that their simplicity disguises the use of sophisticated methodology. A home pregnancy test method involves an elegant application of monoclonal antibody technology to detect the human chorionic gonadotrophin (HCG), which is produced by the developing embryo (Fig. 2). The test is simple to carry out; a few drops of urine are placed in the sample window, and the result is shown within 5 minutes. The addition of the urine solubilizes a monoclonal antibody for HCG, which is covalently bound to tiny blue beads. A second monoclonal antibody specific for another region of the HCG molecule, is firmly attached in a line at the result window. If HCG is present in the sample it is bound by the first antibody, forming a blue bead–antibody–HCG complex. As the urine diffuses through the strip, any HCG present becomes bound at the second antibody site and this concentrates the blue bead complex in a line – a positive result. A third antibody recognizes the constant

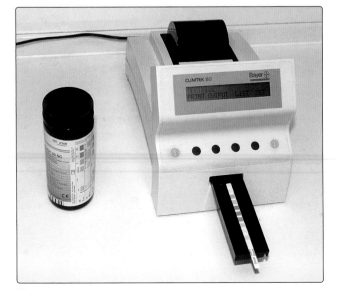

Fig. 1 **A portable bench analyser.**

region of the first antibody and binds the excess, thus providing a control to show that sufficient urine had been added to the test strip, the most likely form of error.

General problems

The obvious advantages in terms of time saving and convenience to both patient and clinician must be balanced by a number of possible problems in the use of these tests. They include:

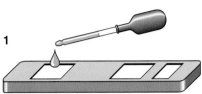

1

A urine sample is applied to the test strip.

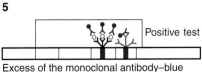

2

HCG   Anti HCG antibody
2nd HCG specific antibodies
3rd antibody

Urine saturates absorbent pad and begins to move along test strip.

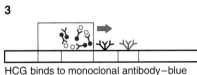

3

HCG binds to monoclonal antibody–blue bead complex, which then moves along the plate as the urine diffuses.

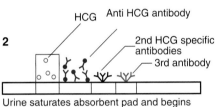

4   attached to blue beads

The HCG–antibody–blue bead complex binds to a 2nd HCG specific antibody fixed to the plate along a straight line. This produces a blue line on the plate.

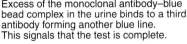

5   Positive test

Excess of the monoclonal antibody–blue bead complex in the urine binds to a third antibody forming another blue line.
This signals that the test is complete.

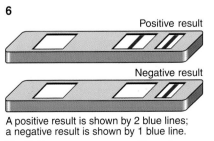

6   Positive result

Negative result

A positive result is shown by 2 blue lines; a negative result is shown by 1 blue line.

Fig. 2 **How a pregnancy test kit works.**

- *Cost.* Many of these tests are expensive alternatives to the traditional methods used in the laboratory. This additional expense must be justified, for example, on the basis of convenience or speed of obtaining the result.
- *Responsibility.* The person performing the assay outside the laboratory (the operator) must assume a number of responsibilities that would normally be those of the laboratory staff. There is the responsibility to perform the assay appropriately and to provide an answer that is accurate, precise and meaningful. The operator must also record the result, so that others may be able to find it (e.g. in the patient's notes), and interpret the result in its clinical context.

Analytical problems

Many problems under this heading will have little to do with the assay technology but will be due to operator errors. Tests designed for use outside the laboratory are robust but are by no means foolproof. Most operators will not be trained laboratory technicians but patients, nurses or clinicians. If an assay is to be performed well these individuals must be trained in its use. This may require the reading of a simple set of instructions (e.g. a home pregnancy test) or attending short training sessions (e.g. the ward-based blood gas analyser). The most commonly encountered analytical errors arise because of failure to:

- calibrate an instrument
- clean an instrument
- use quality control materials
- store reagents or strips in appropriate conditions.

All of these problems can be readily overcome by following instructions carefully. Regular maintenance of the equipment may be necessary, and simple quality control checks should be performed. It should always be possible to arrange simple quality control cross checks with the main biochemistry laboratory.

Interpretive problems

Even when analytically correct results are obtained, there are other problems which must be overcome before the exercise can be considered a success. The general appropriateness of the test must be considered. If an assay is performed in an individual of inappropriate age, sex, or at the wrong time of day, or month, then the result may be clinically meaningless. Similarly, the nature of the sample collected for analysis should be considered when interpreting the result. Where the results seem at odds with the clinical situation, interference from contaminants (e.g. detergents in urine containers) should be considered as should cross reactivity of the assay with more than one analyte (e.g. haemoglobin and myoglobin).

Any biochemical assay takes all these potential problems into account. However, with extra-laboratory testing, correct interpretation of the result is no longer the laboratory's responsibility but that of the operator.

The future

There is no doubt that in the future, biochemical testing of patients at the point of care will become practical for many of the analytes currently measured in the laboratory. There is, however, likely to be much debate about costs and the clinical usefulness of such non-laboratory-based analyses.

Case history 2

At a village fete, a local charity group was fundraising by performing certain sideroom tests. An 11-year-old boy was found to have a blood glucose of 14.4 mmol/L. His family was concerned, and an hour later his cousin, a recently diagnosed diabetic, confirmed the hyperglycaemia with his home monitoring equipment, and found glycosuria +++.

- What is the significance of these findings?

Comment on page 162.

Point of care testing

- Many biochemical tests are performed outside the normal laboratory setting, for the convenience of patient and clinician.
- Although apparently simple, such tests may yield erroneous results because of operator errors.
- It is important that advice be readily available to interpret each result in the clinical context.

Reference intervals

Below is a list of reference intervals for a selection of tests that are performed in clinical biochemistry laboratories. The intervals shown are those used at Glasgow Royal Infirmary and may differ elsewhere. Ideally, individual laboratories should use reference intervals that are based on values obtained from subjects appropriately selected from local populations, but this is not always feasible. For some analytes, e.g. glucose and cholesterol, conversion factors are supplied to allow different units to be compared. The list is not intended to be comprehensive; it is merely provided for guidance in answering the cases and examples in this book. Please note that age- and sex-specific reference intervals (not shown) are available for a range of analytes including alkaline phosphatase, creatinine, and urate. Glucose, insulin and triglyceride all rise postprandially and should, where possible, be measured in the fasting state.

ALPHABETICAL LIST OF REFERENCE INTERVALS – GENERAL

(All reference intervals listed are for serum measurements in adults unless otherwise stated)

Alanine aminotransferase (ALT)	3–55 U/L	Iron binding capacity (IBC)	45–77 µmol/L
Albumin	40–52 g/L	Lactate	0.7–1.8 mmol/L
Alkaline phosphatase (ALP)	80–280 U/L	Lactate dehydrogenase (LDH)	230–525 U/L
Aspartate aminotransferase (AST)	12–48 U/L		1.0–8.6 U/L (adult
Amylase	70–300 U/L		males up to
Bicarbonate	21–28 mmol/L		60 years)
Bilirubin (total)	3–22 µmol/L		2–33 U/L (adult males
Calcium (corrected)	2.2–2.6 mmol/L		>60 years)
Chloride	95–105 mmol/L	Magnesium	0.7–1.0 mmol/L
Cholesterol (total plasma)	<5 mmol/L (divide by	Osmolality	275–295 mmol/kg
	0.02586 to convert		(serum)
	to mg/dL)		50–1400 mmol/kg
C-reactive protein (CRP)	0–10 mg/L		(urine)
Creatine kinase (CK)	<150 U/L	PCO_2 (arterial blood)	4.6–6.0 kPa
Creatinine	40–130 µmol/L	pH (arterial blood)	7.35–7.45
γ-glutamyl transpeptidase (γGT)	<36 U/L	Phosphate	0.7–1.4 mmol/L
Glucose (blood)	4.0–5.5 mmol/L (divide	PO_2 (arterial blood)	10.5–13.5 kPa
	by 0.05551 to convert	Potassium	3.5–5.0 mmol/L
	to mg/dL)	Protein	62–82 g/L
Glycated haemoglobin (HbA$_{1c}$)	6–7% taken to indicate	Sodium	135–145 mmol/L
	good diabetic	Triglyceride	<2.5 mmol/L
	control	Urate	0.1–0.4 mmol/L
Hydrogen ion (H$^+$)(arterial blood)	35–45 nmol/L	Urea	2.5–8.0 mmol/L
Iron	10–40 µmol/L		

ALPHABETICAL LIST OF REFERENCE INTERVALS – ENDOCRINE

(All reference intervals listed are for serum measurements in adults unless otherwise stated)

Cortisol	280–720 nmol/L (morning)		500–1500 pmol/L (mid-cycle)
	60–340 nmol/L (evening)		440–880 pmol/L (luteal phase)
			<200 pmol/L (postmenopausal)
			<150 pmol/L (males)
Follicle-stimulating hormone (FSH)	3–13 U/L (follicular phase)	Parathyroid hormone (PTH)	1–6 pmol/L
	9–18 U/L (mid-cycle)	Progesterone	>30 nmol/L in luteal phase taken to
	1–10 U/L (luteal phase)		indicate ovulation
	1–12 U/L (males)		
Free androgen index (FAI)	36–156 (males)		
	<7 (females)	Prolactin	60–500 mU/L (females)
			60–360 mU/L (males)
Growth hormone (GH)	<10 mU/L	Sex hormone-binding globulin	30–120 nmol/L (females)
Human chorionic gonadotrophin (HCG)	<5 U/L except in pregnancy	(SHBG)	
		Testosterone	1.0–3.2 nmol/L (females)
Insulin	<13 mU/L (multiply by 7.175		11–36 nmol/L (males)
	to convert to pmol/L)	Thyroid-stimulating hormone (TSH)	0.35–5.0 mU/L
Luteinizing hormone (LH)	0.8–9.8 U/L (follicular phase)	Thyroxine (T$_4$)	55–144 nmol/L
	17.9–49.0 U/L (mid-cycle)	Tri-iodothyronine (total T$_3$)	0.9–2.6 nmol/L
	0.6–10.8 U/L (luteal phase)		
Oestradiol	180–1000 pmol/L		
	(follicular phase)		

Core Biochemistry

Fluid and electrolyte balance: concepts and vocabulary

Fluid and electrolyte balance is central to the management of any patient who is seriously ill. Measurement of serum sodium, potassium, urea and creatinine, frequently with chloride and bicarbonate, is the most commonly requested biochemical profile and yields a great deal of information about a patient's fluid and electrolyte status and renal function. A typical report is shown in Figure 1.

Body fluid compartments

The major body constituent is water. An 'average' person, weighing 70 kg, contains about 42 litres of water in total. Two-thirds (28 L) of this is intracellular fluid (ICF) and one-third (14 L) is extracellular fluid (ECF). The ECF can be further subdivided into plasma (3.5 L) and interstitial fluid (10.5 L).

A schematic way of representing fluid balance is a water tank model that has a partition and an inlet and outlet (Fig. 2). The inlet supply represents fluids taken orally or by intravenous infusion, while the outlet is normally the urinary tract. Insensible loss can be thought of as surface evaporation.

Selective loss of fluid from each of these compartments gives rise to distinct signs and symptoms.

Intracellular fluid loss, for example, causes cellular dysfunction, which is most notably evident as lethargy, confusion and coma. Loss of blood, an ECF fluid, leads to circulatory collapse, renal shutdown and shock. Loss of total body water will eventually produce similar effects. However, the signs of fluid depletion are not seen at first since the water loss, albeit substantial, is spread across both ECF and ICF compartments.

The water tank model illustrates the relative volumes of each of these compartments and can be used to help visualize some of the clinical disorders of fluid and electrolyte balance. It is important to realize that the assessment of the *volume* of body fluid compartments is not the undertaking of the biochemistry laboratory. The patient's state of hydration, i.e. the volume of the body fluid compartments, is assessed on clinical grounds. The term 'dehydration' simply means that fluid loss has occurred from body compartments. Overhydration occurs when fluid accumulates in body compartments. Figure 3 illustrates dehydration and overhydration by reference to the water tank model. When interpreting electrolyte results it may be useful to construct this 'biochemist's picture' to visualize what is wrong with the patient's fluid balance

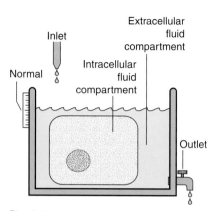

Fig. 2 **Water tank model of body fluid compartments.**

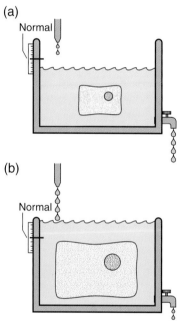

Fig. 3 **The effect of volume depletion and volume expansion on the water tank model of body compartments. (a)** Dehydration: loss of fluid in ICF and ECF due to increased urinary losses. **(b)** Overhydration: increased fluid in ICF and ECF due to increased intake.

and what needs to be done to correct it. The principal features of disordered hydration are shown in Table 1. Clinical assessments of skin turgor, eyeball tension and the mucous membranes are not always reliable. Ageing affects skin elasticity and the oral mucous membranes may appear dry in patients breathing through their mouths.

Electrolytes

Sodium (Na^+) is the principal extracellular cation, and potassium (K^+), the principal intracellular cation. Inside cells the main anions are protein

BIOCHEMISTRY DEPARTMENT   GLASGOW ROYAL INFIRMARY

Name: M   D.o.b. 31/7/25   Hospital GRI   Ward B10Ch

Address: INSTITUTE OF BIOCHEMISTRY   Consultant SHEPHERD   Received 12/10   1222   Hospital Number 246810 R

Accession Number 365586 F

Clinical Information C.R.F.

Date	Time	Sodium 135-145 mmol/l	Potassium 3.5-5.0 mmol/l	Chloride 97-107 mmol/l	CO₂ Content 23-35 mmol/l	Urea 2.5-8.0 mmol/l	Creatinine 40-130 µmol/l	Osmolality 270-295 mmol/kg	Urine Osmolality mmol/kg	Glucose (fasting) 4.0-5.5 mmol/l	Amylase 70-200 U/l	Comment (see Overleaf)
4/10	1130	132	4.2	100	17	36.7	541					
5/10	0900	133	4.4	99	19	32.1	672				435	
6/10	1545	134	3.3	98	21	38.0	580					
7/10	0900	130	4.2	104	18	33.8	534			6.5		
8/10	0900	130	4.1	100	15	36.4	560			8.0		
9/10	0955	135	4.0	101	17	37.2	550					
10/10	1010	132	4.5	100	18	35.9	574					
12/10	1222	132	4.6	101	18	36.9	600					

COMMENT   ISSUED AT 16:28:52 ON 13/10

Note: Reference values given are for general guidance, are not differentiated by age and sex, and are not suitable for publication.

Fig. 1 **A cumulative report form showing electrolyte results in a patient with chronic renal failure.**

Table 1 **The principal clinical features of severe hydration disorders**		
Feature	Dehydration	Overhydration
Pulse	Increased	Normal
Blood pressure	Decreased	Normal or increased
Skin turgor	Decreased	Increased
Eyeballs	Soft/sunken	Normal
Mucous membranes	Dry	Normal
Urine output	Decreased	May be normal or decreased
Consciousness	Decreased	Decreased

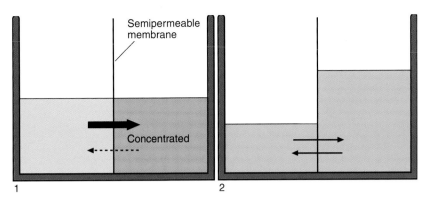

Fig. 4 **Osmolality changes and water movement in body fluid compartments.** The osmolality in different body compartments must be equal. This is achieved by the movement of water across semipermeable membranes in response to concentration changes.

and phosphate, whereas in the ECF chloride (Cl⁻) and bicarbonate (HCO₃⁻) predominate.

A request for measurement of serum 'electrolytes' usually generates values for the concentration of sodium and potassium ions, together with chloride and bicarbonate ions. Sodium ions are present at the highest concentration and hence make the largest contribution to the total plasma osmolality (see later). Although potassium ion concentrations in the ECF are low compared with the high concentrations inside cells, changes in plasma concentrations are very important and may have life-threatening consequences (see pp. 22–23).

Urea and creatinine concentrations provide an indication of renal function, with increased concentrations indicating a decreased glomerular filtration rate (see pp. 28–29).

Concentration

Remember that a concentration is a ratio of two variables: the amount of solute (e.g. sodium), and the amount of water. A concentration can change because either or both variables have changed. For example, a sodium concentration of 140 mmol/L may become 130 mmol/L because the amount of sodium in the solution has fallen or because the amount of water has increased (see p. 6).

Osmolality

Body fluids vary greatly in their composition. However, while the concentration of substances may vary in the different body fluids, the overall number of solute particles, the osmolality, is identical. Body compartments are separated by semipermeable membranes through which water moves freely. Osmotic

pressure must always be the same on both sides of a cell membrane, and water moves to keep the osmolality the same, even if this water movement causes cells to shrink or expand in volume (Fig. 4). The osmolality of the ICF is *normally the same as the ECF*. The two compartments contain isotonic solutions.

The osmolality of a solution is expressed in mmol solute per kilogram of solvent, which is usually water. In man, the osmolality of serum (and all other body fluids except urine) is around 285 mmol/kg.

Osmolality of a serum or plasma sample can be measured directly, or it may be calculated if the concentrations of the major solutes are already known. There are many formulae used to calculate the serum osmolality. Clinically, the simplest is:

$$\text{Serum osmolality} = 2 \times \text{serum [sodium]}$$
$$[\text{mmol/kg}] \qquad\qquad [\text{mmol/L}]$$

This simple formula only holds if the serum concentration of urea and glucose are within the reference intervals. If either or both are abnormally high, the concentration of either or both (in mmol/L) must be added in to give the calculated osmolality. Sometimes there

is an apparent difference between the measured and calculated osmolality. This is known as the *osmolal gap* (p. 17).

Oncotic pressure

The barrier between the intravascular and interstitial compartments is the capillary membrane. Small molecules move freely through this membrane and are, therefore, not osmotically active across it. Plasma proteins, by contrast, do not and they exert a colloid osmotic pressure, known as oncotic pressure (the protein concentration of interstitial fluid is much less than blood). The balance of osmotic and hydrostatic forces across the capillary membrane may be disturbed if the plasma protein concentration changes significantly (see p. 48).

> *Clinical note*
> When water moves across cell membranes, the cells may shrink or expand. When this happens in the brain, neurological signs and symptoms may result.

> **Fluid and electrolyte balance: concepts and vocabulary**
> - The body has two main fluid compartments, the intracellular fluid and the extracellular fluid.
> - The ICF is twice as large as the ECF.
> - Water retention will cause an increase in the volume of both ECF and ICF.
> - Water loss (dehydration) will result in a decreased volume of both ECF and ICF.
> - Sodium ions are the main ECF cations.
> - Potassium ions are the main ICF cations.
> - The volumes of the ECF and ICF are estimated from knowledge of the patient's history and by clinical examination.
> - Serum osmolality can be measured directly or calculated from the serum sodium, urea and glucose concentrations.

Water and sodium balance

Body water and the electrolytes it contains are in a state of constant flux. We drink, we eat, we pass urine and we sweat; during all this it is important that we maintain a steady state. A motor car's petrol tank might hold about 42 L, similar to the total body water content of the average 70 kg male. If 2 L were lost quickly from the tank it would hardly register on the fuel indicator. However, if we were to lose the same volume from our intravascular compartment we would be in serious trouble. We are vulnerable to changes in our fluid compartments, and a number of important homeostatic mechanisms exist to prevent or minimize these. Changes to the electrolyte concentration are also kept to a minimum.

To survive, multicellular organisms must maintain their ECF volume. Humans deprived of fluids die after a few days from circulatory collapse as a result of the reduction in the total body water. Failure to maintain ECF volume, with the consequence of impaired blood circulation, rapidly leads to tissue death due to lack of oxygen and nutrients, and failure to remove waste products.

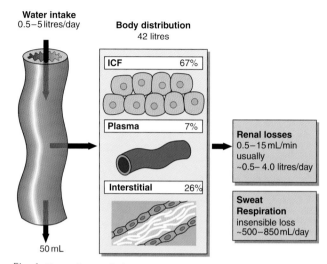

Fig. 1 **Normal water balance.**

Water

Normal water balance is illustrated in Figure 1.

Water intake largely depends on social habits and is very variable. Some people drink less than half a litre each day, and others may imbibe more than 5 L in 24 hours without harm. Thirst is rarely an overriding factor in determining intake in Western societies.

Water losses are equally variable and are normally seen as changes in the volume of urine produced. The kidneys can respond quickly to meet the body's need to get rid of water. The urine flow rate can vary widely in a very short time. However, even when there is need to conserve water, man cannot completely shut down urine production. Total body water remains remarkably constant in health despite massive fluctuations in intake. Water excretion by the kidney is very tightly controlled by arginine vasopressin (AVP; also called antidiuretic hormone, ADH).

The body is also continually losing water through the skin as perspiration, and from the lungs during respiration. This is called the 'insensible' loss. This water loss amounts to between 500 and 850 mL/day. Water may also be lost in disease from fistulae, or in diarrhoea, or because of prolonged vomiting.

AVP and the regulation of osmolality

Specialized cells in the hypothalamus sense differences between their intracellular osmolality and that of the extracellular fluid, and adjust the secretion of AVP from the posterior pituitary gland. A rising osmolality promotes the secretion of AVP while a declining osmolality switches the secretion off (Fig. 2). AVP causes water to be retained by the kidneys. Fluid deprivation results in the stimulation of endogenous AVP secretion, which reduces the urine flow rate to as little as 0.5 mL/minute in order to conserve body water. However, within an hour of drinking 2 L of water, the urine flow rate may rise to 15 mL/minute as AVP secretion is shut down. Thus, by regulating water excretion or retention, AVP maintains normal electrolyte concentrations within the body.

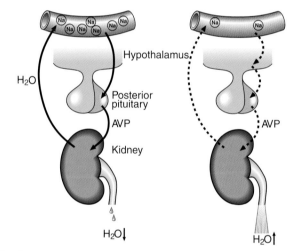

Fig. 2 **The regulation of water balance by AVP and osmolality.**

Sodium

The total body sodium of the average 70 kg man is approximately 3700 mmol, of which approximately 75% is exchangeable (Fig. 3). A quarter of the body sodium is termed non-exchangeable, which means it is incorporated into tissues such as bone and has a slow turnover rate. Most of the exchangeable sodium is in the extracellular fluid. In the ECF, which comprises both the plasma and the interstitial fluid, the sodium concentration is tightly regulated at around 140 mmol/L.

Sodium intake is variable, a range of less than 100 mmol/day to more than 300 mmol/day being encountered in Western societies. In health, total body sodium does not change even if intake falls to as little as 5 mmol/day or is greater than 750 mmol/day.

Sodium losses are just as variable. In practical terms, urinary sodium excretion matches sodium intake. Most sodium excretion is via the kidneys. Some sodium is lost in sweat (approximately 5 mmol/day) and in the faeces (approximately 5 mmol/day). In disease the gastrointestinal

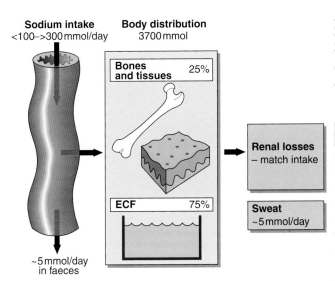

Fig. 3 **Normal sodium balance.**

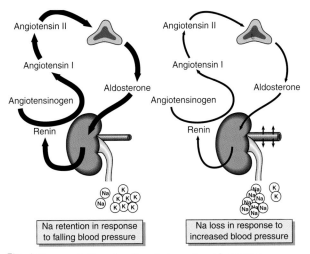

Fig. 4 **The regulation of sodium balance by aldosterone.**

tract is often the major route of sodium loss. This is a very important clinical point, especially in paediatric practice, as infantile diarrhoea may result in death from salt and water depletion.

Urinary sodium output is regulated by two hormones:

- aldosterone
- atrial natriuretic peptide.

Aldosterone

Aldosterone decreases urinary sodium excretion by increasing sodium reabsorption in the renal tubules at the expense of potassium and hydrogen ions. Aldosterone also stimulates sodium conservation by the sweat glands and the mucosal cells of the colon, but in normal circumstances these effects are trivial. A major stimulus to aldosterone secretion is the volume of the ECF. Specialized cells in the juxtaglomerular apparatus of the nephron sense decreases in blood pressure and secrete renin, the first step in a sequence of events that leads to the secretion of aldosterone by the glomerular zone of the adrenal cortex (Fig. 4).

Atrial natriuretic peptide

Atrial natriuretic peptide is a polypeptide hormone predominantly secreted by the cardiocytes of the right atrium of the heart. It increases urinary sodium excretion. The

physiological role, if any, of this hormone is unclear, but it probably only plays a minor role in the regulation of ECF volume and sodium concentration. To date, no disease state can be attributed to a primary disorder in the secretion of atrial natriuretic peptide.

Regulation of volume

It is important to realize that water will only remain in the extracellular compartment if it is held there by the osmotic effect of ions. As sodium (and accompanying anions, mainly chloride) are largely restricted to the extracellular compartment, the amount of sodium in the ECF determines what the volume of the compartment will be. This is an important concept.

Aldosterone and AVP interact to maintain normal volume and concentration of the ECF. Consider a patient who has been vomiting and has diarrhoea from a gastrointestinal infection. With no intake the patient becomes fluid depleted. Water and sodium have been lost. Because the ECF volume is low, aldosterone secretion is high. Thus, as the patient begins to take fluids orally, any salt ingested is maximally retained. As this raises the ECF osmolality, AVP action then ensures that water is retained too. Thus, aldosterone and AVP interaction continues until ECF fluid volume and composition return to normal.

Case history 3

A man is trapped in a collapsed building after an earthquake. He has sustained no serious injuries or blood loss. He has no access to food or water until he is rescued after 72 hours.

■ What will have happened to his body fluid compartments?

Comment on page 162.

Clinical note

Assessment of the volumes of body fluid compartments is not carried out in the clinical biochemistry laboratory. This must be done clinically by history taking and examination.

Water and sodium balance

- Water is lost from the body as urine and as obligatory 'insensible' losses from the skin and lungs.
- Sodium may be lost from the body in urine or from the gut, e.g. prolonged vomiting, diarrhoea and intestinal fistulae.
- Arginine vasopressin (AVP) regulates renal water loss and thus causes changes in the osmolality of body fluid compartments.
- Aldosterone regulates renal sodium loss and controls the sodium content of the ECF.
- Changes in sodium content of the ECF cause changes in volume of this compartment because of the combined actions of AVP and aldosterone.

Hyponatraemia: pathophysiology

Hyponatraemia is defined as a serum sodium concentration below the reference interval of 135–145 mmol/L. It is the abnormality most frequently encountered in clinical biochemistry.

Development of hyponatraemia

The serum concentration of sodium is simply a ratio, of sodium (in millimoles) to water (in litres), and hyponatraemia can arise either because of loss of sodium ions or retention of water.

- *Loss of sodium.* Sodium is the main extracellular cation and plays a critical role in the maintenance of blood volume and pressure, by osmotically regulating the passive movement of water. Thus when significant sodium depletion occurs, water is lost with it, giving rise to the characteristic clinical signs associated with ECF compartment depletion. Primary sodium depletion should *always* be actively considered if only to be excluded; failure to do so can have fatal consequences.
- *Water retention.* Retention of water in the body compartments dilutes the constituents of the extracellular space including sodium, causing hyponatraemia. Water retention occurs much more frequently than sodium loss, and where there is no evidence of fluid loss from history or examination, water retention as the mechanism becomes a near-certainty.

Water retention

The causes of hyponatraemia due to water retention are shown in Figure 1. Water retention usually results from impaired water excretion and rarely from increased intake (compulsive water drinking). Most patients who are hyponatraemic due to water retention have the so-called syndrome of inappropriate antidiuresis (SIAD). The SIAD is encountered in many conditions, e.g. infection, malignancy, chest disease, and trauma (including surgery); it can also be drug-induced. SIAD results from the inappropriate secretion of AVP. Whereas in health the AVP concentration fluctuates between 0 and 5 pmol/L due to changes in osmolality, in SIAD huge (non-osmotic) increases (up to 500 pmol/L) can be seen. Powerful non-osmotic stimuli include hypovolaemia and/or hypotension, nausea and vomiting, hypoglycaemia, and pain. The frequency with which SIAD occurs in clinical practice mirrors the widespread prevalence of these stimuli.

AVP has other effects in the body aside from regulating renal water handling (Table 1).

Sodium loss

The causes of hyponatraemia due to sodium loss are shown in Figure 1. Sodium depletion is extremely rare and effectively occurs only when there is pathological sodium loss, either from the gastrointestinal tract or in urine. Gastrointestrinal losses (Table 2) commonly include those from vomiting and diarrhoea; in patients with fistulae due to bowel

Table 1 **Actions of AVP, other than renal water regulation**
■ Potent vasoconstrictor
■ Potent hormonal stimulator of hepatic glycogenolysis
■ Increases the plasma concentration of Factor VIII – hence the use of the AVP analogue DDAVP in mild haemophilia
■ Augments ACTH secretion from the anterior pituitary thus increasing cortisol production

Table 2 **A guide to the electrolyte composition of gastrointestinal fluids**

Fluid	Concentration		
	Na^+	K^+	Cl^-
		mmol/L	
Gastric juice	70	10	110
Small intestinal fluid	120	10	100
Diarrhoea	50	30	50
Rectal mucus	100	40	100
Bile, pleural and peritoneal fluids	140	5	100

disease, losses may be severe. Urinary loss may result from mineralocorticoid deficiency (especially aldosterone) or from drugs that antagonize aldosterone, e.g. spironolactone.

Initially in all of the above situations, sodium loss is accompanied by water loss and the serum sodium concentration remains normal. As sodium and water loss continue, the reduction in ECF and blood volume stimulates AVP secretion non-osmotically, overriding the osmotic control mechanism. The increase in AVP secretion causes water retention and thus patients become hyponatraemic. Another reason why sodium-losing patients may become hyponatraemic is because a deficit of isotonic sodium-containing fluid is replaced only by water.

As indicated above, when significant sodium depletion occurs water is lost with it, giving rise to the clinical signs characteristic of ECF and blood volume depletion. In the context of hyponatraemia these findings are diagnostic of sodium depletion; the clinical findings are evidence of fluid (water) depletion, whilst the hyponatraemia indicates that the ratio of sodium to water is reduced.

Sodium depletion – a word of caution

Not all patients with sodium depletion are hyponatraemic. Patients with sodium loss due to an osmotic

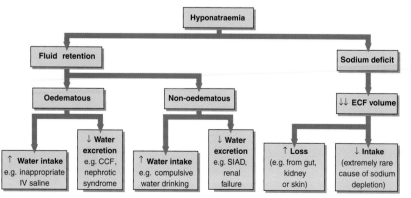

Fig. 1 **The causes of hyponatraemia.**

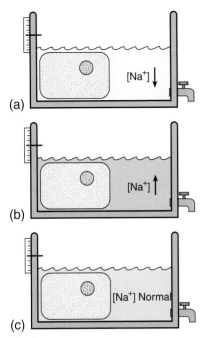

(a)

(b)

(c)

Fig. 2 **Water tank models showing that reduced ECF volume may be associated with reduced, increased or normal serum [Na⁺].**

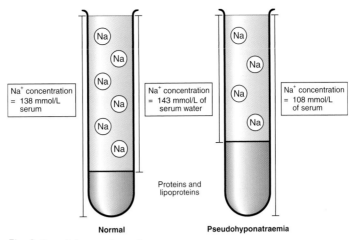

Fig. 3 **Pseudohyponatraemia.**

diuresis may become hypernatraemic if more water than sodium is lost. Life-threatening sodium depletion can also be present with a normal serum sodium concentration. In short, the serum sodium concentration does not of itself provide any information about the presence or severity of sodium depletion (Fig. 2). The history and clinical examination are much more useful in this regard.

Pseudohyponatraemia

Hyponatraemia is sometimes reported in patients with severe hyperproteinaemia or hyperlipidaemia. In such patients, the increased amounts of protein or lipoprotein occupy more of the plasma volume than usual, and the water less (Fig. 3). Sodium and the other electrolytes are distributed in the water fraction only, and these patients have a normal sodium concentration in their plasma water. However, many of the methods used in analytical instruments measure the sodium concentration in the total plasma volume, and take no account of a water fraction that occupies less of the total plasma volume than usual. An artefactually low sodium result may thus be obtained in these circumstances. Such *pseudohyponatraemia* should be suspected if there is a discrepancy between the degree of apparent

hyponatraemia and the symptoms that one might expect due to the low sodium concentration (see pp. 18–19), e.g. a patient with a sodium concentration of 110 mmol/L who is completely asymptomatic. The serum osmolality is unaffected by any changes in the fraction of the total plasma volume occupied by proteins or lipids, since they are not dissolved in the water fraction and, therefore, do not make any contribution to the osmolality. A normal serum osmolality in a patient with severe hyponatraemia is, thus, strongly suggestive of pseudohyponatraemia. This can be assessed formally by

calculating the osmolal gap, the difference between the *measured* osmolality and the *calculated* osmolality.

Clinical note
Oedema is not just a consequence of secondary hyperaldosteronism. In some situations, the factors that cause the expansion of the ECF compartment (such as inflammation or restricted venous return) are localized.

Case history 4

A 64-year-old woman was admitted with anorexia, weight loss and anaemia. Carcinoma of the colon was diagnosed. She was normotensive and did not have oedema. The following biochemical results were obtained shortly after admission.

Na⁺	K⁺	Cl⁻	HCO₃⁻	Urea	Creatinine
		— mmol/L —			μmol/L
123	3.9	86	22	6.2	115

Serum osmolality was measured as 247 mmol/kg; urine osmolality was 178 mmol/kg.

- How may this patient's hyponatraemia be explained?
- What contribution does the urine osmolality make to the diagnosis?

Comment on page 162.

Hyponatraemia: pathophysiology

- Hyponatraemia because of water retention is the commonest biochemical disturbance encountered in clinical practice. In many patients the non-osmotic regulation of AVP overrides the osmotic regulatory mechanism and this results in water retention, which is a non-specific feature of illness.

- Hyponatraemia may occur in the patient with gastrointestinal or renal fluid losses that have caused sodium depletion. The low sodium concentration in serum occurs because water retention is stimulated by increased AVP secretion.

Hyponatraemia: assessment and management

Clinical assessment

Clinicians assessing a patient with hyponatraemia should ask themselves several questions.

- Am I dealing with dangerous (life-threatening) hyponatraemia?
- Am I dealing with water retention or sodium loss?
- How should I treat this patient?

To answer these questions, they must use the patient's history, the findings from clinical examination, and the results of laboratory investigations. Each of these may provide valuable clues.

Severity

In assessing the risk of serious morbidity or mortality in the patient with hyponatraemia, several pieces of information should be used:

- the serum sodium concentration
- how quickly the sodium concentration has fallen from normal to its current level
- the presence of signs or symptoms attributable to hyponatraemia
- evidence of sodium depletion.

The serum sodium concentration itself gives some indication of dangerous or life-threatening hyponatraemia. Many experienced clinicians use a concentration of 120 mmol/L as a threshold in trying to assess risk (the risk declines at concentrations significantly greater than 120 mmol/L, and rises steeply at concentrations less than 120 mmol/L). However, this arbitrary cut-off should be applied with caution, particularly if it is not known how quickly the sodium concentration has fallen from normal to its current level. A patient whose serum sodium falls from 145 to 125 mmol/L in 24 hours may be at great risk.

Often, the clinician must rely exclusively on history and, especially, clinical examination to assess the risk to the patient. Symptoms due to hyponatraemia reflect neurological dysfunction resulting from cerebral overhydration induced by hypo-osmolality. They are non-specific and include nausea, malaise, headache, lethargy and a reduced level of consciousness. Seizures, coma and focal neurological signs are not usually seen until the sodium concentration is less than 110 to 115 mmol/L.

If there is clinical evidence of sodium depletion (see below), there is a high risk of mortality if treatment is not instituted quickly.

Mechanism

History

Fluid loss, e.g. from gut or kidney, should always be sought as a possible pointer towards primary sodium loss. Even if there is no readily identifiable source of loss, the patient should be asked about symptoms that may reflect sodium depletion, such as dizziness, weakness and light-headedness.

If there is no history of fluid loss, water retention is likely. Many patients will not give a history of water retention as such; history taking should instead be aimed at identifying possible causes of the SIAD. For example, rigors may point towards infection, or weight loss towards malignancy.

Clinical examination

The clinical signs characteristic of ECF and blood volume depletion are shown in Figure 1. These signs should always be looked for; in hyponatraemic patients they are diagnostic of sodium depletion. If they are present in the recumbent state, severe life-threatening sodium depletion is present and urgent treatment is needed. In the early phases of sodium depletion postural hypotension may be the only sign. By contrast, even when water retention is strongly suspected, there may be no clinical evidence of water overload. There are two good reasons for this. Firstly, water retention due to the SIAD (the most frequent explanation) occurs gradually, often over weeks or even months. Secondly, the retained water is distributed evenly over all body compartments; thus the increase in the ECF volume is minimized.

Biochemistry

Sodium depletion is diagnosed largely on clinical grounds, whereas in patients with suspected water retention, history and examination may be unremarkable. However, both sodium depletion and SIAD produce a similar biochemical picture (Table 1) with reduced serum osmolality reflecting hyponatraemia, and a high urine osmolality reflecting AVP secretion. In sodium depletion, AVP secretion is appropriate to the hypovolaemia resulting from sodium and water loss; in SIAD it is

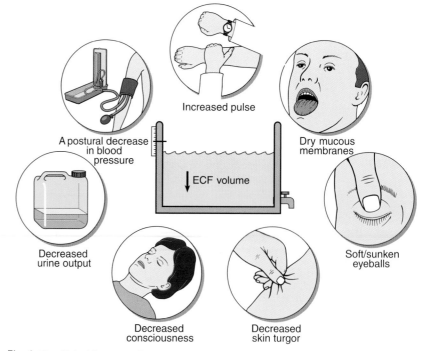

Increased pulse

A postural decrease in blood pressure

↓ECF volume

Dry mucous membranes

Decreased urine output

Soft/sunken eyeballs

Decreased consciousness

Decreased skin turgor

Fig. 1 **The clinical features of ECF compartment depletion.**

Table 1 **Biochemical picture for sodium depletion and SIAD**

	Sodium depletion	Water retention
Symptoms*	Often present, e.g. dizziness, light-headedness, collapse	Usually absent
Signs*	Often present. Signs of volume depletion, e.g. hypotension (see Fig. 1)	Usually absent Oedema
Clinical value of signs	Diagnostic of sodium depletion if present	Oedema narrows differential diagnosis
Clinical course	Rapid	Slow
Serum osmolality	Low	Low
Urine osmolality	High	High
Urinary sodium excretion	Low if gut/skin loss of sodium Variable if kidney loss	Variable but usually increased
Water balance	Too little	Too much
Sodium balance	Too little	Normal Too much if oedema
Treatment aim	Replace sodium	Restrict water Natriuresis if oedema

*Relating specifically to the mechanism. There may well be symptoms/signs relating to the underlying cause

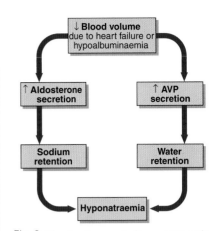

Fig. 3 **The development of hyponatraemia in the oedematous patient.**

inappropriate (non-osmotic). Urinary sodium excretion is often increased in SIAD (a hypervolaemic state). It may be low or high in sodium depletion depending on whether the pathological loss is from gut or kidney.

Oedema

Oedema is an accumulation of fluid in the interstitial compartment. It is readily elicited by looking for pitting in the lower extremities of ambulant patients (Fig. 2), or in the sacral area of recumbent patients. It arises from a reduced effective circulating blood volume, due either to heart failure or hypoalbuminaemia.

The response to this is secondary hyperaldosteronism. Aldosterone causes sodium (and water) retention, thus expanding the ECF volume. Patients with oedema become hyponatraemic despite sodium retention because the effective hypovolaemia also stimulates AVP secretion, resulting in additional water retention (Fig. 3).

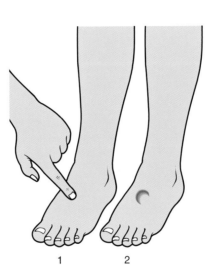

Fig. 2 **Pitting oedema.** After depressing the skin firmly for a few seconds an indentation or pit is seen.

Clinical note

The use of oral glucose and salt solutions to correct sodium depletion in infective diarrhoea is one of the major therapeutic advances of the last century and is life-saving, particularly in developing countries.

Family practitioners, nurses and even parents are able to treat sodium depletion using these oral salt solutions, without making biochemical measurements.

Treatment

Hypovolaemic patients are sodium-depleted and should be given sodium. Normovolaemic patients are likely to be retaining water and should be fluid restricted. Oedematous patients have an excess of both total body sodium and water; they should be given a diuretic to induce natriuresis, and be fluid restricted. More aggressive treatment (usually requiring hypertonic saline) may be indicated if symptoms attributable to hyponatraemia are present, or the sodium concentration is less than 110 mmol/L.

Case history 5

A 42-year-old man was admitted with a 2-day history of severe diarrhoea with some nausea and vomiting. During this period his only intake was water. He was weak, unable to stand and when recumbent his pulse was 104/minute and blood pressure was 100/55 mmHg. On admission, his biochemistry results were:

Na⁺	K⁺	Cl⁻	HCO₃⁻	Urea	Creatinine
		mmol/L			μmol/L
131	3.0	86	19	17.8	150

■ What is the most appropriate treatment for this patient?

Comment on page 162.

Hyponatraemia: clinical assessment and management

■ Patients with hyponatraemia because of sodium depletion show clinical signs of fluid loss such as hypotension. They do not have oedema.

■ Treatment of hyponatraemia, due to sodium depletion, should be with sodium and water replacement, preferably orally.

■ Hyponatraemic patients without oedema, who have normal serum urea and creatinine and blood pressure, have water overload. This may be treated by fluid restriction.

■ Hyponatraemic patients with oedema are likely to have both water and sodium overload. These patients may be treated with diuretics and fluid restriction.

Hypernatraemia

Hypernatraemia is an increase in the serum sodium concentration above the reference interval of 135–145 mmol/L. Just as hyponatraemia develops because of sodium loss or water retention, so hypernatraemia develops either because of water loss or sodium gain.

Water loss

Pure water loss may arise from decreased intake or excessive loss. Severe hypernatraemia due to poor intake is most often seen in elderly patients, either because they have stopped eating and drinking voluntarily, or because they are unable to get something to drink, e.g. the unconscious patient after a stroke. The failure of intake to match the ongoing insensible water loss is the cause of the hypernatraemia. Less commonly there is failure of AVP secretion or action, resulting in water loss and hypernatraemia. This is called diabetes insipidus; it is described as central if it results from failure of AVP secretion, or nephrogenic if the renal tubules do not respond to AVP.

Water and sodium loss can result in hypernatraemia if the water loss exceeds the sodium loss. This can happen in osmotic diuresis, as seen in the patient with poorly controlled diabetes mellitus, or due to excessive sweating or diarrhoea, especially in children. However, loss of body fluids because of vomiting or diarrhoea usually results in *hyponatraemia* (see pp. 16–17).

Sodium gain

Hypernatraemia due to sodium gain (often referred to generically as 'salt poisoning' even where there is no suggestion of malicious or self-induced harm) is much less common than water loss. It is easily missed precisely because it may not be suspected. It can occur in several clinical contexts, each very different. Firstly, sodium bicarbonate is sometimes given to correct life-threatening acidosis. However, it is not always appreciated that the sodium concentration in 8.4% sodium bicarbonate is 1000 mmol/L. A less concentrated solution (1.26%) is available and is preferred. Secondly,

near-drowning in salt-water may result in the ingestion of significant amounts of brine, the sodium concentration of which is once again vastly in excess of physiological. Thirdly, infants are susceptible to hypernatraemia if given high-sodium feeds either accidentally or on purpose. For example, the administration of one tablespoon of NaCl to a newborn can raise the plasma sodium by as much as 70 mmol/L.

The pathophysiological parallel to the administration of sodium is the rare condition of primary hyperaldosteronism (Conn's syndrome), where there is excessive aldosterone secretion and consequent sodium retention by the renal tubules. Similar findings may be made in the patient with Cushing's syndrome, where there is excess cortisol production. Cortisol has weak mineralocorticoid activity. However, in both these conditions the serum sodium concentration rarely rises above 150 mmol/L. The mechanisms of hypernatraemia are summarized in Figure 1.

Clinical features

Hypernatraemia may be associated with a decreased, normal or expanded ECF volume (Fig. 2). The clinical context is all-important. With mild hypernatraemia (sodium <150 mmol/L), if the patient has obvious clinical features of dehydration (Fig. 3), it is likely that the ECF volume is reduced and that one is dealing with loss of both water and sodium. With more severe hypernatraemia (sodium 150 to 170 mmol/L), pure water loss is likely if the clinical signs of dehydration are mild in relation to the severity of the hypernatraemia. This is because pure water loss is distributed evenly throughout all body compartments (ECF and ICF). (The sodium content of the ECF is unchanged in pure water loss.) With gross hypernatraemia (sodium >180 mmol/L), one should suspect salt poisoning if there is little or no clinical evidence of dehydration; the amount of water that would need to be lost to elevate the sodium to this degree should be clinically obvious,

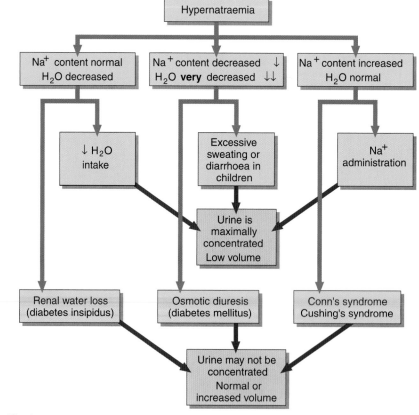

Fig. 1 **The causes of hypernatraemia.**

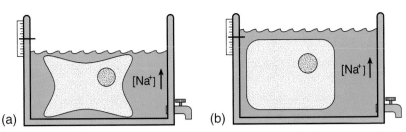

(a)   (b)

Fig. 2 **Hypernatraemia is commonly associated with a contracted ECF volume, and less commonly with an expanded compartment.**
(a) Volumes of ECF and ICF are reduced.
(b) ECF volume is shown here to be slightly expanded; ICF volume is normal.

irrespective of whether there has been concomitant sodium loss. Salt gain may present with clinical evidence of overload, such as raised jugular venous pressure or pulmonary oedema.

Treatment

Patients with hypernatraemia due to pure water loss need free water; this may be given orally, or intravenously as 5% dextrose. If there is clinical evidence of dehydration indicating probable loss of sodium as well, sodium should also be administered. Salt poisoning is a difficult clinical problem to manage. The sodium overload can be treated with diuretics and the natriuresis replaced with water. Caution must be exercised with the use of intravenous dextrose in salt-poisoned patients – they are volume-expanded already and susceptible to pulmonary oedema.

Other osmolality disorders

A high plasma osmolality may sometimes be encountered for reasons other than hypernatraemia. Causes include:

- increased urea in renal disease
- hyperglycaemia in diabetes mellitus
- the presence of ethanol or some other ingested substance.

A large discrepancy between the measured osmolality and the calculated osmolality is called the osmolal gap (see p. 13) and suggests the presence of a significant contributor to the osmolality unaccounted for in the calculation. In practice, this is almost always due to the presence of ethanol in the blood. Very occasionally, however, it may be due

to other substances such as methanol or ethylene glycol from the ingestion of antifreeze. The calculation of the osmolal gap can be clinically very useful in the assessment of comatose patients.

The consequences of disordered osmolality are due to the changes in volume that arise as water moves in or out of cells to maintain osmotic balance. Note that of the three examples above, only glucose causes significant fluid movement. Glucose cannot freely enter cells, and an increasing ECF concentration causes water to move out of cells and leads to intracellular dehydration. Urea and ethanol permeate cells and do not cause such fluid shifts, as long as concentration changes occur slowly.

Clinical note

Patients often become hypernatraemic because they are unable to complain of being thirsty. The comatose patient is a good example. He or she will be unable to communicate his/her needs, yet insensible losses of water will continue from lungs/skin and need to be replaced.

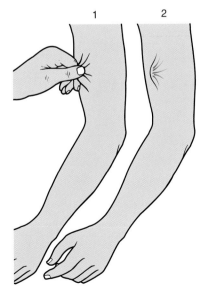

1   2

Fig. 3 **Decreased skin turgor.** This sign is frequently unreliable in the elderly, who have reduced skin elasticity. In the young it is a sign of severe dehydration with fluid loss from the ECF.

Case history 6

A 76-year-old man with depression and very severe incapacitating disease was admitted as an acute emergency. He was clinically dehydrated. His skin was lax and his lips and tongue were dry and shrivelled looking. His pulse was 104/min, and his blood pressure was 95/65 mmHg. The following biochemical results were obtained on admission:

Na^+	K^+	Cl^-	HCO_3^-	Urea	Creatinine
		— mmol/L —			μmol/L
172	3.6	140	18	22.9	155

- Comment on these biochemical findings.
- What is the diagnosis?

Comment on page 162.

Hypernatraemia

- Hypernatraemia is most commonly due to water loss (e.g. because of continuing insensible losses in the patient who is unable to drink).
- Failure to retain water as a result of impaired AVP secretion or action may cause hypernatraemia.
- Hypernatraemia may be the result of a loss of both sodium and water as a consequence of an osmotic diuresis, e.g. in diabetic ketoacidosis.
- Excessive sodium intake, particularly from the use of intravenous solutions, may cause hypernatraemia. Rarely, primary hyperaldosteronism (Conn's syndrome) may be the cause.
- A high plasma osmolality may be due to the presence of glucose, urea or ethanol, rather than sodium.

Hyperkalaemia

Potassium disorders are commonly encountered in clinical practice. They are important because of the role potassium plays in determining the resting membrane potential of cells. Changes in plasma potassium mean that 'excitable' cells, such as nerve and muscle, may respond differently to stimuli. In the heart (which is largely muscle and nerve), the consequences can be fatal, e.g. arrhythmias.

Serum potassium and potassium balance

Serum potassium concentration is normally kept within a tight range (3.5–5.0 mmol/L). *Potassium intake* is variable (30–100 mmol/day in the UK) and *potassium losses* (through the kidneys) usually mirror intake. A small amount (~5 mmol/day) is lost in the gut. Potassium balance can be disturbed if any of these fluxes is altered (Fig. 1). An additional factor often implicated in hyperkalaemia and hypokalaemia is *redistribution* of potassium. Nearly all of the total body potassium (98%) is inside cells. If, for example, there is significant tissue damage, the contents of cells, including potassium, leak out into the extracellular compartment, causing potentially dangerous increases in serum potassium (see below).

Hyperkalaemia

Hyperkalaemia is one of the commonest electrolyte emergencies encountered in clinical practice. If severe (>7.0 mmol/L), it is immediately life-threatening and must be dealt with as an absolute priority; cardiac arrest may be the first manifestation. ECG changes seen in hyperkalaemia (Fig. 2) include the classic tall 'tented' T-waves and widening of the QRS complex, reflecting altered myocardial contractility. Other symptoms include muscle weakness and paraesthesiae, again reflecting involvement of nerves and muscles.

Hyperkalaemia can be categorized as due to increased intake, redistribution or decreased excretion.

Increased intake

Failure to appreciate sources of potassium intake may result in dangerous hyperkalaemia, particularly in patients with impaired renal function. For example, many oral drugs are administered as potassium salts. Potassium may also be given intravenously. *Intravenous potassium should not be given faster than 20 mmol/hour except in extreme cases.* Occasionally, blood products may give rise to hyperkalaemia (stored red blood cells release potassium down its concentration gradient). The risk of this is reduced by using relatively fresh blood (less than 5 days old) and/or by 'washing' units prior to transfusing.

Redistribution out of cells

- *Metabolic acidosis.* There is a reciprocal relationship between potassium and hydrogen ions. As the concentration of hydrogen ions increases with the development of metabolic acidosis, so potassium ions inside cells are displaced from the cell by hydrogen ions in order to maintain electrochemical neutrality (Fig. 3). These hydrogen ion changes

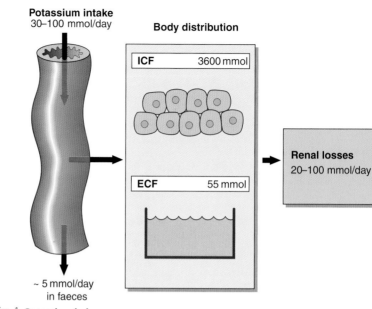

Fig. 1 **Potassium balance.**

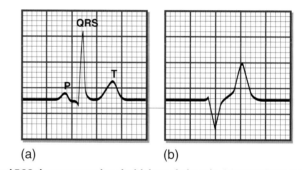
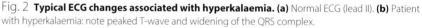

Fig. 2 **Typical ECG changes associated with hyperkalaemia. (a)** Normal ECG (lead II). **(b)** Patient with hyperkalaemia: note peaked T-wave and widening of the QRS complex.

cause marked alterations in serum potassium.

- *Potassium release from damaged cells.* The potassium concentration inside cells (~140 mmol/L) means that cell damage can give rise to marked hyperkalaemia. This occurs in rhabdomyolysis (where skeletal muscle is broken down), extensive trauma, or rarely tumour lysis syndrome, where malignant cells break down.
- *Insulin deficiency.* Insulin stimulates cellular uptake of potassium, and plays a central role in treatment of severe hyperkalaemia. Where there is insulin deficiency or severe resistance to the actions of insulin, as in diabetic ketoacidosis (see pp. 64–65), hyperkalaemia is an associated feature.
- *Hyperkalaemic periodic paralysis.* This is a rare familial disorder with autosomal dominant inheritance. It presents typically as recurrent attacks of muscle weakness or paralysis, often precipitated by rest after exercise.

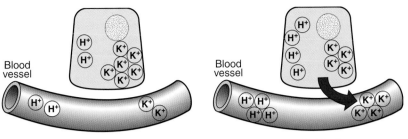

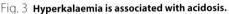

Fig. 3 **Hyperkalaemia is associated with acidosis.**

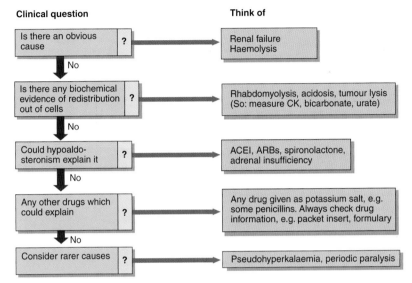

Fig. 4 **The evaluation of hyperkalaemia.**

Pseudohyperkalaemia

This refers to elevation in the measured potassium due to potassium movement out of cells during or after the drawing of the blood specimen. The commonest cause is haemolysis. This is characterized by the release of haemoglobin as well as potassium from red blood cells; the resultant red tint of the serum means that haemolysis is usually evident, and the serum potassium result can therefore be deleted, or commented on.

A small amount of potassium is released from white blood cells and platelets during normal clotting. In patients with grossly elevated white cell or platelet counts, the amount released may be much greater. Such results are usually recognized as spurious when the patient is not acutely unwell, and there is no other obvious cause of hyperkalaemia.

Formal investigation of suspected pseudohyperkalaemia should include simultaneous collection and processing of serum and plasma specimens (the anticoagulant in plasma specimens prevents clotting). Varying the time of sample centrifugation may also provide evidence, in the form of a progressive steep rise in serum potassium seen with delayed centrifugation.

Treatment

Insulin plays a central role in treatment of severe hyperkalaemia. It is infused along with glucose; otherwise correction of hyperkalaemia would give way promptly to dangerous hypoglycaemia. Calcium gluconate may also be given intravenously. This does not correct the hyperkalaemia but does help to counteract its effects on nerve and muscle cells. Slower rises in potassium may be stopped by oral administration of cation exchange resins; these can be given orally as a powder, or rectally as an enema. Finally, dialysis may be required for severe refractory hyperkalaemia.

■ *Pseudohyperkalaemia.* This should be considered when the cause of hyperkalaemia is not readily apparent. Indeed, it is important largely because it can lead to diagnostic dilemmas. It is dealt with in detail below.

Decreased excretion

■ *Renal failure.* The kidneys may not be able to excrete a potassium load when the glomerular filtration rate is very low, and hyperkalaemia is a central feature of reduced glomerular function. It is exacerbated by the associated metabolic acidosis, due to the accumulation of organic ions that would normally be excreted.
■ *Hypoaldosteronism.* Aldosterone stimulates sodium reabsorption in the renal tubules at the expense of potassium and hydrogen (see p. 15). This *mineralocorticoid* activity is shared by many steroid molecules. Deficiency, antagonism or resistance results in loss of sodium, with associated retention of potassium and hydrogen. In clinical practice, hyperkalaemia due to hypoaldosteronism is most often seen with the use of angiotensin-converting enzyme (ACE) inhibitors and angiotensin receptor blockers (ARBs) to treat hypertension; spironolactone and other potassium-sparing diuretics also antagonize the effect of aldosterone. Less frequently, adrenal insufficiency is responsible (see pp. 94–95).

Figure 4 describes an approach to the evaluation of hyperkalaemia.

Clinical note
Some oral drugs are administered as potassium salts. Unexplained, persistent hyperkalaemia should always prompt review of the drug history.

Hyperkalaemia

■ Most potassium in the body is intracellular.
■ The commonest cause of hyperkalaemia is renal impairment.
■ Severe hyperkalaemia is immediately life-threatening and death may occur with no clinical warning signs.
■ Sometimes hyperkalaemia is artefactual – pseudohyperkalaemia.

Hypokalaemia

The factors affecting potassium balance have been described previously (p. 22). Hypokalaemia may be due to reduced potassium intake, but much more frequently results from increased losses or from redistribution of potassium into cells. As with hyperkalaemia, the clinical effects of hypokalaemia are seen in 'excitable' tissues like nerve and muscle. Symptoms include muscle weakness, hyporeflexia and cardiac arrhythmias. Figure 1 shows the changes that may be found on ECG in hypokalaemia.

Diagnosis

The cause of hypokalaemia can usually be determined from the history. Common causes include vomiting and diarrhoea, and diuretics. Where the cause is not immediately obvious, urine potassium measurement may help to guide investigations. Increased urinary potassium excretion in the face of potassium depletion suggests urinary loss rather than redistribution or gut loss. Equally, low or undetectable urinary potassium in this context indicates the opposite.

Reduced intake

This is a rare cause of hypokalaemia. Renal retention of potassium in response to reduced intake ensures that hypokalaemia occurs only when intake is severely restricted. Since potassium is present in meat, fruit and some vegetables, marked potassium restriction is difficult to maintain. Hypokalaemia should, however, be a consideration when severely hypocaloric diets are prescribed to bring about rapid weight loss.

Redistribution into cells

■ *Metabolic alkalosis.* The reciprocal relationship between potassium and hydrogen ions means that in just the same way as metabolic acidosis is associated with hyperkalaemia, so metabolic alkalosis is associated with hypokalaemia. As the concentration of hydrogen ions decreases, so potassium ions move inside cells in order to maintain electrochemical neutrality (Fig. 2).

■ *Treatment with insulin.* Insulin stimulates cellular uptake of potassium, and plays a central role in treatment of severe hyperkalaemia (see pp. 22–23). It should come as no surprise therefore that when insulin is given in the treatment of diabetic ketoacidosis (see pp. 64–65), there is a risk of hypokalaemia. This is well recognized, and virtually all treatment protocols for diabetic ketoacidosis take this into account.

■ *Refeeding.* The so-called 'refeeding syndrome' was first described in prisoners of war. It occurs when previously malnourished patients are fed with high carbohydrate loads. The result is a rapid fall in phosphate, magnesium and potassium, mediated by insulin as it moves glucose into cells. Vulnerable groups include those with anorexia nervosa, cancer, alcoholism and postoperative patients. Many of the complications of this result from hypophosphataemia rather than hypokalaemia.

■ β-*Agonism.* Acute physiological stress can cause potassium to move into cells, an effect mediated by catecholamines through their actions on β_2-receptors. β-agonists like salbutamol (used to treat asthma) or dobutamine (heart failure) predictably induce a similar effect.

■ *Treatment of anaemia.* Folic acid or vitamin B_{12} for megaloblastic anaemia often produce hypokalaemia in the first couple of days of treatment, due to the uptake of potassium by the new blood cells. Treatment of iron deficiency anaemia results in a much slower rate of new blood cell production and is therefore rarely implicated.

■ *Hypokalaemic periodic paralysis.* Like its hyperkalaemic counterpart, hypokalaemic periodic paralysis can be inherited (as an autosomal dominant trait), and be precipitated by rest after exercise. However, it can also be acquired as a result of thyrotoxicosis (possibly due to increased sensitivity to catecholamines), especially in Chinese males. It resembles refeeding in that both can be precipitated by carbohydrate loads and both are associated with low phosphate and magnesium as well.

Increased losses
Gastrointestinal

Gastrointestinal loss of potassium is not usually a diagnostic dilemma. The common causes (diarrhoea and vomiting) are obvious, and the risk of hypokalaemia well recognized. In cholera (associated with massive fluid loss from the gut), daily potassium losses may exceed 100 mmol, compared with ~5 mmol normally. Less frequently, chronic laxative abuse may be responsible. However, this should

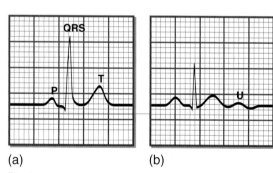

Fig. 1 **Typical ECG changes associated with hypokalaemia. (a)** Normal ECG (lead II). **(b)** Patient with hypokalaemia: note flattened T-wave. U-waves are prominent in all leads.

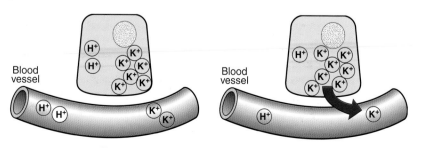

Fig. 2 **Hypokalaemia is associated with alkalosis.**

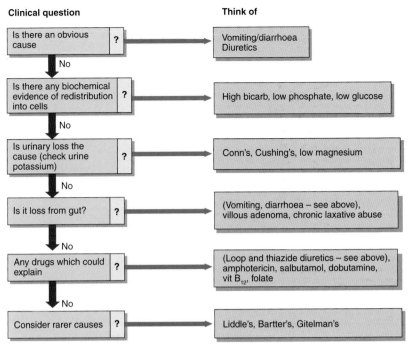

Clinical question

Is there an obvious cause	?

No

Is there any biochemical evidence of redistribution into cells	?

No

Is urinary loss the cause (check urine potassium)	?

No

Is it loss from gut?	?

No

Any drugs which could explain	?

No

Consider rarer causes	?

Think of

Vomiting/diarrhoea
Diuretics

High bicarb, low phosphate, low glucose

Conn's, Cushing's, low magnesium

(Vomiting, diarrhoea – see above), villous adenoma, chronic laxative abuse

(Loop and thiazide diuretics – see above), amphotericin, salbutamol, dobutamine, vit B$_{12}$, folate

Liddle's, Bartter's, Gitelman's

Fig. 3 **The evaluation of hypokalaemia.**

normally be considered only when more likely causes of hypokalaemia have been excluded.

Urinary

■ *Diuretics.* Both loop diuretics and thiazide diuretics produce hypokalaemia. Various mechanisms are implicated, including increased flow of water and sodium to the site of distal potassium secretion, and secondary hyperaldosteronism induced by the loss of volume. Loop diuretics also interfere with potassium reabsorption in the loop of Henle.

■ *Mineralocorticoid excess.* We have indicated previously (p. 15) that aldosterone increases sodium reabsorption in the renal tubules at the expense of potassium and hydrogen ions. This *mineralocorticoid* effect is shared by many steroid molecules, and hypokalaemia is a predictable and frequent consequence of mineralocorticoid excess. Overproduction of steroid hormones is dealt with in more detail on pp. 96–97. Less frequently, renal artery stenosis drives the renin–angiotensin–aldosterone axis (Fig. 4 on p. 15), resulting in hypokalaemia associated with severe, refractory hypertension.

■ *Tubulopathies.* A small number of inherited defects in tubular function produce hypokalaemia by various mechanisms. They may need to be considered in cases of persistent unexplained hypokalaemia.

■ *Hypomagnesaemia.* Hypomagnesaemia from any cause can produce

hypokalaemia, an effect thought to be mediated by interference with renal potassium reabsorption.

Investigation

Figure 3 provides a framework for investigation of hypokalaemia. Often the cause is obvious e.g. vomiting,

> **Clinical note**
> Alcoholic patients are especially prone to hypokalaemia through various mechanisms.

diarrhoea, and further investigations are not required. Some of the causes of hypokalaemia listed above are well recognized as such by clinicians and hypokalaemia is not a diagnostic dilemma, e.g. diuretics, gut loss, insulin treatment. Other causes are infrequently implicated (treatment of anaemia), or are simply very rare (hypokalaemic periodic paralysis), and may not be considered. Where the cause is not immediately evident, it may help to go back to first principles by classifying potential causes into the three broad categories outlined above: reduced intake, redistribution, and increased loss. Measurement of urinary potassium excretion may help to identify (or exclude) renal loss as the likely mechanism. Diagnoses which can be difficult to pin down include laxative abuse(because it is sometimes intermittent) and the eponymous tubulopathies (again, because their phenotypic expression can vary over time).

Treatment

Potassium salts are unpleasant to take orally and are usually given prophylactically in an enteric coating. Severe potassium depletion often has to be treated by intravenous potassium. Intravenous potassium should not be given faster than 20 mmol/hour except in extreme cases and under ECG monitoring.

Case history 7

Mrs MM, a 67-year-old patient with extensive vascular disease, attends the hypertension clinic and is on five different antihypertensive drugs. At her most recent clinic visit, blood pressure was 220/110 mmHg, and a set of U & Es showed the following:

Na$^+$	K$^+$	Cl$^-$	HCO$_3$$^-$	Urea	Creatinine
		mmol/L			μmol/L
139	2.7	106	33	21.7	254

■ What would explain the coexistent hypertension and hypokalaemia in this patient?

Comment on page 162.

Hypokalaemia

■ Decreased intake of potassium rarely causes hypokalaemia because potassium is present in most foods.

■ Bicarbonate should always be measured in the presence of unexplained hypokalaemia.

■ Increased mineralocorticoid activity from various causes leads to hypokalaemia.

■ Low magnesium should be suspected in the presence of persistent hypokalaemia.

Intravenous fluid therapy

Intravenous (IV) fluid therapy is an integral part of clinical practice in hospitals. Every hospital doctor should be familiar with the principles underlying the appropriate administration of intravenous fluids. Each time fluids are prescribed, the following questions should be addressed:

- Does this patient need IV fluids?
- Which fluids should be given?
- How much fluid should be given?
- How quickly should the fluids be given?
- How should the fluid therapy be monitored?

Does this patient need IV fluids?

The easiest and best way to give fluids is orally. The use of oral glucose and salt solutions may be life-saving in infective diarrhoea. However, patients may be unable to take fluids orally. Often the reason for this is self-evident, e.g. because the patient is comatose, or has undergone major surgery, or is vomiting. Sometimes the decision is taken to give fluids intravenously even if the patient is able to tolerate oral fluids. This can be because there is clinical evidence of fluid depletion, or biochemical evidence of electrolyte disturbance, that is felt to be severe enough to require rapid correction (more rapid than could easily be achieved orally).

Which IV fluids should be given?

The list of intravenous fluids that is available for prescription in many hospital formularies is long and potentially bewildering. However, with a few exceptions, many of these fluids are variations on the three basic types of fluid shown in Figure 1.

- *Plasma, whole blood, or plasma expanders.* These replace deficits in the vascular compartment only. They are indicated where there is a reduction in the blood volume due to blood loss from whatever cause. Such solutions are sometimes referred to as 'colloids' to distinguish them from 'crystalloids'. Colloidal particles in solution cannot pass through the (semipermeable) capillary membrane, in contrast with crystalloid particles like sodium and chloride ions, which can. This is why they are confined to the vascular compartment, whereas sodium chloride ('saline') solutions are distributed throughout the entire ECF.
- *Isotonic sodium chloride (0.9% NaCl).* It is called isotonic because its effective osmolality, or tonicity, is similar to that of the ECF. Once it is administered it is confined to the ECF and is indicated where there is a reduced ECF volume, as, for example, in sodium depletion.
- *Water.* If pure water were infused it would haemolyse blood cells as it enters the vein. Water should instead be given as 5% dextrose (glucose), which, like 0.9% saline, is isotonic with plasma initially. The dextrose is rapidly metabolized. The water that remains is distributed evenly through all body compartments and contributes to both ECF and ICF. Five per cent dextrose is, therefore, designed to replace deficits in total body water, e.g. in most hypernatraemic patients, rather than those specifically with reduced ECF volume.

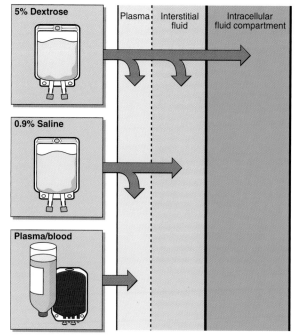

Fig. 1 **The three types of fluid usually used in intravenous fluid therapy are shown here with the different contributions they make to the body fluid compartments.**

How much fluid should be given?

This depends on the extent of the losses that have already occurred of both fluid and electrolytes, and on the losses/requirements anticipated over the next 24 hours. The latter depends, in turn, on both insensible losses and measured losses.

Existing losses

It may not be possible to calculate the exact deficit of water or electrolytes. This is not as critical as one might expect. Even where there is a severe deficit of water or sodium, it is important not to replace too quickly if complications of over-rapid correction are to be avoided. Unless there are severe ongoing losses it is the duration rather than the rate of fluid replacement that varies.

Anticipated losses

It is useful to know what 'normality' is, i.e. what the fluid and electrolyte requirements would be for a healthy subject if for some reason they were unable to eat or drink orally. Most textbooks quote a water throughput of between 2 and 3 L daily, a sodium throughput of 100 to 200 mmol/day, and a potassium throughput that varies from 20 to 200 mmol/day. These figures include the insensible losses (those that occur from skin, respiration and faeces); these are not normally measured and, for water, amount to about 800 mL/day. In artificial ventilation or excessive sweating insensible losses may increase greatly.

How quickly should the fluids be given?

The appropriate rate of fluid replacement varies enormously according to the clinical situation. For example, a patient with trauma-induced diabetes insipidus can lose as much as 15 L urine daily. The two very different clinical scenarios below illustrate the importance of the rate of IV fluid replacement.

Perioperative patient

It might be expected that intravenous fluid therapy for a patient undergoing elective surgery would be based simply on 'normality' (see above) and that an appropriate daily regimen should include between 2.0 and 3.0 L isotonic fluids, of which 1.0 L should be 0.9% saline (which will provide ~155 mmol sodium), with potassium supplementation. However, this approach does not take account of the metabolic response to trauma, which provides a powerful non-osmotic stimulus to AVP secretion, with resultant water retention, or of the response to physiological stress, which both reduces sodium excretion and increases potassium excretion, or of the redistribution of potassium that occurs as a result of tissue damage. In the immediate postoperative period, a daily regimen that includes 1.0 to 1.5 L IV fluid containing 30 to 50 mmol sodium and no potassium will often be adequate.

Hyponatraemia

Patients with severe hyponatraemia are vulnerable to demyelination if the serum sodium is raised acutely. The mechanism may involve osmotic shrinkage of axons, which leads to severing of the links with their myelin sheaths. Osmotic demyelination is especially likely in the pons (*central pontine myelinolysis*) and results in severe neurological disorders or death. For this reason, it is recommended that serum sodium should be raised by not more than 10 to 12 mmol/L per day.

How should the fluid therapy be monitored?

The best place to study monitoring of IV fluid replacement in practice is in the intensive care setting. Here, comprehensive monitoring of a patient's fluid and electrolyte balance (Fig. 2) allows the prescribed fluid regimen to be tailored to the patient's individual requirement.

Clinical note

Assessing a patient's fluid and electrolyte status has as much, if not more, to do with clinical skill than biochemical interpretation. Look at the patient in Figure 2 and think about what information is available. Your answer may include consideration of the following:

- case records (details of patient history, examination)
- examination of patient (JVP, CVP, pulse, BP, presence of oedema, chest sounds, skin turgor)
- fluid balance and nursing charts (BP, pulse, temperature, fluid-input and output)
- nasogastric and surgical wound drainage, in addition to urinary catheter bag
- presence of IV fluid therapy (type, volume)
- ambient temperature (wall thermometer).

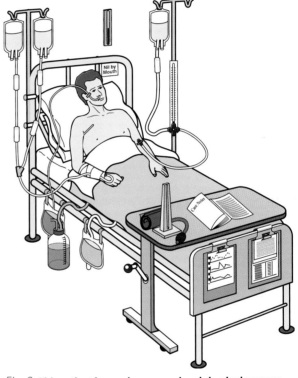

Fig. 2 **This patient has undergone major abdominal surgery and is now 2 days postop.**

Case history 8

Postoperatively, a 62-year-old woman was noted to be getting progressively weaker. There was no evidence of fever, bleeding or infection. Blood pressure was 120/80 mmHg. Before the operation her serum electrolytes were normal, as were her renal function and cardiovascular system. Three days after the operation her electrolytes were repeated.

Na$^+$	K$^+$	Cl$^-$	HCO$_3^-$	Urea	Creatinine
		mmol/L			*μmol/L*
125	4.2	77	32	21.4	145

Random urine osmolality = 920 mmol/kg
Urine [Na$^+$] < 10 mmol/L
Urine [K$^+$] = 15 mmol/L

- What is the pathophysiology behind these findings?
- What other information do you require in order to prescribe the appropriate fluid therapy?

Comment on page 162.

Intravenous fluid therapy

- Intravenous fluid (IV) therapy is commonly used to correct fluid and electrolyte imbalance.
- The simple guidelines for IV fluid therapy are:
  - first assess patient clinically, then biochemically, paying particular attention to cardiac and renal function
  - use simple solutions
  - in prescribing fluids, attempt to make up deficits and anticipate future losses
  - monitor patient closely at all times during fluid therapy.

Investigation of renal function (1)

Functions of the kidney

The functional unit of the kidney is the nephron, shown in Figure 1. The functions of the kidneys include:

- regulation of water, electrolyte and acid–base balance
- excretion of the products of protein and nucleic acid metabolism: e.g. urea, creatinine and uric acid.

The kidneys are also endocrine organs, producing a number of hormones, and are subject to control by others (Fig. 2). Arginine vasopressin (AVP) acts to influence water balance, and aldosterone affects sodium reabsorption in the nephron. Parathyroid hormone promotes tubular reabsorption of calcium, phosphate excretion and the synthesis of 1,25-dihydrocholecalciferol (the active form of vitamin D). Renin is made by the juxtaglomerular cells and catalyses the formation of angiotensin I and ultimately aldosterone synthesis.

It is convenient to discuss renal function in terms of *glomerular* and *tubular* function.

Glomerular function

Serum creatinine

The first step in urine formation is the filtration of plasma at the glomeruli (Fig. 1). The glomerular filtration rate (GFR) is defined as the volume of plasma from which a given substance is completely cleared by glomerular filtration per unit time. This is approximately 140 mL/min in a healthy adult, but varies enormously with body size, and so is usually normalized to take account of this. Conventionally, it is corrected to a body surface area (BSA) of 1.73 m^2 (so the units are mL/min/1.73 m^2).

Historically, measurement of creatinine in serum has been used as a convenient but insensitive measure of glomerular function. Figure 3 shows that GFR has to halve before a significant rise in serum creatinine becomes apparent – a 'normal' serum creatinine does not necessarily mean all is well. By way of example, consider an asymptomatic person who shows a serum creatinine of 130 µmol/L:

- In a young woman this might well be abnormal and requires follow-up.
- In a muscular young man this is the expected result.
- In an elderly person this may simply reflect the physiological decline of GFR with age.

Creatinine clearance

Simultaneous measurement of urinary excretion of creatinine by means of a timed urine collection allows estimation of creatinine clearance. The way this is worked out is as follows. The amount of creatinine excreted in urine over a given period of time is the product of the volume of urine collected (say, V litres in 24 hours) and the urine creatinine concentration (U). The next step is to work out the volume of plasma that would have contained this amount (U × V) of creatinine. This is done by dividing the amount excreted (U × V) by the plasma concentration of creatinine (P):

$$\text{Volume of plasma} = \frac{U \times V}{P}$$

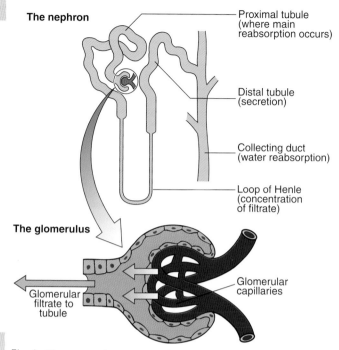

The nephron

- Proximal tubule (where main reabsorption occurs)
- Distal tubule (secretion)
- Collecting duct (water reabsorption)
- Loop of Henle (concentration of filtrate)

The glomerulus

- Glomerular filtrate to tubule
- Glomerular capillaries

Fig. 1   **Diagrammatic representation of a nephron.**

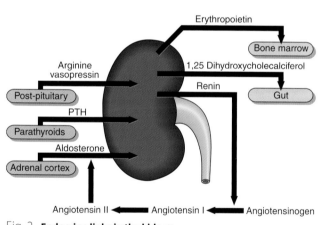

- Erythropoietin
- Bone marrow
- Arginine vasopressin
- 1,25 Dihydroxycholecalciferol
- Renin
- Gut
- Post-pituitary
- PTH
- Parathyroids
- Aldosterone
- Adrenal cortex
- Angiotensin II ← Angiotensin I ← Angiotensinogen

Fig. 2   **Endocrine links in the kidney.**

This is the volume of plasma that would have to be completely 'cleared' of creatinine during the time of collection in order to give the amount seen in the urine. It is known as the *creatinine clearance*. Although it is more sensitive than serum creatinine in detecting reduced GFR it is inconvenient for patients and imprecise, and has now been largely superseded by the so-called prediction equations which estimate GFR.

Estimated GFR (eGFR)

The relatively poor inverse correlation between serum creatinine and GFR can be improved by taking into account some of the confounding variables, such as age, sex, ethnic origin and body weight. The formula developed by Cockcroft and Gault, and the four-variable equation derived from the Modification of Diet in Renal Disease (MDRD) Study are the most widely used of these prediction equations. These are compared in Table 1.

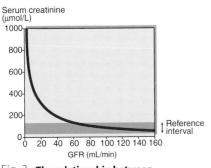

Fig. 3 The relationship between glomerular filtration rate and serum creatinine concentration. Glomerular filtration rate may fall considerably before serum creatinine is significantly increased.

Table 1 **Cockcroft–Gault versus four-variable ('simplified') MDRD equation**	
Cockcroft–Gault	**Four-variable ('simplified') MDRD equation**
Developed in the mid-1970s	Developed in the late 1990s
Incorporates age, sex and weight	Incorporates age, sex and ethnicity*
Widely used to calculate drug dosages	Widely used on biochemistry reports
Developed in a population with reduced GFR	Developed in a population with reduced GFR

*But has only been validated in some ethnic groups, e.g. Caucasians, Afro-Caribbeans.

Limitations of eGFR

Although prediction equations are an improvement on serum creatinine, and creatinine clearance, they are merely *estimates* of GFR and should be interpreted with caution. For example, they are more likely to be inaccurate in subjects with relatively normal GFR. For this reason, many hospital laboratories do not report a specific result when the GFR is greater than 60 mL/min/1.73 m². Other patient groups where eGFR is less accurate include those with abnormal body shape or mass, e.g. muscle wasting, amputees. Finally, there is evidence that the GFR estimated by the MDRD formula is affected by consumption of meat.

eGFR – additional observations

It is worth putting the limitations of eGFR outlined in the previous section into their proper context. Estimates of GFR e.g. the four-variable MDRD formula, are undoubtedly better than serum creatinine on its own at identifying reduced glomerular function, simply because they take some of the confounding variables into account (see Table 1). The Cockcroft–Gault formula requires weight in addition to age and sex (and creatinine) in order to be applied. It is therefore much easier to apply the MDRD formula which incorporates age, sex and ethnicity, but not weight. This is one of the reasons why the MDRD equation is widely used. However, Cockcroft–Gault is still widely used to calculate drug dosages.

Reduced glomerular function, e.g. eGFR 50–60 mL/min/1.73 m², is known to be associated with cardiovascular risk and subsequent progression to more severe renal failure, but much remains to be clarified about this group of patients, e.g. the time-course of progression. This is an area of active research.

Other measures

Cystatin C is a low-molecular-weight protein, the serum concentrations of which, like creatinine, correlate inversely with GFR. However, unlike creatinine, the concentration of cystatin C is independent of weight and height, muscle mass, adult age or sex and is largely unaffected by intake of meat or non-meat-containing foods. Thus it has been studied as a potential alternative method of assessment.

Various other markers may be used to estimate clearance, but are too costly and labour-intensive to be widely applied. They include inulin, and radioisotopic markers such as ^{51}Cr-EDTA. Inulin clearance is widely regarded as the most accurate (gold standard) estimate of GFR.

Proteinuria

Another aspect of glomerular function is its 'leakiness'. The glomerular basement membrane does not usually allow passage of albumin and large proteins. A small amount of albumin, usually less than 25 mg/24 hours, is found in urine. When larger amounts, in excess of 250 mg/24 hours, are detected, significant damage to the glomerular membrane has occurred.

Albumin excretion in the range 25–300 mg/24 hours is termed microalbuminuria (p. 63). Tubular proteinuria is discussed on pages 30–31.

Clinical note
The glomerular filtration rate, like the heart and respiration rates, fluctuates throughout the day. A change in the GFR of up to 20% between two consecutive creatinine clearances may not indicate any real change in renal function.

Case history 9

A man aged 35 years presenting with loin pain has a serum creatinine of 150 µmol/L. A 24-hour urine of 2160 mL is collected and found to have a creatinine concentration of 7.5 mmol/L.

■ Calculate the creatinine clearance and comment on the results.

An error in the timed collection was subsequently reported by the nursing staff, and collection time was reported to be 17 hours.

■ How does this affect the result and its interpretation.

Comment on page 163.

Investigation of renal function (1)

■ Serum creatinine concentration is an insensitive index of renal function, as it may not appear to be elevated until the GFR has fallen below 50% of normal.

■ eGFR is an improvement on serum creatinine but is an estimate and should be interpreted cautiously.

■ Proteinuria may be used as a marker of renal damage and predicts its progression.

Investigation of renal function (2)

Renal tubular function

The glomeruli provide an efficient filtration mechanism for ridding the body of waste products and toxic substances. To ensure that important constituents, such as water, sodium, glucose and amino acids, are not lost from the body, tubular reabsorption must be equally efficient. For example, 180 L of fluid pass into the glomerular filtrate each day, and more than 99% of this is recovered. Compared with the GFR as an assessment of glomerular function, there are no easily performed tests that measure tubular function in a quantitative manner.

Tubular dysfunction

Some disorders of tubular function are inherited, for example some patients are unable to reduce their urine pH below 6.5, because of a failure of hydrogen ion secretion. However, renal tubular damage is much more frequently secondary to other conditions or insults. Any cause of acute renal failure may be associated with renal tubular failure.

Investigation of tubular function

Osmolality measurements in plasma and urine

The renal tubules perform a bewildering array of functions. However, in practice, the urine osmolality serves as a proxy or general marker of tubular function. This is because of all the tubular functions, the one most frequently affected by disease is the ability to concentrate the urine. If the tubules and collecting ducts are working efficiently, and if AVP is present, they will be able to reabsorb water. Just how well can be assessed by measuring urine concentration. This is conveniently done by determining the osmolality, and then comparing this to the plasma. If the urine osmolality is 600 mmol/kg or more, tubular function is usually regarded as intact. When the urine osmolality does not differ greatly from plasma (urine:plasma osmolality ratio ~1), the renal tubules are not reabsorbing water.

The water deprivation test

The causes of polyuria are summarized in Table 1. Renal tubular dysfunction is one of several causes of disordered water homeostasis. Where measurement of baseline urine osmolality is inconclusive, formal water deprivation may be indicated. The normal physiological response to water deprivation is water retention, which minimizes the rise in plasma osmolality that would otherwise be observed. The body achieves this water retention by means of AVP, the action of which on the renal tubules may be inferred from a rising urine osmolality. In practice, if the urine osmolality rises to 600 mmol/kg or more in response to water deprivation, diabetes insipidus is effectively excluded. A flat urine osmolality response is characteristically seen in diabetes insipidus where the hormone AVP is lacking. In compulsive water drinkers, a normal (rising) response is usually seen.

It should be noted that the water deprivation test is unpleasant for the patient. It is also potentially dangerous if there is severe inability to retain water. The test must be terminated if more than 3 L of urine is passed. An alternative approach, which is sometimes used first (or instead of), is to fluid restrict overnight (8pm–10am) and measure the osmolality of urine voided in the morning. If the urine osmolality fails to rise in response to water deprivation, desmopressin (DDAVP), a synthetic analogue of AVP, is administered. The subsequent urine osmolality response allows central diabetes insipidus to be distinguished from nephrogenic diabetes insipidus. In the former, the renal tubules respond normally to the DDAVP and the urine osmolality rises. Nephrogenic diabetes insipidus is characterized by failure of the tubules to respond; the urine osmolality response remains flat.

Urine pH and the acid load test

Renal tubular acidosis (RTA) may be characterized as follows:

- *Type I*. There is a defective hydrogen ion secretion in the distal tubule that may be inherited or acquired.
- *Type II*. The capacity to reabsorb bicarbonate in the proximal tubule is reduced.
- *Type III*. Is a paediatric variant of type I renal tubular acidosis.
- *Type IV*. Bicarbonate reabsorption by the renal tubule is impaired as a consequence of aldosterone deficiency, aldosterone receptor defects, or drugs which block aldosterone action.

The first step in making a diagnosis of RTA is to establish the presence of a persistent unexplained metabolic acidosis. If RTA is suspected after other diagnoses have been considered and excluded, a *fresh* urine specimen

Table 1 **Causes of polyuria**		
Cause	Urine osmolality	Plasma osmolality
	mmol/kg	
Increased osmotic load, e.g. due to glucose	~500	~310
Increased water ingestion	<200	~280
Diabetes inspidius	<200	~300
Nephrogenic diabetes insipidus	<200	~300

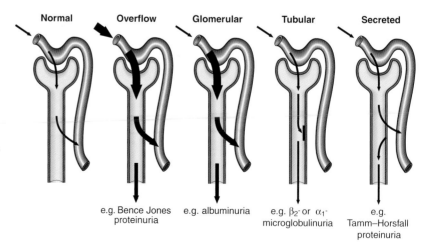

Fig. 1 **The classification of proteinuria**.

Normal   Overflow   Glomerular   Tubular   Secreted

e.g. Bence Jones proteinuria   e.g. albuminuria   e.g. β₂- or α₁-microglobulinuria   e.g. Tamm–Horsfall proteinuria

should be collected for measurement of urine pH. (If the specimen is not fresh, urease-splitting bacteria may alkalinize the specimen post collection giving a falsely high urine pH.) The normal response to a metabolic acidosis is to increase acid excretion, and a urine pH of less than 5.3 makes diagnosis of RTA unlikely as the cause of the acidosis. Where the urine pH is not convincingly acidic, an acid load test may be indicated. This involves administering ammonium chloride (which makes the blood more acidic) and measuring the urine pH in serial samples collected hourly for about 8 hours afterwards. Rarely, the excretion rates of titratable acid and ammonium ion, and the serum bicarbonate concentration, may have to be measured in order to make the diagnosis. This test should not be performed in patients who are already severely acidotic or who have liver disease.

Specific proteinuria

Causes of proteinuria are summarized in Figure 1. Mention has already been made of protein in urine as an indicator of leaky glomeruli (p. 29). β_2-microglobulin and α_1-microglobulin are small proteins that are filtered at the glomeruli and are usually reabsorbed by the tubular cells. An increased concentration of these proteins in urine is a sensitive indicator of renal tubular cell damage.

Glycosuria

The presence of glucose in urine when blood glucose is *normal* usually reflects the inability of the tubules to reabsorb glucose because of a specific tubular lesion. Here, the renal threshold (the capacity for the tubules to reabsorb the substance in question) has been reached. This is called renal glycosuria and is a benign condition. Glycosuria can also present in association with other disorders of tubular function – the Fanconi syndrome.

Case history 10

RS, a 30-year-old woman, fractured her skull in an accident. She had no other major injuries, no significant blood loss, and her cardiovascular system was stable. She was unconscious for 2 days after the accident. On the 4th day of her admission to hospital she was noted to be producing large volumes of urine and complaining of thirst. Biochemical findings were:

Na+	K+	Cl–	HCO₃–	Urea	Creatinine	Glucose
		— mmol/L —			µmol/L	mmol/L
150	3.6	106	25	5.5	80	5.4

Serum osmolality = 310 mmol/kg
Urine osmolality = 110 mmol/kg
Urine volume = 8 litres/24 h

■ Is a water deprivation test required to make the diagnosis in this patient?

Comment on page 163.

Aminoaciduria

Normally, amino acids in the glomerular filtrate are reabsorbed in the proximal tubules. They may be present in urine in excessive amount either because the plasma concentration exceeds the renal threshold, or because there is specific failure of normal tubular reabsorptive mechanisms. The latter may occur in the inherited metabolic disorder cystinuria, or more commonly because of acquired renal tubular damage.

Specific tubular defects

The Fanconi syndrome

The Fanconi syndrome is a term used to describe the occurrence of generalized tubular defects such as renal tubular acidosis, aminoaciduria and tubular proteinuria. It can occur as a result of heavy metal poisoning, or from the effects of toxins and inherited metabolic diseases such as cystinosis.

Renal stones

Renal stones (calculi) produce severe pain and discomfort, and are common causes of obstruction in the urinary tract (Fig. 2). Chemical analysis of renal stones is important in the investigation of why they have formed. Types of stone include:

Clinical note

Orthostatic, or postural, proteinuria is common in teenagers. It is a benign condition in which proteinuria occurs only when the subjects are standing upright, and is a result of an increase in the hydrostatic pressure in the renal veins.

- *Calcium phosphate*: may be a consequence of primary hyperparathyroidism or renal tubular acidosis.
- *Magnesium, ammonium and phosphate*: are often associated with urinary tract infections.
- *Oxalate*: may be a consequence of hyperoxaluria.
- *Uric acid*: may be a consequence of hyperuricaemia (see pp. 142–143).
- *Cystine*: these are rare and a feature of the inherited metabolic disorder cystinuria (see p. 158).

Urinalysis

Examination of a patient's urine is important and should not be restricted to biochemical tests. (see pp. 32–33).

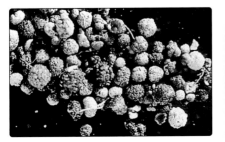

Fig. 2 **Renal calculi.**

Investigation of renal function (2)

- Chemical examination of urine is one aspect of urinalysis.
- A comparison of urine and serum osmolality measurements will indicate if a patient has the ability to concentrate urine.
- Specific tests are available to measure urinary concentrating ability and the ability to excrete an acid load.
- The presence of specific small proteins in urine indicates tubular damage.
- Chemical analysis of renal stones is important in the investigation of their aetiology.

Urinalysis

Urinalysis is so important in screening for disease that it is regarded as an integral part of the complete physical examination of every patient, and not just in the investigation of renal disease. Urinalysis comprises a range of analyses that are usually performed at the point of care rather than in a central laboratory. Examination of a patient's urine should not be restricted to biochemical tests. Figure 1 summarizes the different ways urine may be examined.

Procedure

Biochemical testing of urine involves the use of commercially available disposable strips (Fig. 2). Each strip is impregnated with a number of coloured reagent 'blocks' separated from each other by narrow bands. When the strip is manually immersed in the urine specimen, the reagents in each block react with a specific component of urine in such a way that (a) the block changes colour if the component is present, and (b) the colour change produced is proportional to the concentration of the component being tested for.

To test a urine sample:

- fresh urine is collected into a clean dry container
- the sample is not centrifuged
- the disposable strip is briefly immersed in the urine specimen; care must be taken to ensure that all reagent blocks are covered

- the edge of the strip is held against the rim of the urine container to remove any excess urine
- the strip is then held in a horizontal position for a fixed length of time that varies from 30 seconds to 2 minutes
- the colour of the test areas are compared with those provided on a colour chart (Fig. 2). The strip is held close to the colour blocks on the chart and matched carefully, and then discarded.

The range of components routinely tested for in commonly available commercial urinalysis strips is extensive and includes glucose, bilirubin, ketones, specific gravity, blood, pH (hydrogen ion concentration), protein, urobilinogen, nitrite and leucocytes (white blood cells).

Urinalysis is one of the commonest biochemical tests performed outside the laboratory. It is most commonly performed by non-laboratory staff. Although the test is simple, failure to follow the correct procedure may lead to inaccurate results. A frequent example of this is where test strips are read too quickly or left too long. Other potential errors may arise because test strips have been stored wrongly or are out of date.

Glucose

The presence of glucose in urine (glycosuria) indicates that the filtered load of glucose exceeds the ability of the renal tubules to reabsorb all of it. This usually reflects hyperglycaemia

and should, therefore, prompt consideration of whether more formal testing for diabetes mellitus is appropriate, e.g. by measuring fasting blood glucose. However, glycosuria is not always due to diabetes. The renal threshold for glucose may be lowered, for example in pregnancy, and glucose may enter the filtrate even at normal plasma concentrations (renal glycosuria).

Blood glucose rises rapidly after a meal, overcoming the normal renal threshold temporarily (alimentary glycosuria). Both renal and alimentary glycosuria are unrelated to diabetes.

Bilirubin

Bilirubin exists in the blood in two forms, conjugated and unconjugated. Only the conjugated form is water-soluble, so bilirubinuria signifies the presence in urine of conjugated bilirubin. This is always pathological. Conjugated bilirubin is normally excreted through the biliary tree into the gut where it is broken down; a small amount is reabsorbed into the portal circulation, taken up by the liver and re-excreted in bile. Interruption of this so-called enterohepatic circulation usually stems from mechanical obstruction, and results in high levels of conjugated bilirubin in the systemic circulation, some of which spills over into the urine.

Urobilinogen

In the gut, conjugated bilirubin is broken down by bacteria to products known collectively as faecal urobilinogen, or stercobilinogen. This too undergoes an enterohepatic circulation. However, unlike bilirubin, urobilinogen is found in the systemic circulation and is often detectable in the urine of normal subjects. Thus the finding of urobilinogen in urine is of less diagnostic significance than bilirubin. High levels are found in any condition where bilirubin turnover is increased, e.g. haemolysis, or where its enterohepatic circulation is interrupted, e.g. by liver damage.

Ketones

Ketones are the products of fatty acid breakdown. Their presence usually indicates that the body is using fat to provide energy rather than storing it for later use. This can occur in

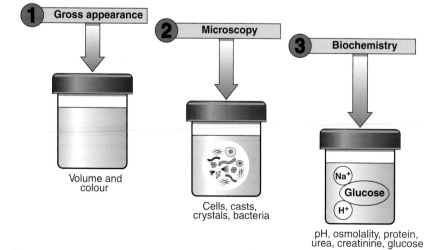

Fig. 1 **The place of biochemical testing in urinalysis.**

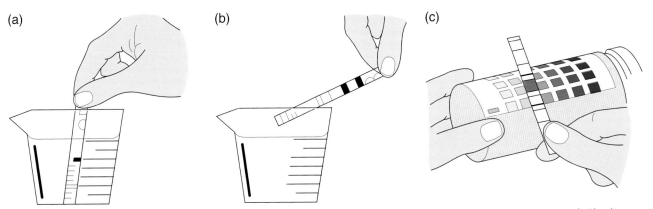

Fig. 2 **Multistix testing of a urine sample: (a)** Immersion of test strip in urine specimen. **(b)** Excess urine removed. **(c)** Test strip is compared with colour chart on bottle label.

uncontrolled diabetes, where glucose is unable to enter cells (diabetic ketoacidosis), in alcoholism (alcoholic ketoacidosis), or in association with prolonged fasting or vomiting.

Specific gravity

This is a semi-quantitative measure of urinary density, which in turn reflects concentration. A higher specific gravity indicates a more concentrated urine. Assessment of urinary specific gravity usually just confirms the impression gained by visually inspecting the colour of the urine. When urine concentration needs to be quantitated, most people will request urine osmolality, which has a much wider working range.

pH (hydrogen ion concentration)

Urine is usually acidic (urine pH substantially less than 7.4 indicating a high concentration of hydrogen ions). Measurement of urine pH is useful either in cases of suspected adulteration, e.g. drug abuse screens, or where there is an unexplained metabolic acidosis (low serum bicarbonate). The renal tubules normally excrete hydrogen ions by mechanisms that ensure tight

regulation of the blood hydrogen ion concentration. Where one or more of these mechanisms fail, an acidosis results (so-called renal tubular acidosis or RTA; see p. 30). Measurement of urine pH may, therefore, be used to screen for RTA in unexplained metabolic acidosis; a pH less than 5.3 indicates that the kidneys are able to acidify urine and are, therefore, unlikely to be responsible.

Protein

Proteinuria may signify abnormal excretion of protein by the kidneys (due either to abnormally 'leaky' glomeruli or to the inability of the tubules to reabsorb protein normally), or it may simply reflect the presence in the urine of cells or blood. For this reason it is important to check that the dipstick test is not also positive for blood or leucocytes (white cells); it may also be appropriate to screen for a urinary tract infection by sending urine for culture.

Blood

The presence of blood in the urine (haematuria) is consistent with various possibilities ranging from malignancy through urinary tract infection to

contamination from menstruation. Dipstick tests for blood are able to detect haemoglobin and myoglobin in addition to red blood cells – the presence in the urine sediment of large numbers of red cells establishes the diagnosis of haematuria. The absence of red cells, despite a strongly positive dipstick test for blood, points towards myoglobinuria or haemoglobinuria.

Nitrite

This dipstick test depends on the conversion of nitrate (from the diet) to nitrite by the action in the urine of bacteria that contain the necessary reductase. A positive result points towards a urinary tract infection.

Leucocytes

The presence of leucocytes in the urine suggests acute inflammation and the presence of a urinary tract infection.

Case history 11

A patient attending the hospital outpatient clinic is found to have proteinuria on dipstick testing. On examination he has pitting oedema of both ankles.

■ What might explain these findings?

Comment on page 163.

Clinical note

Microbiological testing of a urine specimen (usually a mid-stream specimen or MSSU) is routinely performed to confirm the diagnosis of a urinary tract infection. These samples should be collected into sterile containers and sent to the laboratory without delay for culture and antibiotic sensitivity tests.

Urinalysis

■ Urinalysis should be part of the clinical examination of every patient.

■ Chemical analysis of a urine specimen is carried out using commercially available disposable strips.

■ The range of components routinely tested for includes glucose, bilirubin, ketones, specific gravity, blood, pH, protein, urobilinogen, nitrite and leucocytes.

Acute renal failure

Renal failure is the cessation of kidney function. In acute renal failure (ARF), the kidneys fail over a period of hours or days. Chronic renal failure (CRF) develops over months or years and leads eventually to end-stage renal failure (ESRF). ARF may be reversed and normal renal function regained, whereas CRF is irreversible.

Aetiology

ARF arises from a variety of problems affecting the kidneys and/or their circulation. It usually presents as a sudden deterioration of renal function indicated by rapidly rising serum urea and creatinine concentrations. As acute renal failure is common in the severely ill, sequential monitoring of kidney function is important for early detection in this group of patients.

Usually, urine output falls to less than 400 mL/24 hours, and the patient is said to be oliguric. The patient may pass no urine at all, and be anuric. Occasionally urine flow remains high when tubular dysfunction predominates.

Kidney failure or uraemia can be classified as (Fig. 1):

- *Pre-renal*: the kidney fails to receive a proper blood supply.
- *Post-renal*: the urinary drainage of the kidneys is impaired because of an obstruction.
- *Renal*: intrinsic damage to the kidney tissue. This may be due to a variety of diseases, or the renal damage may be a consequence of prolonged pre-renal or post-renal problems.

Diagnosis

In nearly all cases the clinical history and presentation will indicate that a patient has, or may develop, ARF. The first step in assessing the patient with ARF is to identify any pre- or post-renal factors that could be readily corrected and allow recovery of renal function. The history and examination of the patient, including the presence of other severe illness, drug history and time course of the onset of the ARF, may well provide important clues. Factors that precipitate pre-renal uraemia are usually associated with a reduced effective ECF volume and include:

- decreased plasma volume because of blood loss, burns, prolonged vomiting, or diarrhoea
- diminished cardiac output
- local factors, such as an occlusion of the renal artery.

Pre-renal factors lead to decreased renal perfusion and reduction in GFR. Both AVP and aldosterone are secreted maximally and a small volume of concentrated urine is produced.

Biochemical findings in pre-renal uraemia include the following:

- *Serum urea and creatinine are increased.* Urea is increased proportionally more than creatinine because of its reabsorption by the tubular cells, particularly at low urine flow rates. This leads to a relatively higher serum urea concentration than creatinine, which is not so readily reabsorbed.
- *Metabolic acidosis*: because of the inability of the kidney to excrete hydrogen ions.
- *Hyperkalaemia*: because of the decreased glomerular filtration rate and acidosis.
- *A high urine osmolality.*

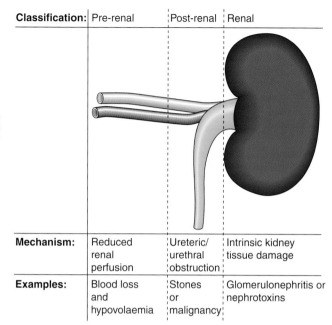

Classification:	Pre-renal	Post-renal	Renal
Mechanism:	Reduced renal perfusion	Ureteric/ urethral obstruction	Intrinsic kidney tissue damage
Examples:	Blood loss and hypovolaemia	Stones or malignancy	Glomerulonephritis or nephrotoxins

Fig. 1 **The classification of acute renal failure.**

Post-renal factors cause decreased renal function, because the effective filtration pressure at the glomeruli is reduced due to the back pressure caused by the blockage. Causes include:

- renal stones
- carcinoma of cervix, prostate, or occasionally bladder.

If these pre- or post-renal factors are not corrected, patients will develop intrinsic renal damage (acute tubular necrosis).

Acute tubular necrosis

Acute tubular necrosis may develop in the absence of pre-existing pre-renal or post-renal failure. The causes include:

- acute blood loss in severe trauma
- septic shock
- specific renal disease, such as glomerulonephritis
- nephrotoxins, such as the aminoglycosides, analgesics or herbal toxins.

Patients in the early stages of acute tubular necrosis may have only modestly increased serum urea and creatinine that then rise rapidly over a period of days, in contrast to the slow increase over months and years seen in chronic renal failure.

It may be difficult to decide the reason for a patient's oliguria. The biochemical features that distinguish pre-renal uraemia from intrinsic renal damage are shown in Table 1.

Management

Important issues in the management of the patient with ARF include:

- *Correction of pre-renal factors, if present, by replacement of any ECF volume deficit.* Care should be taken that the patient does not become fluid overloaded. In cardiac failure, inotropic agents may be indicated.

Table 1 **Biochemical features in the differential diagnosis of the oliguric patient**

Biochemical feature	Pre-renal failure	Intrinsic renal damage
Urine sodium	<20 mmol/L	>40 mmol/L
Urine/serum urea	>10:1	<3:1
Urine/plasma osmolality	>1.5:1	<1.1:1

- *Treatment of the underlying disease* (e.g. to control infection).
- *Biochemical monitoring*. Daily fluid balance charts provide an assessment of body fluid volume. Serum creatinine indicates the degree of impairment of the GFR and the rate of deterioration or improvement. Serum potassium should be monitored closely.
- *Dialysis*. Indications for dialysis include a rapidly rising serum potassium concentration, severe acidosis, and fluid overload.

Recovery

There may be three distinct phases in the resolving clinical course of a patient with acute renal failure (Fig. 2). An initial oliguric phase, where glomerular impairment predominates, is followed by a diuretic phase when urine output is high, as glomerular function improves but tubular function remains impaired. During a recovery phase, complete renal function may return. Careful clinical and biochemical monitoring is necessary throughout the course of the patient's illness.

It should be noted that initially the urea and creatinine may be normal in ARF. The serum potassium usually rises very quickly in catabolic patients, with or without tissue damage, and falls quickly once the urine flow rate increases. The urine volume cannot be related to the GFR. The serum urea and creatinine remain high during the diuretic phase, because the GFR is still low and the large urine volumes reflect tubular damage. In the recovery phase the serum urea and creatinine fall as the GFR improves and the serum potassium concentration returns to normal, as the tubular mechanisms recover.

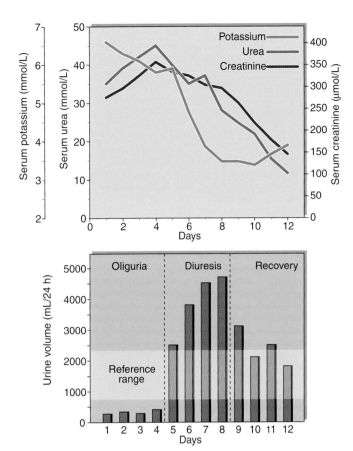

Fig. 2 **The biochemical course of a typical patient with acute renal failure.**

Clinical note

Acute tubular necrosis is the commonest cause of severe life-threatening hyperkalaemia. The rapidly increasing serum potassium is usually the indication to start the patient on dialysis.

Case history 12

A male, aged 50, presented with pyrexia. He was clinically dehydrated and oliguric.

Na⁺	K⁺	Cl⁻	HCO₃⁻	Urea	Creatinine
		mmol/L			*μmol/L*
140	5.9	112	16	22.9	155

Serum osmolality = 305 mmol/kg
Urine osmolality = 629 mmol/kg

- What do these biochemistry results indicate about the patient's condition?

Comment on page 163.

Acute renal failure

- ARF is the failure of renal function over a period of hours or days identified by a rising serum urea and creatinine.
- Acute renal failure may be classified as pre-renal, renal or post-renal.
- Prompt identification of pre- or post-renal factors may allow correction of the problem before damage to nephrons occurs.
- Management of a patient with intrinsic renal damage will include sequential measurement of creatinine, sodium, potassium and bicarbonate in serum, and urine sodium and potassium excretion and osmolality.
- Care should be taken to prevent fluid overload in the treatment of patients with renal disease.
- Life-threatening hyperkalaemia may be a consequence of ARF.

Chronic renal failure

Chronic renal failure (CRF) is the progressive irreversible destruction of kidney tissue by disease which, if not treated by dialysis or transplant, will result in the death of the patient. The aetiology of CRF encompasses the spectrum of known kidney diseases. The end result of progressive renal damage is the same no matter what the cause of the disease may have been. The major effects of renal failure all occur because of the loss of functioning nephrons. It is a feature of CRF that patients may have few if any symptoms until the glomerular filtration rate falls below 15 mL/minute (i.e. to 10% of normal function), and the disease is far advanced.

Consequences of CRF

Sodium and water metabolism
Most CRF patients retain the ability to reabsorb sodium ions, but the renal tubules may lose their ability to reabsorb water and so concentrate urine. Polyuria, although present, may not be excessive because the GFR is so low. Because of their impaired ability to regulate water balance, patients in renal failure may become fluid overloaded or fluid depleted very easily.

Potassium metabolism
Hyperkalaemia is a feature of advanced CRF and poses a threat to life (Fig. 1). The ability to excrete potassium decreases as the GFR falls, but hyperkalaemia may not be a major problem in CRF until the GFR falls to very low levels. Then, a sudden deterioration of renal function may precipitate a rapid rise in serum potassium concentration. An unexpectedly high serum potassium concentration in an outpatient should always be investigated with urgency.

Acid–base balance
As CRF develops, the ability of the kidneys to regenerate bicarbonate and excrete hydrogen ions in the urine becomes impaired. The retention of hydrogen ions causes a metabolic acidosis.

Calcium and phosphate metabolism
The ability of the renal cells to make 1,25-dihydroxy-cholecalciferol falls as the renal tubular damage progresses. Calcium absorption is reduced and there is a tendency towards hypocalcaemia. Parathyroid hormone (PTH) is stimulated in an attempt to restore plasma calcium to normal, and high circulating PTH may have adverse effects on bone if this is allowed to continue (renal osteodystrophy; Fig. 2).

Erythropoietin synthesis
Anaemia is often associated with chronic renal disease. The normochromic normocytic anaemia is due primarily to failure of erythropoietin production. Biosynthesized human erythropoietin may be used to treat the anaemia of CRF.

Clinical features

These are illustrated in Figure 3. Early in chronic renal failure the normal reduction in urine formation when the patient is recumbent and asleep is lost. Patients who do not experience daytime polyuria may nevertheless have nocturia as their presenting symptom.

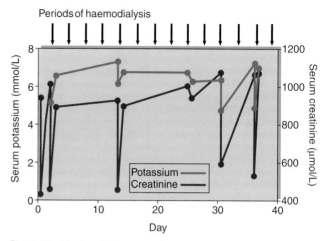

Fig. 1 **The biochemical course of a typical patient with chronic renal failure.** Note that biochemical analyses have not been performed before and after all periods of dialysis.

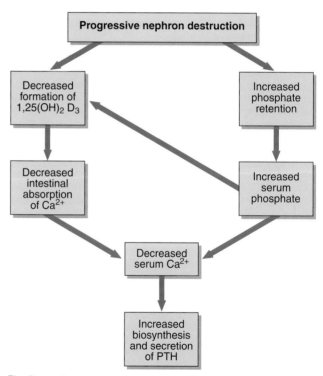

Fig. 2 **How hypocalcaemia and secondary hyperparathyroidism develop in renal disease.**

Management

In some cases it may be possible to treat the cause of the CRF and at least delay the progression of the disease. Conservative measures may be used to alleviate symptoms before dialysis becomes necessary, and these involve much

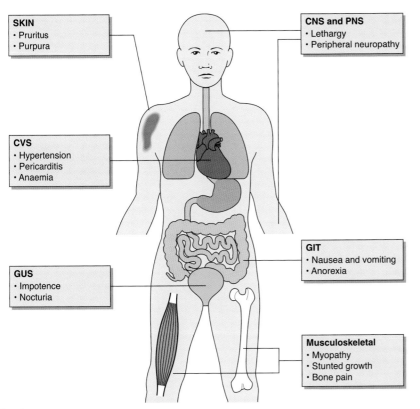

Fig. 3 **The clinical consequences of CRF.**

SKIN
• Pruritus
• Purpura

CVS
• Hypertension
• Pericarditis
• Anaemia

GUS
• Impotence
• Nocturia

CNS and PNS
• Lethargy
• Peripheral neuropathy

GIT
• Nausea and vomiting
• Anorexia

Musculoskeletal
• Myopathy
• Stunted growth
• Bone pain

use of the biochemical laboratory. Important considerations are:

■ Water and sodium intake should be carefully matched to the losses. Dietary sodium restriction and diuretics may be required to prevent sodium overload.
■ Hyperkalaemia may be controlled by oral ion-exchange resins (Resonium A).
■ Hyperphosphataemia may be controlled by oral aluminium or magnesium salts, which act by sequestering ingested phosphate in the gut.
■ The administration of hydroxylated vitamin D metabolites may prevent the development of secondary hyperparathyroidism. There is a risk of hypercalcaemia with this treatment.
■ Dietary restriction of protein, to reduce the formation of nitrogenous waste products, may give symptomatic improvement. A negative nitrogen balance should, however, be avoided.

Most patients with CRF will eventually require dialysis, in which case these conservative measures must be continued. In contrast, after a successful kidney transplant, normal renal function is re-established.

Dialysis

Haemodialysis and peritoneal dialysis will sustain life when other measures can no longer maintain fluid, electrolyte and acid–base balance. The key to dialysis is the provision of a semipermeable membrane through which ions and small molecules, present in plasma at high concentration, can diffuse into the low concentrations of a rinsing fluid. In haemodialysis, an artificial membrane is used. In peritoneal dialysis, the dialysis fluid is placed in the peritoneal cavity, and molecules move out of the blood vessels of the peritoneal wall. Continuous ambulatory peritoneal dialysis (CAPD) is an effective way of removing waste products. The dialysis fluid is replaced every 6 hours.

Note that haemodialysis and peritoneal dialysis may relieve many of the symptoms of chronic renal failure and rectify abnormal fluid and electrolyte and acid–base balance. These treatments do not, however, reverse the other metabolic, endocrine or haematological consequences of chronic renal failure.

Renal transplant

Although transplant of a kidney restores almost all of the renal functions, patients require long-term immunosuppression. For example, ciclosporin is nephrotoxic at high concentrations and monitoring of both creatinine and ciclosporin is necessary to balance the fine line between rejection and renal damage due to the drug.

> **Clinical note**
> Hypertension is both a common cause and a consequence of renal disease. Good blood pressure control is an essential part of treatment and delays the progression of chronic renal failure.

Case history 13

MH is a 40-year-old woman with chronic renal failure who is being treated by haemodialysis. Her serum biochemistry just prior to her last dialysis showed:

Na+	K+	Cl⁻	HCO₃⁻	Urea	Creatinine
		mmol/L			µmol/L
130	5.7	100	16	25.5	1430

■ What is the significance of these results?
■ What other biochemical tests should be performed, and how might the results influence treatment?

Comment on page 163.

Chronic renal failure

■ Chronic renal failure is the progressive irreversible destruction of kidney tissue by disease which, if not treated by dialysis or transplant, will result in the death of the patient.
■ Patients with CRF may be without symptoms until the GFR falls to very low values.
■ Consequences of CRF include disordered water and sodium metabolism, hyperkalaemia, abnormal calcium and phosphate metabolism, and anaemia.

Acid–base: concepts and vocabulary

H+ concentration

Blood hydrogen ion concentration [H+] is maintained within tight limits in health. Normal levels lie between 35 and 45 nmol/L. Values greater than 120 nmol/L or less than 20 nmol/L are usually incompatible with life. In the past, [H+] in blood was described as pH, but now it is more usual for results to be reported in molar concentration units, as nmol/L (Fig. 1).

[H+] nmol/L		pH
160		6.80
150		
140		
130		6.90
120		
110		
100		7.00
90		
80		7.10
70		
60		7.20
50		7.30
40		7.40
30		7.50
		7.60
20		7.70
		7.80
10		

Fig. 1 **The negative logarithmic relationship between [H+] and pH.**

H+ production

Hydrogen ions are produced in the body as a result of metabolism, particularly from the oxidation of the sulphur-containing amino acids of protein ingested as food. The total amount of H+ produced each day in this way is of the order of 60 mmol. If all of this was to be diluted in the extracellular fluid ($\approx$14 L), [H+] would be 4 mmol/L, or 100 000 times more acid than normal! This just does not happen, as all the H+ produced are efficiently excreted in urine. Everyone who eats a diet rich in animal protein passes a urine that is profoundly acidic.

Metabolism also produces CO_2. In solution this gas forms a weak acid. Large amounts of CO_2 are produced by cellular activity each day with the potential to upset acid–base balance, but under normal circumstances all of this CO_2 is excreted via the lungs, having been transported in the blood. Only when respiratory function is impaired do problems occur.

Buffering

A buffer is a solution of the salt of a weak acid that is able to bind H+. Buffering does not remove H+ from the body. Rather, buffers temporarily mop up any excess H+ that are produced, in the same way that a sponge soaks up water. Buffering is only a short-term solution to the problem of excess H+. Ultimately, the body must get rid of the H+ by renal excretion.

The body contains a number of buffers to even out sudden changes in H+ production. Proteins can act as buffers, and the haemoglobin in the erythrocytes has a high capacity for binding H+. In the ECF, bicarbonate buffer is the most important. In this buffer system, bicarbonate (HCO_3^-) combines with H+ to form carbonic acid (H_2CO_3). This buffer system is unique in that the (H_2CO_3) can dissociate to water and carbon dioxide.

Whereas simple buffers rapidly become ineffective as the association of the H+ and the anion of the weak acid reaches equilibrium, the bicarbonate system keeps working because the carbonic acid is removed as carbon dioxide. The limit to the effectiveness of the bicarbonate system is the initial concentration of bicarbonate. Only when all the bicarbonate is used up does the system have no further buffering capacity. The acid–base status of patients is assessed by consideration of the bicarbonate system of plasma.

The association of H+ with bicarbonate occurs rapidly, but the breakdown of carbonic acid to carbon dioxide and water happens relatively slowly. The reaction is accelerated by an enzyme, carbonic anhydrase, which is present particularly where this reaction is most needed, in the erythrocytes and in the kidneys. Buffering by the bicarbonate system effectively removes H+ from the ECF at the expense of bicarbonate. The carbon dioxide that is formed can be blown off in the lungs, and the water mixes with the large body water pool. The extracellular fluid contains a large amount of bicarbonate, around 24 mmol/L. If H+ begins to build up for any reason, the bicarbonate concentration falls as the buffering system comes into play.

H+ excretion in the kidney

All the H+ that is buffered must eventually be excreted from the body via the kidneys, regenerating the bicarbonate used up in the buffering process and maintaining the plasma bicarbonate concentration within normal limits (Fig. 2). Secretion of H+ by the tubular cells serves initially to reclaim bicarbonate from the glomerular filtrate so that it is not lost from the body. When all the bicarbonate has been recovered, any deficit due to the buffering process is regenerated. The mechanisms for bicarbonate *recovery* and for bicarbonate *regeneration* are very similar and are sometimes confused (Fig. 2).

The excreted H+ must be buffered in urine or the [H+] would rise to very high

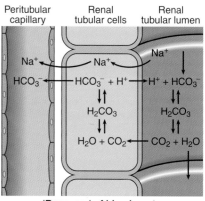

'Recovery' of bicarbonate

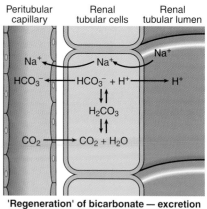

'Regeneration' of bicarbonate — excretion of hydrogen ion

Fig. 2 **The recovery and regeneration of bicarbonate by excretion of H+ in the renal tubular cell.** Note that H+ is actively secreted into the urine while CO_2 diffuses along its concentration gradient.

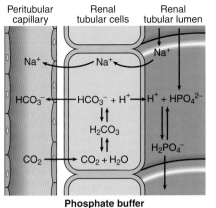

Phosphate buffer

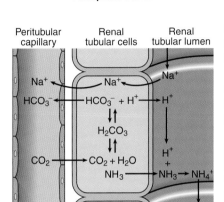

Ammonia buffer

Fig. 3 **Buffering of hydrogen ions in urine.**

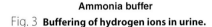

levels. Phosphate acts as one such buffer, while ammonia is another (Fig. 3).

Assessing status

Normal acid–base balance involves the bicarbonate buffer system. In chemical terms, the bicarbonate buffer system can be considered in the same way as any other chemical dissociation.

$$\left[H^+\right]+\left[HCO_3^-\right]\Leftrightarrow\left[H_2CO_3\right]$$

By the law of mass action:

$$\left[H^+\right]=\frac{K\left[H_2CO_3\right]}{\left[HCO_3^-\right]}$$

(where K is the first dissociation constant of carbonic acid)

But the carbonic acid (H_2CO_3) component is proportional to the dissolved carbon dioxide, which is in turn proportional to the partial pressure of the CO_2. Indeed, Henry's law shows that [CO_2] in solution = s.PCO_2, where s is the solubility of the gas in water. [H_2CO_3] can, therefore, be replaced in the mass action equation by PCO_2. At this point, an understanding of the role of the bicarbonate buffer system in assessing clinical acid–base disorders can be achieved simply by reference to the relationship:

$$\left[H^+\right]\text{is proportional to}\frac{PCO_2}{\left[HCO_3^-\right]}$$

which shows that the H^+ concentration in blood varies as the bicarbonate concentration and PCO_2 change. If everything else remains constant:

- Adding H^+, removing bicarbonate or increasing the PCO_2 will all have the same effect; that is, an increase in [H^+].
- Removing H^+, adding bicarbonate or lowering PCO_2 will all cause the [H^+] to fall.

Blood [H^+] is 40 nmol/L and is controlled by our normal pattern of respiration and the functioning of our kidneys.

An indication of the acid–base status of the patient can be obtained by measuring the components of the bicarbonate buffer system.

Acid–base disorders

'Metabolic' acid–base disorders are those that directly cause a change in the bicarbonate concentration. Examples include diabetes mellitus, where altered intermediary metabolism in the absence of insulin causes a build up of H^+ from the ionization of acetoacetic and β-hydroxybutyric acids, or loss of bicarbonate from the extracellular fluid, e.g. from a duodenal fistula.

'Respiratory' acid–base disorders affect directly the PCO_2. Impaired respiratory function causes a build-up of CO_2 in blood, whereas, less commonly, hyperventilation can cause a decreased PCO_2.

Compensation

The simple relationships of the bicarbonate buffer system are complicated by physiological mechanisms that have evolved to try to return a disordered [H^+] to normal.

Where lung function is compromised, the body attempts to increase the excretion of H^+ via the renal route. This is known as *renal compensation* for the primary respiratory disorder. Renal compensation is slow to take effect.

Where there are metabolic disorders, some compensation is possible by the lungs. This is known as *respiratory compensation* for the primary metabolic disorder. Respiratory compensation is quick to take effect.

If compensation is complete, the [H^+] returns to within reference limits, although the PCO_2 and [HCO_3^-] remain grossly abnormal. The acid–base disorder is said to be 'fully compensated'. Compensation is often partial, in which case the [H^+] has not been brought within the reference limits. The actual blood [H^+] at any time in the course of an acid–base disorder is a consequence of the severity of the primary disturbance and the amount of compensation that has occurred.

Terminology

Acidosis and alkalosis are clinical terms that define the primary acid–base disturbance. They can be used even when the [H^+] is within the normal range, i.e. when the disorders are fully compensated. The definitions are:

- *Metabolic acidosis*. The primary disorder is a decrease in bicarbonate concentration.
- *Metabolic alkalosis*. The primary disorder is an increased bicarbonate.
- *Respiratory acidosis*. The primary disorder is an increased PCO_2.
- *Respiratory alkalosis*. The primary disorder is a decreased PCO_2.

'Acidaemia' and 'alkalaemia' refer simply to whether the [H^+] in blood is higher or lower than normal, and the terms are not frequently used.

Acid–base: concepts and vocabulary

- The assessment of acid–base status is carried out by measuring [H^+], [HCO_3^-] and PCO_2, the components of the bicarbonate buffer system in plasma.
- Adding H^+, removing bicarbonate or increasing the PCO_2 will all have the same effect, an increase in [H^+].
- Removing H^+, adding bicarbonate or lowering PCO_2 will all cause the [H^+] to fall.
- Primary problems with H^+ production or excretion are reflected in the [HCO_3^-] and these are called 'metabolic' acid–base disorders.
- Primary problems with CO_2 excretion are reflected in PCO_2; these are called 'respiratory' acid–base disorders.
- The body has physiological mechanisms that try to restore [H^+] to normal. These processes are called 'compensation'.
- The observed [H^+] in any acid–base disorder reflects the balance between the primary disturbance and the amount of compensation.

Metabolic acid–base disorders

Metabolic acid–base disorders are reflected in changes in the ECF bicarbonate concentration that commonly occur because of a build-up or loss of hydrogen ions. Direct loss or gain of bicarbonate will also cause metabolic acid–base disorders. Primary metabolic acid–base disorders are recognized by inspecting the bicarbonate concentration (Fig. 1). Respiratory compensation takes place quickly so patients with metabolic acid–base disorders will usually show some change in blood PCO_2 because of hyperventilation or hypoventilation (Fig. 2).

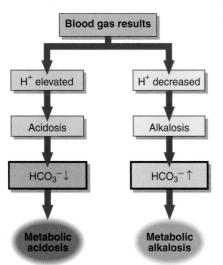

Fig. 1 **Recognizing primary metabolic acid–base disorders by inspecting the HCO_3^- concentration.**

Metabolic acidosis

In a metabolic acidosis the primary problem is a reduction in the bicarbonate concentration of the extracellular fluid. The main causes of a metabolic acidosis are shown in Figure 3. These are:

- increased production of hydrogen ions
- ingestion of hydrogen ions, or of drugs that are metabolized to acids
- impaired excretion of hydrogen ions by the kidneys
- loss of bicarbonate from the gastrointestinal tract or in the urine.

The anion gap

The cause of a metabolic acidosis will nearly always be apparent from the clinical history of the patient, but occasionally knowledge of the anion gap may be helpful. This can be assessed by looking at the serum electrolyte results and calculating the difference between the sum of the two main cations, sodium and potassium, and the sum of the two main anions, chloride and bicarbonate. There is no real gap, of course, as plasma proteins are negatively charged at normal [H+]. These negatively charged amino acid side chains on the proteins account for most of the apparent discrepancy when the measured electrolytes are compared. *The anion gap is thus a biochemical tool that is sometimes of help in assessing acid–base problems. It is not a physiological reality.*

In practice, because the potassium concentration is so small and will vary by so little, it is generally excluded when calculating the anion gap. Thus:

Anion gap = [Na+] − [(Cl−) + (HCO₃−)]

In a healthy person, the anion gap has a value of between 6 and 18 mmol/L. When the bicarbonate concentration rises or falls, other ions must take its place to maintain electrochemical neutrality. If chloride substitutes for bicarbonate, the anion gap does not change. However, the anion gap value will increase in metabolic conditions in which acids, such as sulphuric, lactic or acetoacetic, are produced, or when salicylate is present.

Causes of metabolic acidosis

Metabolic acidosis with an elevated anion gap occurs in:

- *Renal disease.* Hydrogen ions are retained along with anions such as sulphate and phosphate.
- *Diabetic ketoacidosis.* Altered metabolism of fatty acids, as a consequence of the lack of insulin, causes endogenous production of acetoacetic and β-hydroxybutyric acids.
- *Lactic acidosis.* This results from a number of causes, particularly tissue anoxia. *In acute hypoxic states such as respiratory failure or cardiac arrest lactic acidosis develops within minutes and is life-threatening.* Lactic acidosis may also be caused by liver disease. The presence of a lactic acidosis can be confirmed, if necessary, by the measurement of plasma lactate concentration.
- *Certain cases of overdosage or poisoning.* The mechanism common to all of these is the production of acid metabolites. Examples include salicylate overdose where build-up of lactate occurs, methanol poisoning when formate accumulates, or ethylene glycol poisoning where oxalate is formed.

Metabolic acidosis with a *normal* anion gap is sometimes referred to as a 'hyperchloraemic acidosis' because a reduced HCO_3^- concentration is balanced by increased Cl− concentration. It is seen in:

- *Chronic diarrhoea or intestinal fistula.* Fluids containing bicarbonate are lost from the body.

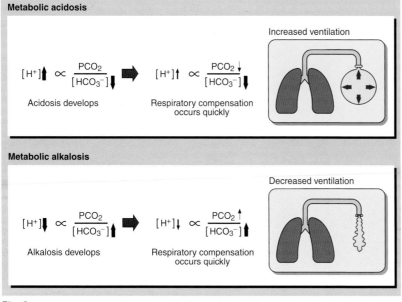

Fig. 2 **Compensation in primary metabolic disorders.**

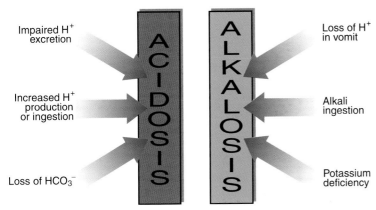

Fig. 3 **Reasons for metabolic acidosis and alkalosis.**

- *Renal tubular acidosis.* Renal tubular cells are unable to excrete hydrogen ions efficiently, and bicarbonate is lost in the urine.

Clinical effects of acidosis

The compensatory response to metabolic acidosis is hyperventilation, since the increased [H⁺] acts as a powerful stimulant of the respiratory centre. The deep, rapid and gasping respiratory pattern is known as Kussmaul breathing. Hyperventilation is the appropriate physiological response to acidosis and it occurs rapidly.

A raised [H⁺] leads to increased neuromuscular irritability. There is a hazard of arrhythmias progressing to cardiac arrest, and this is made more likely by the presence of hyperkalaemia, which will accompany the acidosis (pp. 22–23). Depression of consciousness can progress to coma and death.

Metabolic alkalosis

The causes of a metabolic alkalosis are shown in Figure 3. The condition may be due to:

- *Loss of hydrogen ion in gastric fluid during vomiting.* This is especially seen when there is pyloric stenosis preventing parallel loss of bicarbonate-rich secretions from the duodenum.
- *Ingestion of an absorbable alkali such as sodium bicarbonate.* Very large doses are required to cause a metabolic alkalosis unless there is renal impairment.
- *Potassium deficiency.* In severe potassium depletion, often a consequence of diuretic therapy, hydrogen ions are retained inside cells to replace the missing potassium ions. In the renal tubule more hydrogen ions, rather than potassium, are exchanged for reabsorbed sodium. So, despite there being an alkalosis, the patient passes an acid urine. This is often referred to as a 'paradoxical' acid urine, because in other causes of metabolic alkalosis urinary [H⁺] usually falls.

Clinical effects of alkalosis

The clinical effects of alkalosis include hypoventilation, confusion and eventually coma. Muscle cramps, tetany and paraesthesia may be a consequence of a decrease in the unbound plasma calcium concentration, which is a consequence of the alkalosis.

> ### Clinical note
> A patient who has had prolonged nasogastric suction following surgery will lose gastric fluid in large quantities and may develop a metabolic alkalosis.

Case history 14

A 28-year-old man is admitted to hospital with a week-long history of severe vomiting. He confessed to self-medication of his chronic dyspepsia. He was clinically severely dehydrated and had shallow respiration. Initial biochemical results were:

Arterial blood gases:

H⁺	PCO₂	HCO₃⁻	PO₂
nmol/L	kPa	mmol/L	kPa
28	7.2	43	15

Serum:

Na⁺	K⁺	Cl⁻	HCO₃⁻	Urea	Creatinine
		— mmol/L —			μmol/L
146	2.8	83	41	31	126

A random urine sample was obtained, and had the following biochemical results: osmolality 630 mmol/kg, Na⁺ <20 mmol/L, K⁺ 35 mmol/L, pH 5.

- What is the acid–base disorder and how has it arisen?
- How might the urine results help in the diagnosis?

Comment on page 163.

Metabolic acid–base disorders

- In metabolic acidosis, the blood [H⁺] may be high or normal, but the [HCO₃⁻] is always low. In compensated conditions, PCO₂ is lowered.
- The commonest causes of metabolic acidosis are renal disease, diabetic ketoacidosis and lactic acidosis.
- Consideration of the anion gap may sometimes be helpful in establishing the cause of a metabolic acidosis.
- In metabolic alkalosis, the [H⁺] is depressed and the [HCO₃⁻] is always raised. Respiratory compensation results in an elevated PCO₂.
- The commonest cause of a metabolic alkalosis is prolonged vomiting.

Respiratory and mixed acid–base disorders

In respiratory acid–base disorders the primary disturbance is caused by changes in arterial blood PCO_2 (Fig. 1). Respiratory disorders are related to changes either in the amount of air moving in or moving out of the lungs (ventilation), or in the ability of gases to diffuse across the alveolar membrane (gas exchange). In both cases PCO_2 changes and the carbonic acid concentration rises or falls.

It may appear confusing that carbonic acid can cause an acidosis, since for each hydrogen ion produced, a bicarbonate molecule is also generated. However, the effect of adding one hydrogen ion to a concentration of 40 nmol/L is much greater than that of adding one bicarbonate molecule to a concentration of 26 mmol/L.

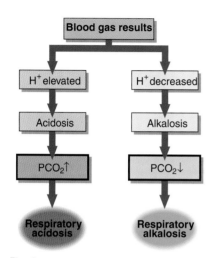

Fig. 1 **Primary respiratory disorders are recognized by inspecting the PCO_2.**

Respiratory acidosis

Respiratory acidosis may be acute or chronic. Acute conditions occur within minutes or hours. They are uncompensated. Renal compensation has no time to develop as the mechanisms that adjust bicarbonate reabsorption take 48–72 hours to become fully effective. The primary problem in acute respiratory acidosis is alveolar hypoventilation. If airflow is completely or partially reduced, the PCO_2 in the blood will rise immediately and the [H^+] will rise quickly (Fig. 2). A resulting low PO_2 and high PCO_2 causes coma. If this is not relieved rapidly, death results.

Examples of acute, and hence uncompensated, respiratory acidosis are:

- choking
- bronchopneumonia
- acute exacerbation of asthma/COAD.

Chronic respiratory acidosis usually results from chronic obstructive airways disease (COAD) and is usually a long-standing condition, accompanied by maximal renal compensation. In a chronic respiratory acidosis the primary problem again is usually impaired alveolar ventilation, but renal compensation contributes markedly to the acid–base picture. Compensation may be partial or complete. The kidney increases hydrogen ion excretion and ECF bicarbonate levels rise. Blood [H^+] tends back towards normal (Fig. 3).

It takes some time for the kidneys to respond to a high PCO_2 and a high [H^+], and therefore compensation will only be maximal some days after the onset of the clinical problem. In many patients with chronic respiratory conditions, extensive renal compensation will keep the blood [H^+] near normal, despite grossly impaired ventilation. In stable chronic bronchitis the [H^+] may be within the reference interval despite a very high PCO_2. This is achieved only by maintaining a plasma bicarbonate concentration twice that of normal. The PO_2 is usually depressed, and becomes more so as lung damage increases with time (pp. 44–45). Examples of chronic respiratory disorders are:

- chronic bronchitis
- emphysema.

The causes of respiratory acidosis are summarized in Figure 4.

$$[H^+] = \frac{K\, PCO_2}{[HCO_3^-]} \qquad PCO_2 = kPa \qquad [HCO_3^-] = mmol/L$$
$$[H^+] = nmol/L \qquad K = 178$$

Normal control

$$[H^+] = 178 \times \frac{PCO_2\ (5.3)}{[HCO_3^-]\,(25)} = 38\ nmol/L$$

Hypoventilating patient: PCO_2 rises by 2kPa

$$[H^+] = 178 \times \frac{PCO_2\ (7.3)}{[HCO_3^-]\,(25)} = 52\ nmol/L$$

Fig. 2 **Why an increased PCO_2 causes an acidosis.**

Respiratory acidosis

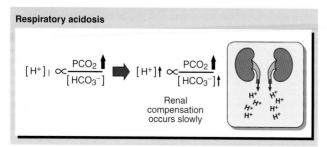

$$[H^+]_I \propto \frac{PCO_2\uparrow}{[HCO_3^-]} \implies [H^+]\uparrow \propto \frac{PCO_2\uparrow}{[HCO_3^-]\uparrow}$$

Renal compensation occurs slowly

Fig. 3 **Renal compensation in primary respiratory acidosis.**

Respiratory alkalosis

Respiratory alkalosis is much less common than acidosis but can occur when respiration is stimulated or is no longer subject to feedback control (Fig. 4). Usually these are acute conditions, and there is no renal compensation. The treatment is to inhibit or remove the cause of the hyperventilation, and the acid–base balance should return to normal. Examples are:

- hysterical overbreathing
- mechanical over-ventilation in an intensive care patient
- raised intracranial pressure, or hypoxia, both of which may stimulate the respiratory centre.

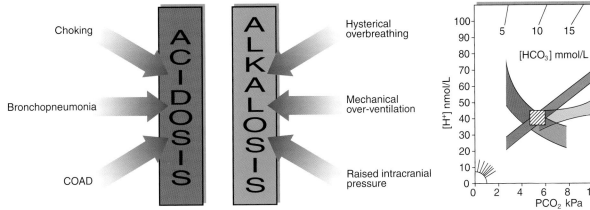

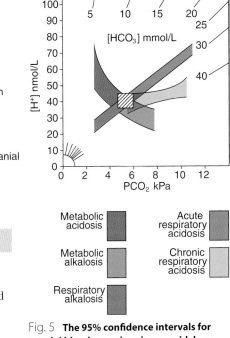

Fig. 4 **Causes of respiratory acidosis and alkalosis.**

Metabolic acidosis · Metabolic alkalosis · Respiratory alkalosis · Acute respiratory acidosis · Chronic respiratory acidosis

Fig. 5 **The 95% confidence intervals for arterial blood gases in primary acid–base disorders.** Arterial [H+] is plotted against PCO_2 with lines of equal [HCO_3^-] radiating from origin. The hatched box shows normal values. Graphs such as these may be used to chart the progress of a patient under treatment to correct an acid–base disorder.

Mixed acid–base disorders

It is not uncommon for patients to have more than one acid–base disorder. A patient may have both a metabolic and respiratory acidosis, such as the chronic bronchitic patient who develops renal impairment. In such a patient with a raised [H+], the PCO_2 will be increased and the bicarbonate concentration will be low, both expected findings in primary respiratory and primary metabolic acidosis.

Where the two acid–base conditions are antagonistic in the way they affect the [H+], one of the disorders may mimic the compensatory response. A patient may present with a metabolic acidosis and a coexistent respiratory alkalosis, as occurs commonly in salicylate overdose. The respiratory disorder may appear, at first sight, to be simply the compensatory response.

Other examples of mixed acid–base disorders commonly encountered are:

- a patient with chronic obstructive airways disease, causing a respiratory acidosis, with thiazide-induced potassium depletion and consequent metabolic alkalosis
- hyperventilation causing a respiratory alkalosis, with prolonged nasogastric suction that causes a metabolic alkalosis
- salicylate poisoning in which respiratory alkalosis occurs due to stimulation of the respiratory centre, together with metabolic acidosis due to the effects of the drug on metabolism.

Care must be taken in the interpretation of the blood gas results in these patients. *Knowledge of the clinical picture is essential.* Theoretically, the limits of the compensatory responses in simple primary acid–base disorders are known (Fig. 5). When compensation apparently falls outside of these expected limits, it is likely that a second acid–base disorder is present.

There is further discussion on the interpretation of blood gas results on pages 46–47.

Case history 15

Miss AM was admitted to hospital with a crushed chest. On admission her arterial blood gases were:

H+	HCO_3^-	PCO_2	PO_2
nmol/L	mmol/L	kPa	kPa
63	29	10.1	6.4

- What do these results indicate?

Comment on page 163.

Clinical note

When interpreting acid–base results, the patient's clinical history is the most important factor in determining the nature of the disorder, or indeed in deciding if more than one disorder might be present. Biochemical measurements are the only means of quantifying the severity of the disorder(s) and the degree of compensation.

Respiratory and mixed acid–base disorders

- In respiratory acidosis the blood [H+] is usually high, but may be within the reference interval. The PCO_2 is always raised. In compensated conditions, [HCO_3^-] is also raised.

- Acute respiratory acidosis is a medical emergency and needs to be dealt with by removing the source of the respiratory problem.

- In contrast to respiratory compensation in metabolic disorders, the renal compensating mechanisms are much slower to take effect.

- In chronic respiratory disorders the [H+] often settles at a new steady state, within the reference interval, at which compensation is maximal.

- Respiratory alkalosis is uncommon and can be a result of mechanical over-ventilation or hysterical overbreathing.

- The interpretation of mixed acid–base disorders may be confusing if one of the disorders mimics the expected compensation. Knowledge of the clinical picture is important if the correct interpretation is to be placed on the results.

Oxygen transport

Normal oxygen transport

The total blood oxygen content is the sum of the dissolved oxygen and that bound to haemoglobin. Only a small fraction (2%) of the total oxygen in blood is in solution, and this dissolved oxygen is directly proportional to the arterial PO_2. The arterial PO_2 is also an important factor affecting the amount of oxygen that is bound to haemoglobin, as oxyhaemoglobin. The relationship is shown in the oxygen–haemoglobin dissociation curve (Fig. 1).

Measurement of blood *oxygen saturation*, the percentage of the total haemoglobin present as oxyhaemoglobin, may be used to assess the ability of blood to carry oxygen to the tissues. This clearly depends on the relative amounts of both oxygen and haemoglobin, as well as their ability to bind together. Delivery of oxygen to the tissues also depends on blood flow, which is in turn influenced by other factors (Table 1).

When arterial PO_2 is high (above 10 kPa), the blood haemoglobin is almost fully saturated with oxygen and measurements of oxygen saturation are not normally required. Indeed, measurements of oxygen saturation are not widely available outside of intensive therapy units. In patients exposed to carbon monoxide following smoke inhalation, the PO_2 may give a misleading indication of the amount of oxygen being carried in the blood because carbon monoxide binds to haemoglobin with greater affinity than does oxygen (Fig. 1).

When metabolic needs exceed the supply of oxygen, cells switch to anaerobic glycolysis to provide ATP, and produce lactic acid. Measurement of serum lactate concentration can provide additional evidence of the adequacy of tissue oxygenation.

In practice, tissue perfusion is more important than blood oxygen content in ensuring that aerobic metabolism can continue.

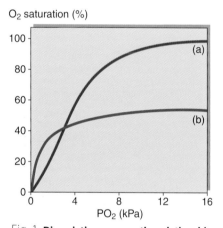

O$_2$ saturation (%)

Fig. 1 **Dissociation curves – the relationship between PO$_2$ and oxygen binding to haemoglobin. (a)** The normal oxygen haemoglobin dissociation curve. **(b)** The effect of 50% CO.

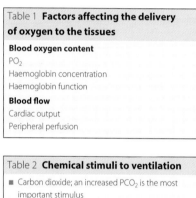

Table 1 **Factors affecting the delivery of oxygen to the tissues**
Blood oxygen content
PO$_2$
Haemoglobin concentration
Haemoglobin function
Blood flow
Cardiac output
Peripheral perfusion

Table 2 **Chemical stimuli to ventilation**
■ Carbon dioxide; an increased PCO$_2$ is the most important stimulus
■ [H$^+$]: a rise in hydrogen ion concentration stimulates ventilation; in respiratory disease [H$^+$] and PCO$_2$ rise together
■ Oxygen: a decreased PO$_2$ increases ventilation, but is of less importance unless PO$_2$ falls below 8 kPa

Respiratory failure

Figure 2 shows how the partial pressures of oxygen and carbon dioxide change as blood flows to the tissues and returns to the lungs. The mechanical process of moving air into and out of the respiratory tract is called ventilation. Carbon dioxide diffuses through alveolar membranes much more efficiently than oxygen, even though there is only a small pressure gradient. The PCO_2 of arterial blood is thus identical to the PCO_2 within the alveoli, and the arterial PCO_2 is therefore a measure of alveolar ventilation. If ventilation is impaired, alveolar PO_2 falls and alveolar PCO_2 rises. Arterial blood reflects these changes. The main chemical stimuli to ventilation are shown in Table 2.

It is possible to calculate the alveolar–arterial PO_2 gradient to determine the extent of defective gas exchange (Fig. 3), but in practice it is rarely necessary to do this.

An arterial PO_2 less than 8.0 kPa in a patient breathing room air at rest is known as 'respiratory failure'. Classically, hypoxia with carbon dioxide retention is called type 2 respiratory failure. Hypoxia without carbon dioxide retention is type 1 respiratory failure.

Two processes contribute to the blood gas pattern in those patients with hypoxia, where PCO_2 is not elevated (type 1 respiratory failure). These are:

■ impaired diffusion
■ ventilation/perfusion imbalance.

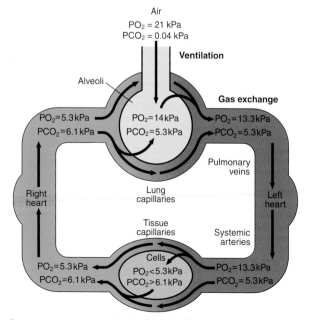

Fig. 2 **Normal gas pressures are maintained by ventilation and gas exchange.**

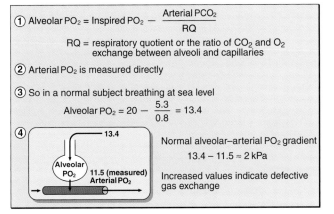

① Alveolar PO₂ = Inspired PO₂ − $\dfrac{\text{Arterial PCO}_2}{\text{RQ}}$

RQ = respiratory quotient or the ratio of CO_2 and O_2 exchange between alveoli and capillaries

② Arterial PO₂ is measured directly

③ So in a normal subject breathing at sea level

Alveolar PO₂ = 20 − $\dfrac{5.3}{0.8}$ = 13.4

④

13.4

Alveolar PO₂

11.5 (measured) Arterial PO₂

Normal alveolar–arterial PO₂ gradient

13.4 − 11.5 ≈ 2 kPa

Increased values indicate defective gas exchange

Fig. 3 **How to calculate the alveolar–arterial PO₂ difference.**

Clinical note
Pulse oximetry is an accurate non-invasive way of assessing oxygen saturation. Oxygenated and reduced haemoglobin absorb light at different wavelengths. If light of these wavelengths is passed through a blood vessel, the proportion of oxygenated haemoglobin can be calculated. Pulse oximetry allows these measurements in 'pulsing' blood only, producing results that approximate to arterial values.

Impaired diffusion

Here the presence of fluid, as in pulmonary oedema, or thickened alveolar walls, such as occurs in pulmonary fibrosis, inhibits oxygen diffusion, although carbon dioxide passage is more readily accomplished. PO₂ is low but PCO₂ may be within reference limits.

Ventilation/perfusion imbalance

In patients with a *lobar* pneumonia, some of the blood perfusing the lungs does not come into contact with functional alveoli and retains its carbon dioxide, and is not oxygenated. In blood reaching other parts of the lungs, gas exchange takes place efficiently. Arterial blood is a mixture of that exiting both regions. The increased PCO₂ stimulates ventilation and ensures that the functioning alveoli are worked harder to restore PCO₂ to normal. The blood gas results will show normal or even low PCO₂ as a result of this hyperventilation (Fig. 4). However, increased ventilation cannot dramatically raise alveolar PO₂ as long as the patient is breathing air.

Blood passing from the right side of the heart directly to the arterial circulation without being exposed to the inspired gas in the ventilated alveoli is an extreme example of ventilation/perfusion imbalance. This right to left 'shunting' occurs in cyanotic congenital heart disease.

Hypoxia with raised PCO₂ (type 2 respiratory failure) indicates diminished ventilation and impaired gas exchange, and may be seen in patients with bronchial pneumonia or chronic bronchitis.

Oxygen therapy

In all respiratory diseases, oxygen therapy is a vital aspect of patient management but there is one caution.

Some patients with chronic bronchitis become insensitive to respiratory stimulation by carbon dioxide. This insensitivity may develop over many years, and only the existing hypoxia keeps respiration going. Treating such patients with high concentrations of oxygen only serves to reduce respiration further. PCO₂ rises, acidosis worsens and the patient may become comatose.

Case history 16

A 58-year-old man was admitted with a history of chronic obstructive airways disease for many years. On examination he was cyanosed, breathless and there was marked systemic oedema. A blood sample gave the following results:

Arterial blood gases:

H⁺	PCO₂	HCO₃⁻	PO₂
nmol/L	kPa	mmol/L	kPa
44	9.3	40	4.0

- Describe the acid–base disorder.
- What type of respiratory problem is present?

Comment on page 163.

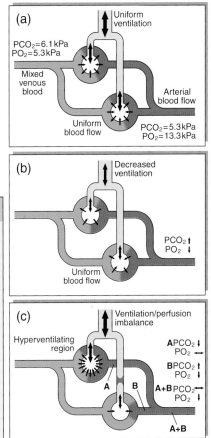

Fig. 4 **Blood gases in (a) normal circumstances, (b) hypoventilation and (c) where there is a ventilation/perfusion imbalance.**

Oxygen transport

- Oxygen is carried in blood mostly bound to haemoglobin. Arterial blood PO₂ determines how much oxygen is bound to haemoglobin, although above a PO₂ of 10 kPa the haemoglobin is usually fully saturated.
- Measurements of haemoglobin and blood oxygen saturation are necessary to assess oxygen availability where the patient is anaemic, or if factors affecting the ability of the haemoglobin to bind oxygen, such as carbon monoxide, are present.
- Delivery of oxygen to the tissues also depends on cardiac output and peripheral perfusion.
- Respiratory failure is defined as an arterial PO₂ of less than 8 kPa in a patient breathing air.
- Hypoxia with CO₂ retention is seen where there is impaired ventilation.
- Hypoxia without CO₂ retention is seen commonly when there is ventilation/perfusion imbalance.

Acid–base disorders: diagnosis and management

Specimens for blood gas analysis

$[H^+]$ and PCO_2 are measured directly in an *arterial* blood sample. This is usually taken from the brachial or radial arteries into a syringe that contains a small volume of heparin as an anticoagulant. It is important to exclude air from the syringe before and after the blood is collected. Any air bubbles in the syringe when the sample has been taken should be expelled before the syringe is capped for immediate transport to the laboratory. Ideally, the syringe and its contents should be placed in ice during transit.

Acid–base problems may be discussed by referring to the three 'components' of the bicarbonate buffer system. In practice, blood gas analysers measure the $[H^+]$ of the sample and its PCO_2. There is no need to measure the third variable, the bicarbonate. By the law of mass action:

$$[H^+] \propto \frac{PCO_2}{[HCO_3^-]}$$

If any two of the variables are known, the third can always be calculated. Indeed, blood gas analysers (Fig. 1) are programmed to provide this information, which is printed out on the report form and usually includes the measured PO_2 as well. There are a multitude of other calculated values on some blood gas analyser printouts, such as base excess and standard bicarbonate. These may be mostly disregarded in the routine assessment of a patient's acid–base balance.

In many laboratories, bicarbonate concentration is also determined directly as part of the electrolyte profile of tests on the laboratory's main analyser, usually on a serum specimen obtained from a venous blood sample. These results (described as 'total CO_2') are not identical to the printout from the blood gas analyser nor should this be expected since they include dissolved carbon dioxide, carbonic acid and other carbamino compounds. However, the results should not differ by more than 3 mmol/L. They may, therefore, be interpreted in the same way. A low bicarbonate in an electrolyte profile will usually indicate the presence of a metabolic acidosis.

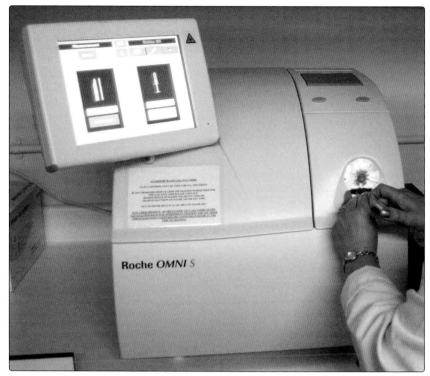

Fig. 1 **Blood gas analyser.**

Interpreting results

The predicted compensatory responses in $[HCO_3^-]$ or PCO_2 when $[H^+]$ changes as a result of primary acid–base disorders are shown in Table 1.

A practical approach to the interpretation of blood gas results is shown in Figure 2. The steps in classifying the acid–base disorder are:

- Look first at the $[H^+]$. Decide if an acidosis or an alkalosis is present.
- If the $[H^+]$ is elevated, decide what is the primary cause of the acidosis. Look at the PCO_2. If this is elevated, then there is a respiratory acidosis. Look at the bicarbonate. If this is decreased, there is a metabolic acidosis.
- If the $[H^+]$ is decreased, decide what is the primary cause of the alkalosis. Look at the PCO_2. If low, then there is a respiratory alkalosis. Look at the bicarbonate. If this is high, then there is a metabolic alkalosis.

- Having decided on the primary acid–base disorder, look to see if there is compensation. There will be a change in the other component (the one which was not used to determine the primary disorder), in the direction which 'compensates' for the primary disorder. If there is not, the acid–base disorder may be uncompensated. If the change is in the opposite direction then a second acid–base disorder may be present. Even if there is compensation consider the possibility that there is a second acid–base problem that mimics the compensatory response.
- If there is compensation, decide if the disorder is fully compensated or partially compensated. If fully compensated, the resulting $[H^+]$ will be within the reference limits.

Clinical cases

The above practical advice is best illustrated by four case examples.

- A patient with chronic bronchitis. Blood gas results are: $[H^+] = 44$ nmol/L; $PCO_2 = 9.5$ kPa; $[HCO_3^-] = 39$ mmol/L. *A compensated respiratory acidosis* is present.
- A patient who has had an acute asthmatic attack. Blood gas results are: $[H^+] = 24$ nmol/L; $PCO_2 = 2.5$ kPa;

Table 1 **Primary acid–base disorders and compensatory responses**	
Primary disorder	**Compensatory response**
↑PCO_2 (Respiratory acidosis)	↑HCO_3^-
↓PCO_2 (Respiratory alkalosis)	↓HCO_3^-
↓HCO_3^- (Metabolic acidosis)	↓PCO_2
↑HCO_3^- (Metabolic alkalosis)	↑PCO_2

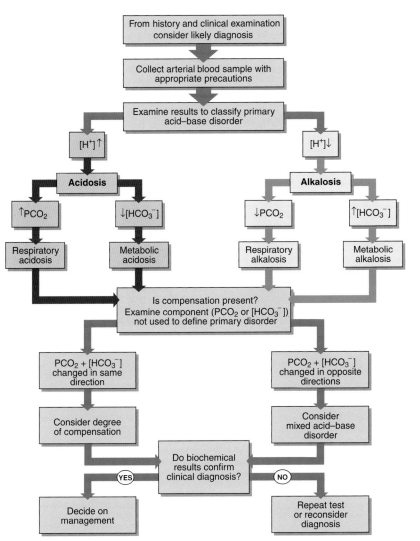

Fig. 2 **Acid–base disorders: diagnosis and management.**

acid–base disorder is to treat the underlying illness. This may involve:

- fluid therapy and insulin in diabetic ketoacidosis
- artificial ventilation by intermittent positive pressure ventilation (IPPV) in acute status asthmaticus
- improvement of GFR by restoring blood volume in a patient with acute blood loss.

In cases where there is a life-threatening acidosis (e.g. $[H^+]$ >100 nmol/L), the infusion of sodium bicarbonate may be considered. The circumstances when this might be appropriate include severe diabetic ketoacidosis. Sodium bicarbonate must always be used with caution. Careful monitoring of the patient by repeatedly measuring the blood gases may be necessary. It should be noted, however, that once sodium bicarbonate has been administered, arterial blood gas results can be very difficult to interpret.

Clinical note
Overcompensation of an acid–base disorder does not occur physiologically but may be induced by the inappropriate use of artificial ventilation or intravenous bicarbonate solutions.

$[HCO_3^-]=20$ mmol/L. An acute, and hence *uncompensated, respiratory alkalosis* is present.

- A young man with a history of dyspepsia and excessive alcohol intake who gives a 24-hour history of vomiting. Blood gas results are $[H^+]=28$ nmol/L; $PCO_2 = 7.2$ kPa; $[HCO_3^-]=48$ mmol/L. This is a *partially compensated metabolic alkalosis*.
- A 50-year-old man with a 2-week history of vomiting and diarrhoea. On examination he is dehydrated and his breathing is deep and noisy. Blood gas results are: $[H^+] = 64$ nmol/L; $PCO_2 = 2.8$ kPa; $[HCO_3^-]=8$ mmol/L. These results show a *partially compensated metabolic acidosis*.

Management of acid–base disorders

Many acid–base disorders are secondary to some other disorder. In most cases the management of an

Case history 17

A 56-year-old woman was admitted seriously ill and confused. The patient had systemic oedema and was being treated with furosemide (frusemide). On admission the following biochemical results were obtained:

Na$^+$	K$^+$	Cl$^-$	HCO$_3^-$	Urea	H$^+$	PCO$_2$	PO$_2$
		mmol/L			nmol/L	kPa	kPa
135	2.6	59	53	6.8	33	9.3	12

- What is the evidence that this patient has a mixed acid–base disorder? Identify the components.
- Explain the aetiology of the present blood gas and electrolyte results.
- How should the patient be treated?

Comment on page 164.

Acid–base disorders: diagnosis and management

- Care should be taken to exclude air from the arterial blood sample taken for blood gas analysis, and speedy transportation to the laboratory should be arranged.
- Blood gas analysers measure $[H^+]$ and PCO_2 directly and calculate $[HCO_3^-]$. This calculated bicarbonate is similar but not identical to the bicarbonate concentration obtained from the electrolyte profile in a serum sample.
- Acid–base disorders can be classified as acidosis or alkalosis, compensated or uncompensated, fully or partially compensated.
- The clinical status of the patient and the blood gas results should always match up.
- Management of acid–base disorders should be directed towards the correction of the underlying illness.

Proteins and enzymes

Plasma proteins

The biochemistry laboratory routinely measures 'total protein' and 'albumin' concentrations, usually in a serum specimen, and reports the 'globulin' fraction as the difference between the first two results. Some proteins (e.g. immunoglobulins) are measured as classes, and immunochemical methods are available for measuring specific proteins and hormones. Enzymes are measured both by determining their activity and by immunochemical methods to assess their mass.

Total protein

Changes in total protein concentration are common. An elevated total protein concentration may mean the presence of a paraprotein. A decreased total protein usually means that the albumin concentration is low.

Albumin

Albumin is the major plasma protein and is synthesized and secreted by the liver. It accounts for about 50% of the total hepatic protein production. Albumin has a biological half-life in plasma of about 20 days. Albumin makes the biggest contribution to the plasma oncotic pressure. If the albumin concentration falls very low, oedema is the result (Fig. 1). There are four main reasons for the occurrence of a low plasma albumin concentration:

- *Abnormal distribution.* Albumin can move into the interstitial space as a result of increased capillary permeability in the acute phase response.
- *Decreased synthesis.* Due to malnutrition (common in developing countries), malabsorption or advanced chronic liver disease.
- *Dilution.* Hypoalbuminaemia can be induced by overhydration.
- *Abnormal excretion or degradation.* The causes include the nephrotic syndrome, protein-losing enteropathies, burns, haemorrhage and catabolic states.

Although serum albumin measurements have been used to monitor a patient's response to long-term nutritional support, they are unreliable and insensitive.

Specific proteins

Measurement of a number of specific proteins gives useful information in the diagnosis and management of disease (Table 1). Characteristic changes in the concentration of

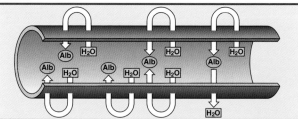

Normal

Low albumin

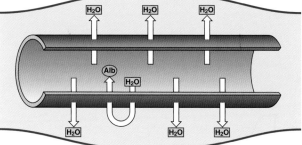

Fig. 1 **Pathogenesis of oedema in hypoalbuminaemia**.

certain plasma proteins are seen following surgery or trauma, or during infection or tumour growth. The proteins involved are called acute phase reactants (pp. 108–109). These acute phase proteins may be used to monitor progress of the condition or its treatment.

Enzymes

Serum enzymes in disease

Enzymes may be classified in two groups. Some, such as the enzymes of the coagulation cascade, have a defined function in blood. Others appear in the blood incidentally and their measurement is of value in diagnosis. Damage to the tissues of origin, or proliferation of the cells from which these enzymes arise, will lead to an increase in the activity of these enzymes in plasma (Fig. 2). It should be noted that increases in serum enzyme activity are only roughly proportional to the extent of tissue damage.

Enzymes that have been shown to have a diagnostic value are:

- *Alanine aminotransferase (ALT):* an indicator of hepatocellular damage.

Table 1 **Specific proteins that are measured in serum**		
Protein name	**Function**	**Reason for assay**
α_1-antitrypsin	Protease inhibitor	Reduced in α_1-antitrypsin deficiency
β_2-microglobulin	A subunit of the HLA antigen	Raised in renal tubular dysfunction on all cell membranes
Caeruloplasmin	Oxidizing enzyme	Reduced in Wilson's disease
C-reactive protein (CRP)	Involved in immune response	Increased in acute illness, especially infection
Ferritin	Binds iron in tissues	Gives an indication of body iron stores
Haptoglobin	Binds haemoglobin	Reduced in haemolytic conditions
Thyroid-binding globulin (TBG)	Thyroid hormone binding	Investigation of thyroid disease
Sex hormone binding globulin	Binds testosterone and oestradiol	Investigation of androgen excess and/or insulin resistance
Transferrin	Iron transport	Assessment of iron status and/or response to nutritional support

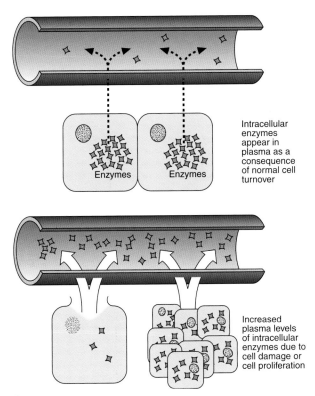

Fig. 2 **Plasma levels of intracellular enzymes.**

■ *Alkaline phosphatase*: increases in cholestatic liver disease and a marker of osteoblast activity in bone disease.
■ *Amylase*: an indicator of cell damage in acute pancreatitis.

■ *Aspartate aminotransferase (AST)*: an indicator of hepatocellular damage, or a marker of muscle damage, such as a myocardial infarction (MI).
■ *Creatine kinase*: a marker of muscle damage and acute MI.
■ *γ-Glutamyl transpeptidase*: a sensitive but non-specific marker of liver disease.
■ *Lipase*: an indicator of cell damage in acute pancreatitis.

A further enzyme of practical interest is cholinesterase. Cholinesterase, normally involved in the process of neuromuscular conduction, incidentally hydrolyses suxamethonium (succinylcholine), a muscle-relaxing drug used in anaesthesia. Patients with abnormal cholinesterase may fail to hydrolyse the drug normally and as a result suffer prolonged paralysis after anaesthesia. This is called scoline apnoea. Cholinesterase measurements are also useful in the diagnosis of poisoning with pesticides that are cholinesterase inhibitors.

Isoenzyme determination

Some enzymes are present in the plasma in two or more molecular forms. These variants are known as isoenzymes and, although they have different structures, they perform the same catalytic function. Different isoenzymes may arise from different tissues and their specific detection may give clues to the site of pathology. Alkaline phosphatase isoenzymes may distinguish between bone and liver disease, especially in patients in whom metastases of bone or liver are suspected. A specific isoenzyme of creatine kinase (CK-MB) is useful in the early detection of myocardial infarction. Heart muscle contains proportionally more of this isoenzyme than skeletal muscle, and raised levels of CK-MB indicate that a myocardial infarction has occurred.

 Clinical note

The only non-specific index of the presence of disease, comparable to C-reactive protein (CRP), is the erythrocyte sedimentation rate (ESR). This, in part, reflects the intensity of the acute phase response. The rate of change of ESR is much less than that of CRP and it reflects the clinical status of the patient less well. It is also affected by the number and morphology of the red cells. CRP can now be measured with relative ease and its determination is preferred over ESR in most pathological conditions. ESR as a non-specific indicator of disease may be helpful, for example in the investigation of paraproteinaemias which do not necessarily provoke an acute phase response.

Case history 18

Eight months after an attack of acute glomerulonephritis, a 38-year-old woman was hospitalized for investigation of progressive bilateral leg oedema. On examination, she was normotensive and exhibited pitting oedema of both ankles and dullness over her lung bases. Her face was pale and puffy and she admitted to frequent minor intercurrent infections.

■ What is your tentative diagnosis?
■ What biochemical analyses would you request, and in what order?
■ What results would be consistent with your diagnosis?

Comment on page 164.

Proteins and enzymes

■ An increase in total protein concentration in a serum specimen is usually due to an increase in the globulin fraction and may indicate the presence of a paraprotein.

■ A decreased total protein concentration is usually due to hypoalbuminaemia.

■ Albumin is the main determinant of plasma oncotic pressure. A very low albumin leads to oedema.

■ Increased enzyme activities in serum indicate either cell damage or increased cell proliferation.

■ Isoenzymes are forms of an enzyme that are structurally different but have similar catalytic properties. Measurement of the isoenzymes of alkaline phosphatase and creatine kinase is of clinical value.

Immunoglobulins

Immunoglobulins, or antibodies, are proteins produced by the plasma cells of the bone marrow as part of the immune response. The plasma cells are B lymphocytes transformed after exposure to a foreign (or occasionally an endogenous) antigen.

Structure

All immunoglobulins have the same basic structure and consist of two identical 'light' and two identical 'heavy' polypeptide chains, held together by disulphide bridges (Fig. 1). The light chains may be either of two types: kappa or lambda. The heavy chains may be of five types: alpha, gamma, delta, epsilon and mu. The immunoglobulins are named after their heavy chain type, as IgA, IgG, IgD, IgE and IgM.

The molecules are characterized by two functional areas:

- The *Fab*, or *variable* end is the area that recognizes and binds to the antigen.
- The *Fc end* is responsible for interaction with other components of the immune system, e.g. complement and T-helper cells.

The various classes of immunoglobulins have different tertiary structure and functions (Table 1). The major antibodies in the plasma are IgG, IgA and IgM.

Electrophoresis of serum proteins

Electrophoresis may be carried out to study a number of protein abnormalities. The normal pattern is shown in Figure 2(a). Immunoglobulins are detected primarily in the gamma globulin area on electrophoresis. Serum should be used for electrophoresis, as the fibrinogen of plasma (consumed during clotting) gives a discrete band that can easily be mistaken for a paraprotein. Electrophoresis can show gross deficiency or excess of immunoglobulins and the presence of discrete bands (paraproteins) (Figs 2b and c). A quantitative measure of each protein class may be obtained by scanning the electrophoresis strip (Fig. 3).

Measurement

Immunoglobulins may be measured in a number of ways, the necessity for the request often being triggered by an observed increase in the 'globulin' fraction (p. 48). If an abnormality is detected, then the particular type of immunoglobulin, or indeed of light or heavy chains where these are produced alone, may be confirmed by immunofixation or quantitatively by other means.

Increased immunoglobulins

Immunoglobulins may be increased non-specifically in a wide variety of infections and also in autoimmune disease. This increased synthesis comes from a number of cell lines, each producing its own specific immunoglobulin. The response is therefore said to be 'polyclonal' and results in a diffuse increase in protein mass throughout the gamma globulin region on electrophoresis. In contrast, cells from a single clone all make identical antibodies. As the cells multiply

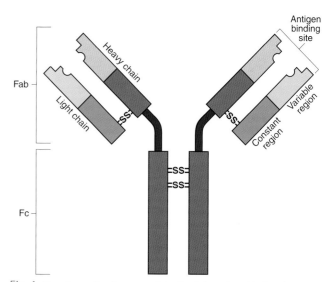

Fig. 1 **Structure of an immunoglobulin.** Fab, antigen binding fragment; Fc, constant fragment.

Table 1 **Classes of immunoglobulin**

Immunoglobulin	Sructure	Location	Action
IgG	Monomer	ECF	Neutralizes toxins, activates complement
IgA	Dimer	ECF+secretions	Antimicrobial
IgM	Pentamer	Mainly intravascular	First to be made in immune response
IgD	Monomer	ECF+cell membrane	Cell surface antigen receptors
IgE	Monomer	ECF	Antiallergenic, antiparasitic

the immunoglobulin production becomes large enough to be observed on electrophoresis as a single discrete band. This may be an intact immunoglobulin or a fragment and is called a paraprotein.

Paraproteins

Paraproteins are found in multiple myeloma, in Waldenström's macroglobulinaemia and in heavy chain diseases. These are malignant conditions. The paraproteins may arise from any of the immunoglobulin classes. Monoclonal light chains are produced in excess of heavy chains in 50% of cases of myeloma, and in 15% of cases only light chains are found. These light chains are small enough to spill into the urine where they are known as Bence Jones protein. Serum electrophoresis may not show the presence of light chains, and urine electrophoresis after concentration may be required to demonstrate the paraprotein.

Myeloma is characterized by osteolytic lesions (Fig. 4), and bone pain is often the presenting symptom. In the face of increasing synthesis of abnormal immunoglobulins, other bone marrow functions are reduced, and there is a decline in red and white cell and platelet formation and decreased production of normal immunoglobulins. Anaemia and susceptibility to infection are the consequences. Treatment of myeloma involves the use of bone marrow suppressive drugs. The increased serum paraprotein may cause renal damage leading to renal failure. Hypercalcaemia is also a feature of myeloma.

Occasionally, paraproteins are found in patients in whom there is no associated pathology. This is called benign

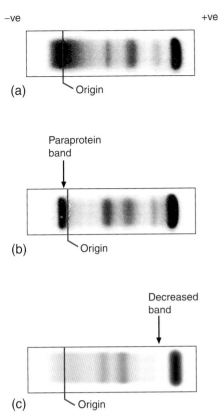

(a) Origin

Paraprotein band

(b) Origin

Decreased band

(c) Origin

Fig. 2 **Electrophoresis of serum proteins.**
(a) Normal pattern; (b) paraprotein band;
(c) α_1-antitrypsin deficiency.

−ve +ve

paraproteinaemia, but such a diagnosis should be made only after the possibility of myeloma has been excluded by the failure of the disease to progress, as gauged by no increase in the concentration of the paraprotein in serum with time. Regular and careful follow-up of such patients is required.

Deficiencies or absence of immunoglobulins

Deficiencies or absence of immunoglobulins can occur as a result of infection, genetic abnormalities or the effects of therapy (Table 2). Where the situation is irreversible, replacement therapy has been used, either by addition of immunoglobulin-rich plasma or by the transplantation of bone-marrow-containing competent plasma cells.

Table 2 **Causes of hypogammaglobulinaemia**

Type	Specific causes
Physiological	Levels of IgA and IgM are low at birth
Genetic	Bruton's X-linked agammaglobulinaemia
	Severe combined immunodeficiency (SCID)
Acquired	Malnutrition
	Malignancy
	Infections, e.g. HIV, measles
	Immunosuppressant drugs, e.g. azathioprine, ciclosporin

Case history 19

A 45-year-old man presented with severe back pain and malaise. He had lost 3 kg weight in 3 months. His blood film showed many primitive RBCs and WBCs. His bone marrow biopsy showed an excess of plasma cells. He did not have a paraprotein band on serum electrophoresis. Analysis of concentrated urine revealed an excess of free monoclonal light chains.

■ What is the diagnosis?

Comment on page 164.

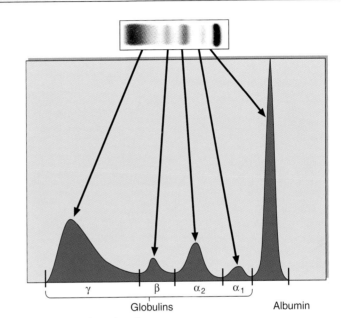

γ β α_2 α_1
Globulins Albumin

Fig. 3 **Scan of an electrophoresis strip.**

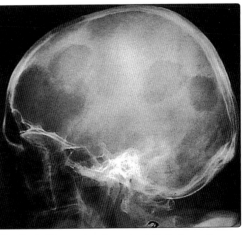

Clinical note
The diagnosis of myeloma requires that two of the following are present:

■ a paraprotein in serum or urine
■ plasma cell infiltration in bone marrow
■ radiological evidence of bone lesions (Fig. 4).

Fig. 4 **Skull X-ray showing osteolytic lesions of myeloma**.

Immunoglobulins

■ Electrophoresis of serum may confirm the presence of a paraprotein in a specimen from a patient with a raised globulin fraction.

■ Some myelomas produce immunological light chains only. These are best demonstrated by urine electrophoresis.

■ Immunoglobulin measurements can give information on:
  – immune deficiency
  – response to infection.

■ Serial study of immunoglobulin levels can be of help in following the progression of disease or in monitoring of treatment.

Myocardial infarction

Infarction is defined as the process by which *necrosis* (cell or tissue death) results from *ischaemia* (loss of blood supply). Infarction of cardiac muscle (myocardial infarction or MI) is one of the commonest causes of morbidity and mortality in adults living in industrialized societies.

Pathology

The underlying pathology in MI is atherosclerosis, an inflammatory process located within the arterial wall in the form of atheromatous plaques (Fig. 1). These cause narrowing of the arterial lumen, resulting in reduced coronary perfusion, the clinical manifestation of which is chest pain (angina pectoris). If an unstable plaque ruptures, the released contents precipitate the formation of a clot. This process, known as thrombosis, may result in sudden complete occlusion of the affected artery and infarction of the area of myocardium it supplies.

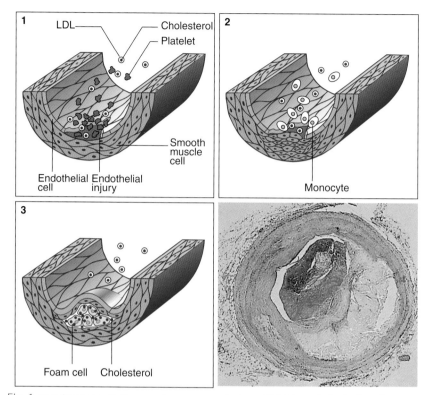

Fig. 1 **Development of atheroma in coronary arteries, with histopathological section (bottom right).**

Diagnosis

The essential components of diagnosis are the history, the characteristic ECG changes and the detection in blood of biochemical markers of myocardial injury. Patients experiencing MI classically complain of severe crushing central chest pain. However, such a characteristic history is not always obtained, and a minority of patients may even have a 'silent' MI. When present, the characteristic ECG changes (Fig. 2) are specific to MI, but they are equivocal or absent in up to 30% of patients. It is in this group of patients that cardiac markers are most useful.

Cardiac markers

'Cardiac enzymes'

When myocardial cells die, they break up and release their contents. This is the basis for the role of cardiac markers in MI diagnosis. Historically, the 'cardiac enzymes' commonly used to diagnose MI included creatine kinase (CK), aspartate aminotransferase (AST) and an isoenzyme of lactate dehydrogenase (LDH_1), also known as hydroxybutyrate dehydrogenase. The activities of these enzymes in serum following an MI are shown in Figure 3. It can be seen from this figure that these enzymes are relatively late risers, limiting their usefulness in the acute context.

CK-MB and myoglobin

An isoenzyme of CK, CK-MB, is more specific to the myocardium and rises much earlier following MI (as little as 1–3 hours post MI) compared with the traditional 'cardiac enzymes' (Fig. 3). Its diagnostic utility can be improved further in various ways. These include expressing CK-MB activity as a ratio of total CK activity (this improves diagnostic specificity), and measuring CK-MB mass instead of activity (this improves sensitivity). Some laboratories will measure CK-MB only if myoglobin is detected. Myoglobin is a haem-containing protein that also rises early following MI, with a diagnostic sensitivity approaching 95% at 6 hours. It is not specific to cardiac muscle and is frequently elevated in other conditions. It is most useful when it is not detected (in rapid exclusion of MI), but can also be used as a screening test for CK-MB as indicated above.

Troponins

The troponins are proteins that regulate muscle contraction. Isoforms of two of these proteins, T and I, are specific to myocardium, and the introduction of assays for cardiac troponin T and I represents a major development in the biochemical detection of MI. It is

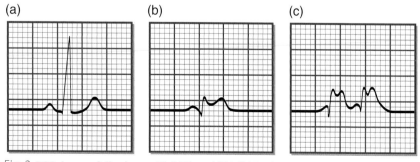

Fig. 2 **ECG changes following an MI. (a)** Normal ECG. **(b)** Two hours after onset of chest pain. Note elevated ST segment. **(c)** Twenty-four hours later the patient had a further episode of chest pain.

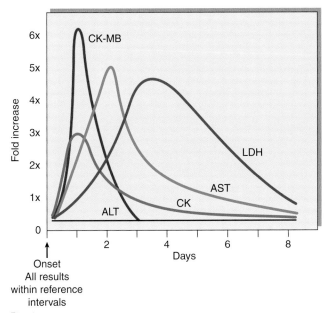

Fig. 3 **Enzymes in serum following an uncomplicated MI.**

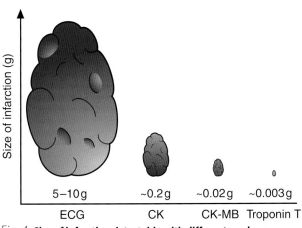

Fig. 4 **Size of infarction detectable with different markers.**

Table 2 **Troponins T and I contrasted**

	Troponin T	**Troponin I**
Molecular weight	37 kDa	22.5 kDa
Nature of protein	Structural	Catalytic
Kinetics of release	Biphasic	Only a single peak
Duration of elevation	Up to 14 days	5–7 days
Number of assays	One	Several
Ontogeny	May be expressed in skeletal muscle in utero	Only ever expressed in myocardium

Clinical note

The classical feature of an MI is crushing chest pain radiating down the left arm. Not all patients with an MI experience this. In addition to the many variants of angina-like pain, it is recognized that a sizeable proportion of MIs are 'silent', and are subsequently only detected by ECG.

In one European heart study, 2% of middle-aged men showed definite ECG evidence of a previously unrecognized MI.

Case history 20

A 52-year-old man presented at the Accident and Emergency department with severe chest pain which had been present for the past hour. He had previously attended the chest pain clinic and had a 2-year history of angina of effort.

- What specific tests would you request from the biochemistry laboratory?

Comment on page 164.

possible with troponins to detect infarctions that are orders of magnitude smaller than those detectable with other cardiac markers (Fig. 4). Crucially, however, any degree of elevation of cardiac troponins implies an impaired clinical outcome for the patient; there is no discernible threshold below which an elevated troponin is deemed harmless.

Troponins are most useful 12 hours or more after an MI, when their diagnostic sensitivity is 100%, i.e. MI can be excluded with confidence with a negative (normal) troponin result if the sample is taken 12 hours or more after the onset of chest pain. However, despite their many potential roles (Table 1) they should not be seen as 'perfect' markers. In the early hours following MI, myoglobin is more sensitive. Also, suspected re-infarction cannot reliably be detected by troponins for as much as 2 weeks, since it takes this length of time for troponins to return to normal following an MI.

Table 2 outlines the main differences between troponin T and troponin I.

The future

The ideal cardiac marker would allow clinicians to make decisions in real time about management of patients with acute coronary syndromes. Point-of-care devices are becoming available that permit simultaneous on-site measurement of myoglobin, CK-MB and cardiac troponin; however, these devices are expensive.

Myocardial infarction

- To make a diagnosis of myocardial infarction (MI), two of the following must be present:
  - severe chest pain
  - ECG changes indicative of MI
  - cardiac enzyme release.

- The cardiac enzymes historically were creatine kinase, aspartate aminotransferase and lactate dehydrogenase.

- A specific CK isoenzyme (CK-MB) is a more specific indicator of cardiac muscle damage than total CK, and can be detected in serum soon after an MI has occurred.

- Cardiac troponins are used as specific markers in MI and unstable angina.

- Early diagnosis of MI is important so that therapy can be started promptly.

Liver function tests

Introduction

The liver plays a major role in protein, carbohydrate and lipid homeostasis (Fig. 1). The metabolic pathways of glycolysis, the Krebs cycle, amino acid synthesis and degradation, and the processes of oxidative phosphorylation are all carried out in the hepatocytes, which are well endowed with mitochondria. The liver contains an extensive reticuloendothelial system for the synthesis and breakdown of blood cells. Liver cells metabolize, detoxify and excrete both endogenous and exogenous compounds. Excretion of water-soluble end products from the metabolism of both nutrients and toxins, and of digestive aids such as bile acids, occurs into the biliary tree.

Liver function tests

What are usually called liver function tests (LFTs) do not assess quantitatively the capacity of that tissue to carry out any of the functions that are described above. 'LFTs' are measurements of blood components that simply provide a lead to the existence, the extent and the type of liver damage. Usually, a request for LFTs will provide results for bilirubin, the aminotransferases and alkaline phosphatase in a serum specimen. Knowledge of the serum albumin concentration may also be of some value in the investigation of liver disease. These biochemical investigations can assist in differentiating the following:

- obstruction to the biliary tract
- acute hepatocellular damage
- chronic liver disease.

Serum total bilirubin concentration and serum alkaline phosphatase activity are indices of cholestasis, a blockage of bile flow. The serum aminotransferase activities are a measure of the integrity of liver cells. The serum albumin concentration is a crude measure of the liver's synthetic capacity, although prothrombin time is preferred (see below).

Bilirubin

Bilirubin is derived from haem, an iron-containing protoporphyrin mainly found in haemoglobin (Fig. 2). An adult normally produces about 450 µmol of bilirubin daily. It is insoluble in water and

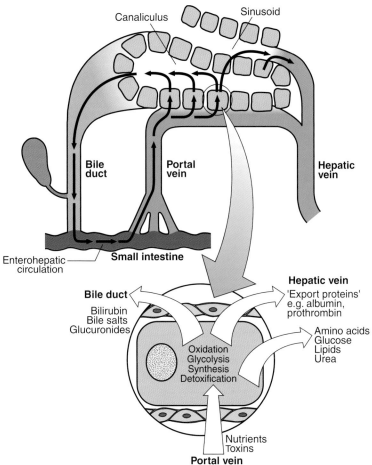

Fig. 1 **Liver functions.**

is transported in plasma almost totally bound to albumin. It is taken up by liver cells and conjugated to form mono- and diglucuronides, which are much more soluble in water than unconjugated bilirubin. The conjugated bilirubin is excreted into the bile. Normal bile contains bilirubin monoglucuronide as 25% and the diglucuronide as 75% of the total, accompanied by traces of unconjugated bilirubin. The main functional constituents of the bile are the bile salts, which are involved in fat digestion and absorption from the small intestine. Serum bile acid concentrations are more sensitive indices of hepatic transport function than are total bilirubin measurements.

In the terminal ileum and colon the bilirubin conjugates are attacked by bacteria to form a group of compounds that are known collectively as *stercobilinogen*, most of which are excreted in faeces. Some are absorbed and eventually re-excreted from the body by way of bile (the enterohepatic circulation). Small amounts of these tetrapyrroles are found in urine in which they are known as *urobilinogen*.

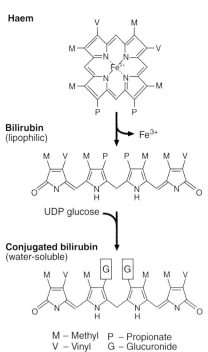

M – Methyl P – Propionate
V – Vinyl G – Glucuronide

Fig. 2 **Structure of bilirubin and conjugated bilirubin.**

When the biliary tract becomes blocked, bilirubin is not excreted and serum concentrations rise. The patient becomes jaundiced. The jaundiced patient is described further on pages 56–57.

The aminotransferases (AST and ALT)

The activities of two aminotransferases, AST and ALT, are widely used in clinical practice as a sensitive, albeit non-specific, index of acute damage to hepatocytes irrespective of its aetiology. Causes of liver damage include hepatitis, no matter the causative agent, and toxic injury, which may accompany any one of a large number of insults to the liver, including drug overdose. Acute liver damage due to shock, severe hypoxia and acute cardiac failure is also seen (see pp. 58–59).

Alkaline phosphatase (ALP)

Increases in alkaline phosphatase activity in liver disease are the result of increased synthesis of the enzyme by cells lining the bile canaliculi, usually in response to cholestasis, which may be either intra- or extrahepatic. Cholestasis, even of short duration, results in an increased enzyme activity to at least twice the upper end of the reference interval. High alkaline phosphatase activity may also occur in infiltrative diseases of the liver, when space-occupying lesions (e.g. tumours) are present. It also occurs in cirrhosis.

Liver is not the sole source of alkaline phosphatase activity. Substantial amounts are present in bone, small intestine, placenta and kidney. In normal blood, the alkaline phosphatase activity is derived mainly from bone and liver, with small amounts from intestine. Placental alkaline phosphatase appears in the maternal blood in the third trimester of pregnancy. Occasionally, the cause of a raised alkaline phosphatase will not be immediately apparent. The liver and bone isoenzymes can be separated by electrophoresis. However, an elevated γGT (see below) would suggest that the liver is the source of the increased alkaline phosphatase.

Gamma-glutamyl transpeptidase (γGT)

γGT is a microsomal enzyme that is widely distributed in tissues including liver and renal tubules. The activity of γGT in plasma is raised whenever there is cholestasis, and it is a very sensitive index of liver pathology. It is also affected by ingestion of alcohol, even in the absence of recognizable liver disease. Alcohol and drugs such as phenytoin induce enzyme activity. In acute hepatic damage, changes in γGT activity parallel those of the aminotransferases.

Plasma proteins

Albumin is the major protein product of the liver. It has a long biological half-life in plasma (about 20 days), and therefore significant falls in albumin concentration are slow to occur if synthesis is suddenly reduced. Hypoalbuminaemia is a feature of advanced chronic liver disease. It can also occur in *severe* acute liver damage.

The total serum globulin concentrations is sometimes used as a crude measure of the severity of liver disease.

Alpha-fetoprotein (AFP) is synthesized by the fetal liver. In normal adults it is present in plasma at low concentrations (<20 µg/L). Measurement of AFP is of value in the investigation of hepatocellular carcinoma in which serum concentrations are increased in 80–90% of cases. AFP is also used as a marker for germ cell tumours (pp. 138–139).

Other proteins, such as α_1-antitrypsin and caeruloplasmin, are measured in the diagnosis of specific diseases affecting the liver (p. 59).

Prothrombin time

The prothrombin time, which is a measure of the activities of certain coagulation factors made by the liver, is sometimes used as an indicator of hepatic synthetic function. Prothrombin has a very short half-life, and an increased prothrombin time may be the earliest indicator of reduced hepatic synthesis.

Case history 21

A 60-year-old woman with a history of breast carcinoma treated by mastectomy 3 years previously is now complaining of general malaise and bone pain. Biochemistry showed that fluid and electrolytes, total protein, albumin and calcium values were all normal. LFTs were as follows:

Bilirubin µmol/L	AST	ALT	Alkaline phosphatase	γGT
		U/L		
7	33	38	890	32

■ Evaluate these results and suggest a likely diagnosis.

Comment on page 164.

Clinical note

Diagnostic imaging techniques are at least as important as biochemical tests in the investigation of liver disease. The arrow highlights an area of defective isotope uptake indicating the presence of a liver metastasis in a patient with disseminated malignant disease.

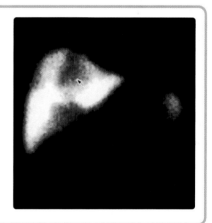

Fig. 3 **Scintiscan of liver.**

Liver function tests

- A request for LFTs will usually generate results for bilirubin, an aminotransferase and alkaline phosphatase.
- Raised activities of the aminotransferases (AST and ALT) indicate hepatocellular damage.
- Increased bilirubin concentration and increased alkaline phosphatase activity indicate the presence of cholestasis, a blockage in bile flow.
- Serial use of LFTs is of most value in following the progress or resolution of liver disease.
- Measurement of γ-glutamyl transpeptidase can give an indication of hepatocellular enzyme induction due to drugs or alcohol.

Jaundice

Jaundice is a yellow discoloration of the skin or sclera (Fig. 1). This is due to the presence of bilirubin in the plasma and is not usually detectable until the concentration is greater than about 50 μmol/L. Normally the bilirubin concentration in plasma is less than 22 μmol/L.

Bilirubin is derived from the tetrapyrrole prosthetic group found in haemoglobin and the cytochromes. It is normally conjugated with glucuronic acid to make it more soluble, and excreted in the bile (Fig. 2). There are three main reasons why bilirubin levels in the blood may rise (Fig. 3).

- *Haemolysis*. The increased haemoglobin breakdown produces bilirubin, which overloads the conjugating mechanism.
- *Failure of the conjugating mechanism within the hepatocyte.*
- *Obstruction in the biliary sytem.*

Both conjugated bilirubin and unconjugated bilirubin may be present in plasma. Conjugated bilirubin is water-soluble. Unconjugated bilirubin is not water-soluble and binds to albumin from which it may be transferred to other proteins such as those in cell membranes. It is neurotoxic, and if levels rise too high in neonates, permanent brain damage can occur.

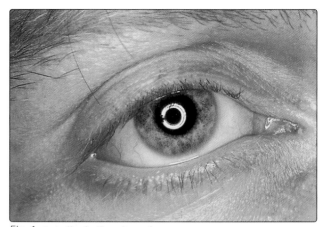

Fig. 1 **Jaundice in the sclera of an eye.**

Biochemical tests

Bilirubin metabolites are responsible for the brown coloration of faeces. If bilirubin does not reach the gut, stools become pale in colour. Bilirubin in the gut is metabolized by bacteria to produce stercobilinogen. This is partly reabsorbed and re-excreted in the urine as urobilinogen, and may be detected by simple biochemical tests. When high levels of conjugated bilirubin are being excreted, urine may be a deep orange colour, particularly if allowed to stand.

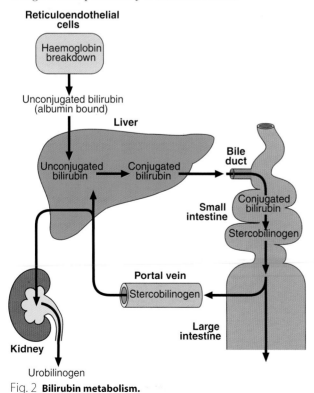

Fig. 2 **Bilirubin metabolism.**

This combination of pale stools and dark urine is characteristic of extrahepatic obstruction of the biliary tract. This is often amenable to surgery, hence the term 'surgical jaundice'.

Differential diagnosis

Jaundice may be a consequence of haemolysis, cholestasis or hepatocellular damage. The causes and features of these are summarized in Figure 3 and Table 1. In addition there are inherited disorders of bilirubin metabolism. Gilbert's disease is the most common and causes a mild unconjugated hyperbilirubinaemia because of defective hepatic uptake of bilirubin. In this condition bilirubin levels rise on fasting.

Haemolysis

Increased bilirubin production caused by haemolysis gives a predominantly unconjugated hyperbilirubinaemia. This, in combination with immature liver function, is commonly encountered in babies. A rapidly rising bilirubin in a neonate should be carefully monitored as it may give rise to brain damage (kernicterus). If the concentration approaches 200 μmol/L, phototherapy should be used to break down the molecule in the skin and reduce the level. If the concentration rises above 300 μmol/L, exchange transfusion may be necessary.

Extrahepatic biliary obstruction

Gallstones can partially or fully block the bile duct. Such a blockage is known as extrahepatic obstruction. If the blockage is complete, both bilirubin and alkaline phosphatase are raised. There is little or no urobilinogen

Table 1	**Laboratory differential diagnosis of jaundice**		
	Haemolytic	**Cholestatic**	**Hepatocellular**
Features	■ Bilirubin usually <75 μmol/L	■ Bilirubin may be ↑↑↑	■ AST + ALT ↑↑
	■ No bilirubin in urine	■ Bilirubin in urine.	■ Bilirubin ↑ later
	■ Reticulocytosis	■ Alkaline phosphatase, usually >3x upper limit of reference range	■ Bilirubin in urine
	■ Haemoglobin ↓		■ Alkaline phosphatase ↑ later
	■ Haptoglobin ↓	■ AST, ALT + LDH usually modestly ↑	
	■ LDH may ↑		

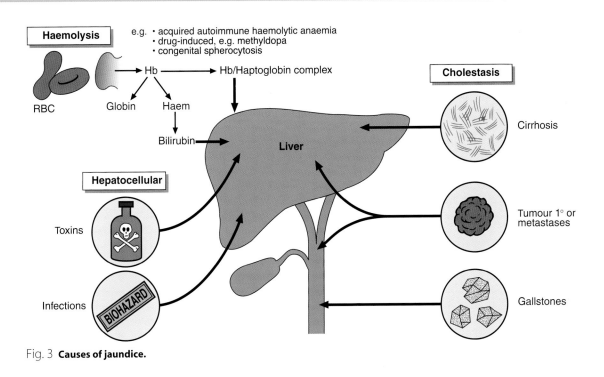

Fig. 3 **Causes of jaundice.**

in urine. Stools will be pale in colour. When the obstruction is removed, the stools regain their colour and urine again becomes positive for urobilinogen. If the blockage is only partial, alkaline phosphatase may be high, although serum bilirubin may well be within the reference interval. This is a classic picture of an isolated secondary neoplasm in the liver, partly disturbing the biliary tree. The normal functioning part of the liver is sufficient to process and excrete the bilirubin. The levels of alkaline phosphatase released into serum will mirror the degree of obstruction. Intrahepatic biliary obstruction is much more difficult to diagnose than extrahepatic obstruction. The bile canaliculi can become blocked due to cirrhosis, liver cancer or infection. This leads to an increased concentration of conjugated bilirubin in serum.

Clinical note

CT scanning is an invaluable tool in the investigation of the jaundiced patient. The dilated bile ducts (arrow) are clearly visible in a CT scan of a patient with extrahepatic obstructive jaundice due to carcinoma of the head of the pancreas (Fig. 4).

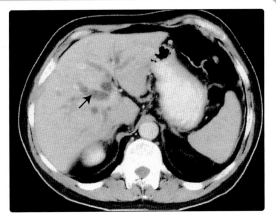

Fig. 4 **CT scan of liver and gall bladder.**

Hepatocellular damage

Obstruction may be secondary to damage to the hepatocytes by infection or toxins, rather than damage to the biliary tract. The most common causes of acute jaundice seen in adults are viral hepatitis and paracetamol poisoning. In these cases, not only are the bilirubin and alkaline phosphatase levels raised, but AST and ALT are elevated indicating hepatocellular damage.

Case history 22

A 65-year-old man came to his GP's surgery with visible jaundice that he had noticed to be deepening in colour. He had no pain but had noticed some weight loss and that his stools were pale. He was a moderate drinker, and was not on any drug therapy. His LFTs were:

Bilirubin µmol/L	AST	ALT	Alkaline phosphatase
		U/L	
250	87	92	850

■ What is the differential diagnosis?
■ What other investigations would be helpful in making a diagnosis?

Comment on page 164.

Jaundice

■ Jaundice indicates that there is an elevated concentration of bilirubin in serum.

■ In neonates it is important to determine the concentration of unconjugated bilirubin in order to decide what treatment is required.

■ In adults, the most common cause of jaundice is obstruction, and this is confirmed by the elevation of both bilirubin and alkaline phosphatase.

Liver disease

Acute liver disease

Acute liver damage occurs for one of three reasons:

- poisoning
- infection
- inadequate perfusion.

Investigation

Biochemical markers of liver disease such as AST and ALT will indicate hepatocyte damage. Elevated serum bilirubin and alkaline phosphatase levels show the presence of cholestasis. Disease progression or recovery can be followed by serial measurements of LFTs.

Poisoning

The best-documented poisons that affect the liver are paracetamol and carbon tetrachloride. These are metabolized by the intact liver in small amounts, but when present at high concentrations they give rise to toxic metabolites, leading to destruction of hepatocytes with massive release of enzymes. The capacity of the liver to withstand an insult is reduced if there is underlying liver damage due to alcohol, malnutrition or other chronic disease.

Some plant and fungal toxins can also cause catastrophic and fatal liver damage within 48 hours (Fig. 1).

A third group of toxins are those that give rise to acute hepatocellular failure only in certain individuals who are susceptible. Important examples include sodium valproate, an anticonvulsant drug that causes toxicity in some children, and halothane, an anaesthetic agent.

Liver infection

Both bacteria and viruses can give rise to infective hepatitis, which causes many deaths worldwide. Hepatitis A, hepatitis B and hepatitis C are the most common.

Outcome

Acute liver damage can progress in three ways:

- It may resolve, as indeed it does in the majority of cases.
- It may progress to acute hepatic failure.
- It may lead to chronic hepatic damage.

Hepatic failure

Acute hepatic failure is a major medical emergency, since the failure of the complex metabolic functions of the liver cannot be compensated for by any other organ. In severe cases, much of the biochemical picture is disrupted. Electrolyte imbalance occurs, and sodium and calcium concentrations may both fall. There may be severe metabolic acid–base disturbances and hypoglycaemia.

Hepatic failure may give rise to renal failure due to exposure of the glomeruli to toxins usually metabolized by the liver. There may be an increase in blood ammonia as a result of the failure to detoxify this to urea. The pattern of abnormalities found in hepatic failure is shown in Figure 2.

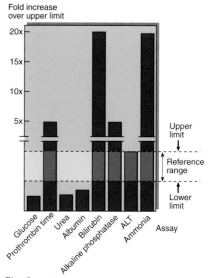

Fig. 2 **Laboratory findings in hepatic failure.**

In acute hepatocellular damage, albumin synthesis is reduced or ceases, eventually leading to hypoalbuminaemia and the development of oedema and/or ascites. The failure of synthesis of clotting factors also leads to an increased tendency to haemorrhage or, in severe cases, to intravascular coagulation.

Recovery from acute hepatocellular damage may take some weeks, during which monitoring of LFTs is helpful in detecting relapse and assisting prognosis.

Chronic liver disease

Three forms of chronic liver damage are:

- alcoholic fatty liver
- chronic active hepatitis
- primary biliary cirrhosis.

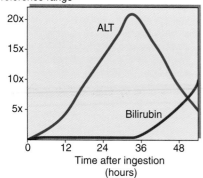

Fig. 1 **Pattern of LFTs following *Amanita phalloides* (a highly poisonous species of mushroom) ingestion.**

Case history 23

A 49-year-old woman attended her GP with an 8-day history of anorexia, nausea and flu-like symptoms. She had noticed that her urine had been dark in colour over the past 2 days. Physical examination revealed tenderness in the right upper quadrant of the abdomen. LFTs were as follows:

Bilirubin	AST	ALT	Alkaline phosphatase	γGT	Total protein	Albumin
μmol/L			—— U/L ——			—— g/L ——
63	936	2700	410	312	68	42

- Comment on these results.
- What is the differential diagnosis?

Comment on page 164.

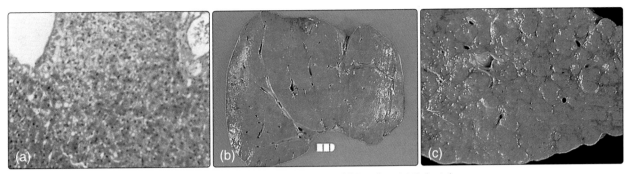

Fig. 3 **Appearance of normal and diseased liver. (a)** Normal liver histology. **(b)** Fatty liver. **(c)** Cirrhotic liver.

All of these conditions may progress to cirrhosis, a disease characterized by extensive liver fibrosis. Fibrosis is the formation of scar tissue, resulting in the disorganization of liver architecture and its shrinkage. (Fig. 3).

Aetiology

Cirrhosis is the terminal stage of chronic liver damage and only occasionally follows an acute course. The most common causes of cirrhosis are:

- chronic excess alcohol ingestion
- viral hepatitis (particularly hepatitis B)
- autoimmune diseases.

Cirrhosis is not reversible, although in alcoholics the preceding stage, that of chronic fatty liver, does respond to abstention from alcohol. For reasons that are not clear, only about 30% of alcoholics progress to cirrhosis.

Clinical features

There are no good biochemical indicators of cirrhosis in the early and stable period, which may last for many years. In the terminal stages the features include:

- developing jaundice
- encephalopathy, which may be related to toxins that are not removed from the plasma
- ascites (see p. 126)
- bleeding tendencies
- terminal liver failure.

However, the cirrhotic liver has a reserve of function despite its macro- and microscopic appearance. The major complaint in cirrhosis may be difficulty in coping with food, especially fatty meals. Patients with cirrhosis have a reduced capacity to metabolize drugs. Some patients with cirrhosis suffer badly from itch, due to the disruption of the biliary architecture and subsequent failure to excrete bile acids, which accumulate in the skin. The immunological response of patients with cirrhosis may well be reduced, leading to increased susceptibility to infection.

Unusual causes of cirrhosis

Cirrhosis can develop in children as a result of α_1-antitrypsin deficiency or Wilson's disease, and in adults due to haemochromatosis. α_1-Antitrypsin deficiency can be detected in newborn infants in whom there may be a prolonged period of jaundice for several weeks. In some cases this progresses to juvenile cirrhosis. Haemochromatosis is a disorder of iron absorption, associated with deposition of iron in the hepatocytes and other tissues, which can lead to liver failure. The diagnosis is by measurement of serum iron, transferrin and ferritin (p. 113). Wilson's disease is an inherited disorder of copper metabolism that leads to failure in copper excretion, low concentrations of caeruloplasmin, and deposition of copper in the liver and other tissues (p. 114). Cirrhosis may also occur following chronic ingestion of pyrrolizidine alkaloids, such as are found in some herbal teas.

Other liver problems

The liver is a common site of secondary metastases from a wide variety of primary tumours, and jaundice may be the first indication of the presence of cancer in some patients.

Primary hepatoma is associated with a number of conditions such as cirrhosis or hepatitis, although a number of causative carcinogens, such as aflatoxins generated by specific fungi infecting foodstuffs, have been identified. Alpha-fetoprotein is a useful marker of primary hepatic tumours (pp. 138–139).

> ### Clinical note
> Liver biopsy is the definitive way of making a specific diagnosis. Before attempting a needle biopsy it is essential that the patient's blood coagulation status is confirmed to be satisfactory.

Liver disease

- Acute liver damage is caused by shock, toxins or infection.
- Biochemical monitoring of liver disease is by sequential measurements of aminotransferases, bilirubin and alkaline phosphatase.
- In acute liver damage there is usually intrahepatic obstruction as well as hepatocellular damage.
- Severe cases of acute liver damage may progress to hepatocellular failure.
- Cirrhosis is the end point of both acute and chronic liver damage, as well as being caused by a number of metabolic and autoimmune diseases.
- Biochemical tests may be of little value in making a specific diagnosis. A liver biopsy is frequently more helpful.

Glucose metabolism and diabetes mellitus

Dietary carbohydrate is digested in the gastrointestinal tract to simple monosaccharides, which are then absorbed. Starch provides glucose directly, while fructose (from dietary sucrose) and galactose (from dietary lactose) are absorbed and also converted into glucose in the liver. Glucose is the common carbohydrate currency of the body. Figure 1 shows the different metabolic processes that affect the blood glucose concentration. This level is, as always, the result of a balance between input and output, synthesis and catabolism.

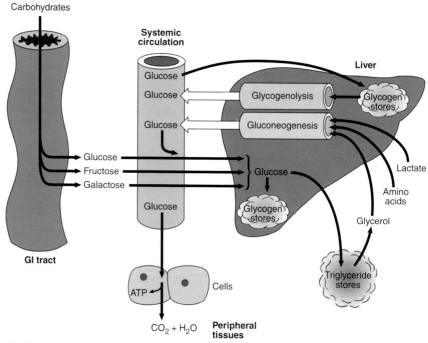

Fig. 1 **Glucose homeostasis.**

Insulin

Insulin is the principal hormone affecting blood glucose levels, and an understanding of its actions is an important prerequisite to the study of diabetes mellitus. Insulin is a small protein synthesized in the beta cells of the islets of Langerhans of the pancreas. It acts through membrane receptors and its main target tissues are liver, muscle and adipose tissue.

Insulin signals the fed state. It switches on pathways and processes involved in the cellular uptake and storage of metabolic fuels, and switches off pathways involved in fuel breakdown (Fig. 2). It should be noted that glucose cannot enter the cells of most body tissues in the absence of insulin.

The effects of insulin are opposed by other hormones, e.g. glucagon, adrenaline, glucocorticoids and growth hormone. These are sometimes called stress hormones, and this explains why patients admitted acutely to hospital often have raised blood glucose.

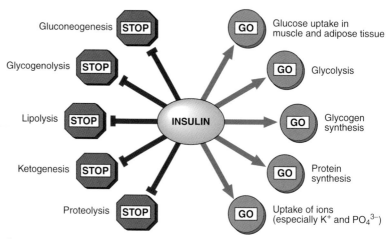

Fig. 2 **The actions of insulin.**

Diabetes mellitus

Diabetes mellitus is the commonest endocrine disorder encountered in clinical practice. It may be defined as a syndrome characterized by hyperglycaemia due to an insulin resistance and an absolute or relative lack of insulin.

Primary diabetes mellitus is generally subclassified into insulin-dependent diabetes mellitus (IDDM) or non-insulin-dependent diabetes mellitus (NIDDM). These clinical entities differ in epidemiology, clinical features and pathophysiology. The contrasting features of IDDM and NIDDM are shown in Table 1.

Secondary diabetes mellitus may result from pancreatic disease, endocrine disease such as Cushing's syndrome, drug therapy, and, rarely, insulin receptor abnormalities.

Insulin-dependent diabetes mellitus (IDDM)

IDDM accounts for approximately 15% of all diabetic patients. It can occur at any age but is most common in the young, with a peak incidence between 9 and 14 years of age. The absolute lack of insulin is a consequence of the autoimmune destruction of insulin-producing beta cells. There may be an environmental precipitating factor such as a viral infection. The presence of islet cell antibodies in serum predicts future development of diabetes.

Non-insulin-dependent diabetes mellitus (NIDDM)

NIDDM accounts for approximately 85% of all diabetic patients and can occur at any age. It is most common between 40 and 80 years but is now being reported in adolescent and even paediatric populations. In this condition there is resistance of peripheral tissues to the actions of

Table 1 Insulin-dependent diabetes mellitus (IDDM) versus non-insulin-dependent diabetes mellitus (NIDDM)

Main features	IDDM	NIDDM
Epidemiology		
Frequency in northern Europe	0.02–0.4%	1–3%
Predominance	N. European	Worldwide
	Caucasians	Lowest in rural areas of developing countries
Clinical characteristics		
Age	<30 years	>40 years
Weight	Low/normal	Increased
Onset	Rapid	Slow
Ketosis	Common	Under stress
Endogenous insulin	Low/absent	Present but insufficient
HLA associations	Yes	No
Islet cell antibodies	Yes	No
Pathophysiology		
Aetiology	Autoimmune destruction of pancreatic islet cells	Impaired insulin secretion and insulin resistance
Genetic associations	Polygenic	Strong
Environmental factors	Viruses and toxins implicated	Obesity, physical inactivity

HDL-cholesterol, and a shift towards smaller, denser LDL) is considered highly atherogenic.

Approximately 60% of diabetic patients die of vascular disease and 35% of coronary heart disease. Blindness is 25 times and chronic renal failure 17 times more common in diabetics. There is increasing evidence that tight glycaemic control delays the onset of these sequelae.

insulin, so that the insulin level may be normal or even high. Obesity is the most commonly associated clinical feature.

underlying mechanisms are unclear, although the (compensatory) hyperinsulinaemia associated with insulin resistance and NIDDM may play a key role. Certainly, the dyslipidaemia seen in these patients (increased triglycerides, decreased

> ### Clinical note
> The clinical symptoms of hyperglycaemia include polyuria, polydipsia, lassitude, weight loss, pruritus vulvae and balanitis. These symptoms are common to both NIDDM and IDDM but are more pronounced in IDDM. It is important to remember that patients with NIDDM may be completely asymptomatic.

Late complications of diabetes mellitus

Diabetes mellitus is not only characterized by the presence of hyperglycaemia but also by the occurrence of late complications:

- *Microangiopathy* is characterized by abnormalities in the walls of small blood vessels, the most prominent feature of which is thickening of the basement membrane. It is associated with poor glycaemic control.
- *Retinopathy* may lead to blindness because of vitreous haemorrhage from proliferating retinal vessels, and maculopathy as a result of exudates from vessels or oedema affecting the macula (Fig. 3).
- *Nephropathy* leads ultimately to renal failure. In the early stage there is kidney hyperfunction, associated with an increased GFR, increased glomerular size and microalbuminuria. In the late stage, there is increasing proteinuria and a marked decline in renal function, resulting in uraemia.
- *Neuropathy* may become evident as diarrhoea, postural hypotension, impotence, neurogenic bladder and neuropathic foot ulcers due to microangiopathy of nerve blood vessels and abnormal glucose metabolism in nerve cells.
- *Macroangiopathy (or accelerated atherosclerosis)* leads to premature coronary heart disease. The exact

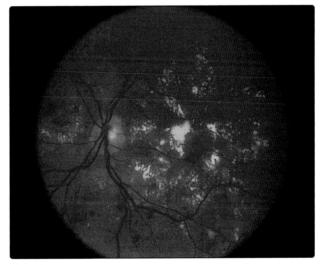

Fig. 3 **Diabetic retinopathy.**

Glucose metabolism and diabetes mellitus

- Glucose is the carbohydrate currency of the body, all other carbohydrates being converted to glucose after digestion and absorption.
- Insulin controls blood glucose by promoting the storage of metabolic fuels.
- Diabetes mellitus is characterized by hyperglycaemia, absolute or relative insulin lack and late complications.
- Insulin-dependent diabetes mellitus (IDDM) is caused by a complete lack of insulin and is most common in the young.
- Non-insulin-dependent diabetes mellitus (NIDDM) accounts for 85% of all diabetics and can occur at any age.
- Late complications of diabetes mellitus are a result of micro- and macroangiopathies.

Diagnosis and monitoring of diabetes mellitus

The diagnosis of diabetes must be made with care since it has far-reaching medical and social consequences. A number of biochemical tests are used in association with clinical assessment for both the initial diagnosis of this condition and long-term monitoring of patients.

Blood glucose

Glucose is routinely measured in blood specimens that have been collected into tubes containing fluoride, an inhibitor of glycolysis. Because of the need sometimes to obtain rapid blood glucose results and the widespread self-monitoring of diabetic patients, blood glucose may also be assessed outside the laboratory using devices as shown in Figure 1.

Diagnosis of diabetes mellitus

The formal diagnosis of diabetes mellitus requires analysis of at least one blood sample. A fasting sample is preferred, but where this is not feasible a random sample may be acceptable. If the diagnosis is not clear from fasting and/or random sampling, a formal oral glucose challenge (oral glucose tolerance test) may be required.

Criteria for diagnosis

The current World Health Organization criteria for diagnosing diabetes mellitus are shown in Table 1. The figures shown apply to the concentrations found in venous plasma; slightly different figures (not shown) apply to whole blood or capillary samples.

Table 1 **Criteria for the diagnosis of diabetes mellitus**

Fasting blood glucose		
Non-diabetic	Impaired fasting glycaemia	Diabetes
<6.0	6.0–6.9	≥7.0
Oral glucose tolerance test		
	Fasting	2-hour
Impaired glucose tolerance	<7.0	7.8–11.0
Diabetes	≥7.0	≥11.1

All figures refer to glucose concentrations (mmol/L) in venous plasma.

The fasting and 2-hour criteria define similar levels of glycaemia above which the risk of diabetic complications increases substantially.

Random blood glucose

If a patient complains of hyperglycaemic (osmotic) symptoms such as thirst, frequency, polyuria, and nocturia, a random blood glucose (RBG) result of ≥11.1 mmol/L may be used to diagnose diabetes. If the patient is asymptomatic, or there is any doubt about the diagnosis, a repeat sample (preferably fasting) is required, e.g. when the result is borderline, there is coexistent disease or the patient is receiving drugs, such as steroids, which might affect the result.

Fasting blood glucose

A fasting blood glucose (FBG) concentration of ≥7.0 mmol/L is regarded as diagnostic of diabetes, whether or not hyperglycaemic symptoms are present. The patient should be fasted overnight (at least 10 hours). If the result falls between 6.0 and 6.9 mmol/L, the patient is said to have 'impaired fasting glycaemia' (see below). Interpretation of fasting glucose results is shown in Table 1.

Oral glucose tolerance test

Sometimes diagnostic confusion still exists even after a repeat sample has been analysed, e.g. borderline or apparently conflicting results. In this situation an oral glucose tolerance test (OGTT) is recommended. A normal diet should have been consumed for at least 3 days prior to the test. A fasting sample is collected immediately before an oral glucose load (75 g of glucose in about 300 mL of water); this should be drunk within 5 minutes or so. A second sample is collected 2 hours later. The patient should be relatively inactive throughout and smoking is prohibited throughout the test. Normal and diabetic responses to an oral glucose load are shown in Figure 2. The interpretation of OGTT results is summarized in Table 1.

Impaired glucose tolerance and impaired fasting glycaemia

Impaired fasting glycaemia (IFG) and impaired glucose tolerance (IGT) are intermediate categories of glycaemia that fall short of the diagnosis of diabetes, but which define an increased risk of developing diabetes. IGT can only be diagnosed after an oral glucose tolerance test. The risks associated with IGT (e.g. risk of developing diabetes) are well-defined and have been characterized over many years. By contrast, IFG is diagnosed from a single fasting sample. Its existence as a diagnostic category arose out of the 1997 recommendation of the American Diabetes Association that oral glucose tolerance tests be abandoned in favour exclusively of fasting samples (this recommendation was not adopted by the World Health Organization when it updated its 1985 diagnostic criteria in 1999). The criteria for IFG are arbitrary and the associated risks less well-defined than for IGT.

IGT and IFG – a word of caution

Patients with IGT or IFG should not simply be reassured that they do not have diabetes and told to return for annual review. They are, in pathogenic terms, quite far down the road to developing diabetes; by definition, their pancreatic secretion of insulin is no

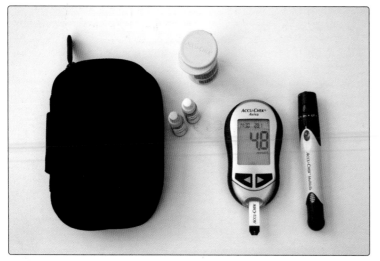

Fig. 1 **Blood glucose testing device.**

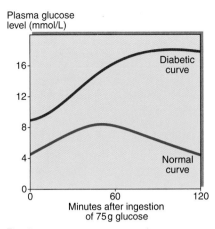

Fig. 2 **Plasma glucose levels following an oral glucose load in normal and diabetic subjects.**

longer fully able to compensate for their insulin resistance. They are also at risk of coronary heart disease, hypertension and dyslipidaemia. These should be screened for and if present should be actively treated at the time, rather than simply waiting for the patient to develop full-blown diabetes mellitus.

Monitoring of diabetes

Self-monitoring

Most diabetic patients are taught how to monitor their own diabetic control. Home urine testing is the simplest form of monitoring and may be acceptable in patients with mild (early) type 2 diabetes. If more accurate monitoring is required, patients may be supplied with a point-of-care glucose monitor. This requires finger-prick whole blood samples (a drop is usually adequate); the patient is usually advised to vary the time of self-testing in order to get an overall picture of their glycaemic control.

Glycated haemoglobin

Hyperglycaemia leads to the non-enzymatic attachment of glucose to a variety of proteins (glycation),

which is virtually irreversible under physiological conditions and the concentration of glycated protein is therefore a reflection of mean blood glucose level during the life of that protein.

Glycated haemoglobin (HbA_{1c}) reflects the mean glycaemia over 2 months prior to its measurement, the half-life of haemoglobin. The HbA_{1c} concentration is expressed as a percentage of the total haemoglobin concentration; 7% or less indicates good glycaemic control. HbA_{1c} is widely used in diabetic clinics and primary care to complement the information from single or even serial blood glucose measurements. Spurious results may sometimes be obtained in patients with inherited structurally abnormal haemoglobins (haemoglobinopathies).

Urine testing

Glycosuria

The presence or absence of glycosuria has no role in the screening or the diagnosis of diabetes. For historical reasons many occupational and other health checks include urine glucose

testing, which may reveal unsuspected diabetes. However, the false-negative rate for this test is unacceptably high.

Ketones in urine or blood

The term 'ketone bodies' refers to acetone and the keto-acids acetoacetate and β-hydroxybutyrate. These are frequently found in uncontrolled diabetes (diabetic ketoacidosis or DKA – see p. 64). They are also found in normal subjects as a result of starvation or fasting, and sometimes in alcoholic patients with poor dietary intake (alcoholic ketoacidosis).

Microalbuminuria

Microalbuminuria may be defined as an albumin excretion rate intermediate between normality (<30 mg/day) and macroalbuminuria (>300 mg/day). It is a marker of early (reversible) diabetic nephropathy and is thus used to screen for renal damage. Albumin excretion at this level varies considerably throughout the day and is best measured in timed (preferably 24-hour) collections; confounders include acute illness, urinary tract infections, cardiac failure and exercise.

Clinical note

The glucose result log book kept by insulin-dependent diabetics who perform home monitoring may at first sight appear to show good and consistent glucose control. This may not always represent the truth. The clinician should determine the true level of control by close questioning and objective assessments such as HbA_{1c} or fructosamine.

Diagnosis and monitoring of diabetes mellitus

■ The diagnosis of diabetes mellitus is made on the basis of blood glucose concentrations either alone or in response to an oral glucose load.

■ In asymptomatic patients the results of an oral glucose tolerance test should be interpreted as diagnostic of diabetes mellitus only when there is an increased 2-hour glucose concentration, and the blood glucose is also equal to or greater than 11.1 mmol/L at some other point during the test.

■ HbA_{1c} and fructosamine are measures of protein glycation and serve as indices of long-term glucose control.

■ Microalbuminuria is a measure of early, reversible, diabetic nephropathy.

Diabetic ketoacidosis

How diabetic ketoacidosis develops

Diabetic ketoacidosis (DKA) is a medical emergency. All metabolic disturbances seen in DKA are the indirect or direct consequences of the lack of insulin (Fig. 1). Decreased glucose transport into tissues leads to hyperglycaemia, which gives rise to glycosuria. Increased lipolysis causes overproduction of fatty acids, some of which are converted into ketones, giving ketonaemia, metabolic acidosis and ketonuria. Glycosuria causes an osmotic diuresis, which leads to the loss of water and electrolytes – sodium, potassium, calcium, magnesium, phosphate and chloride. Dehydration, if severe, produces pre-renal uraemia and may lead to hypovolaemic shock. The severe metabolic acidosis is partially compensated by an increased ventilation rate (Kussmaul breathing). Frequent vomiting is also usually present and accentuates the loss of water and electrolytes. Thus the development of DKA is a series of interlocking vicious circles all of which must be broken to aid the restoration of normal carbohydrate and lipid metabolism.

The most common precipitating factors in the development of DKA are infection, myocardial infarction, trauma or omission of insulin.

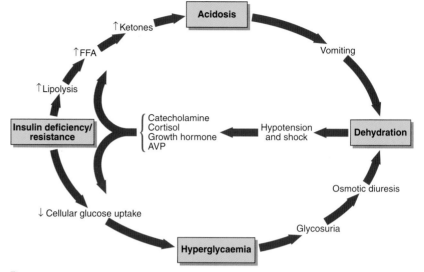

Fig. 1 **The development of diabetic ketoacidosis.**

regimen. The hallmark of good management of a patient with DKA is close clinical and biochemical monitoring.

Laboratory investigations

Initially, urine (if available) should be tested for glucose and ketones, and blood checked for glucose using a test strip. Venous blood should be sent to the laboratory for plasma glucose and serum sodium, potassium, chloride, bicarbonate,

Treatment

The management of DKA requires the administration of three agents:

- *Insulin*. Intravenous insulin is most commonly used. Intramuscular insulin is an alternative when an infusion pump is not available or where venous access is difficult, e.g. in small children.
- *Fluids*. Patients with DKA are usually severely fluid depleted and it is essential to expand their ECF with saline to restore their circulation.
- *Potassium*. Despite apparently normal serum potassium levels, all patients with DKA have whole body potassium depletion that may be severe.

In most cases, rehydration and insulin therapy will correct the metabolic acidosis, and no further therapy is indicated. However, in the most severe cases when the hydrogen ion concentration is greater than 100 nmol/L, IV sodium bicarbonate may be indicated.

The detailed management of diabetic ketoacidosis is shown in Figure 2. The importance of good fluid charts, as in any serious fluid and electrolyte disorder, cannot be over-emphasized. The initial high input of physiological (0.9%) saline is cut back as the patient's fluid and electrolyte deficit improves. Intravenous insulin is given by continuous infusion using an automated pump, and potassium supplements are added to the fluid

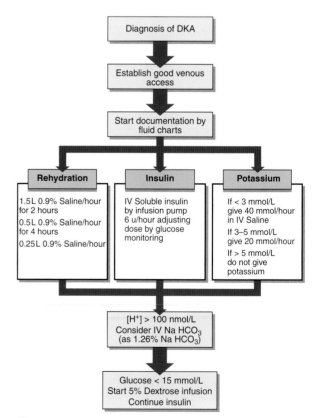

Fig. 2 **A treatment regimen for diabetic ketoacidosis.**

urea and creatinine. An arterial blood sample should also be sent for measurement of blood gases.

It is important to highlight a clinically important consequence of laboratory methodology here. The presence of ketone bodies in serum interferes with creatinine measurement; therefore serum creatinine can be falsely elevated in the acute stage. Reliable creatinine values are obtained only after ketonaemia subsides.

Amylase activity in serum is also increased in diabetic ketoacidosis. Pancreatitis should be considered as a precipitating factor only if there is persistent abdominal pain.

Blood glucose should be monitored hourly at the bedside until less than 15 mmol/L. Thereafter checks may continue 2-hourly. The plasma glucose should be confirmed in the laboratory every 2–4 hours. The frequency of monitoring of blood gases depends on the severity of DKA. In severe cases it should be performed 2-hourly at least for the first 4 hours. The serum potassium level should be checked every 2 hours for the first 6 hours, while urea and electrolytes should be measured at 4-hourly intervals (Fig. 3).

Two other forms of severe metabolic decompensation may occur in diabetics. These are hyperosmolar non-ketotic (HONK) coma and lactic acidosis. Table 1 shows the principal features of these conditions in comparison with DKA.

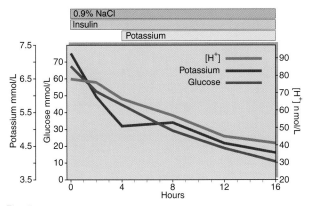

Fig. 3 **Effective treatment of a severe case of diabetic ketoacidosis.**

Table 1 **Principal features of three forms of metabolic decompensation in diabetes**

Features	Diabetic keto-acidosis (DKA)	Hyperosmolar non-ketotic coma (HONK)	Lactic acidosis
Plasma glucose	High	Very high	Variable
Ketones	Present	None	Variable
Acidosis	Moderate/Severe	None	Severe
Dehydration	Prominent	Prominent	Variable
Hyperventilation	Present	None	Present

Case history 25

A 22-year-old patient with diabetes comes to the Accident and Emergency department. She gives a 2-day history of vomiting and abdominal pain. She is drowsy and her breathing is deep and rapid. There is a distinctive smell from her breath.

- What is the most likely diagnosis?
- Which bedside tests could you do to help you to confirm this diagnosis?
- Which laboratory tests would you request?

Comment on page 164.

Hyperosmolar non-ketotic (HONK) coma

Diagnosis
HONK coma occurs mostly in elderly, non-insulin-dependent diabetics, and develops relatively slowly over days or weeks. The level of insulin is sufficient to prevent ketosis but does not prevent hyperglycaemia and osmotic diuresis. Precipitating factors include severe illness, dehydration, glucocorticoids, diuretics, parenteral nutrition, dialysis and surgery. Extremely high blood glucose levels (above 35 mmol/L, and usually above 50 mmol/L) accompany severe dehydration resulting in impaired consciousness.

Treatment
Treatment is similar to that of DKA, with the following modifications. Rehydration should be slower to avoid neurological damage. Dilute (0.45%) saline has been used where the serum sodium level is above 160 mmol/L. However, recent data indicate that in most cases the use of physiological (0.9%) saline is sufficient. The insulin dose requirements are usually lower than in DKA. There is also an increased risk of thromboembolism and prophylactic heparin is recommended.

Lactic acidosis

Diagnosis
Type I lactic acidosis occurs in hypoxic subjects and is due to an excessive production of lactate by peripheral tissues. Hypoxia is not a feature of type II lactic acidosis, which is probably caused by the impaired metabolism of lactate in the liver. Both are characterized by an extreme metabolic acidosis ([H$^+$] above 100 nmol/L). There is a high anion gap with low or absent ketones, and high blood lactate concentrations.

Treatment
Large amounts of intravenous sodium bicarbonate may be required to correct the acidosis. Alternatively the patient may be dialysed against a bicarbonate-containing solution.

Clinical note
Always screen for infections in the diabetic patient presenting with DKA, as this is a common precipitating factor. Blood, urine, sputum and any wound fluids should be sent for culture at the earliest opportunity and certainly before antibiotics are introduced.

Diabetic ketoacidosis

- Diabetic ketoacidosis arises from a number of metabolic problems caused by insulin lack.
- Treatment is by intravenous fluids, insulin and potassium.
- Only in the most severe cases of DKA should sodium bicarbonate be used.
- Close clinical and biochemical monitoring are required to tailor the management protocol to the individual patient.
- Other, much less common, severe metabolic disturbances of carbohydrate metabolism are hyperosmolar non-ketotic coma and lactic acidosis.

Hypoglycaemia

Hypoglycaemia is defined as a low blood glucose concentration. In general, children and adults are not usually symptomatic unless the glucose falls below 2.2 mmol/L. Assessment of hypoglycaemia depends critically on the age of the patient on whether it occurs in the fasting or postprandial state, and on whether the patient has diabetes or not. A detailed drug history is important, and should include over-the-counter and alternative preparations as well as prescribed medications.

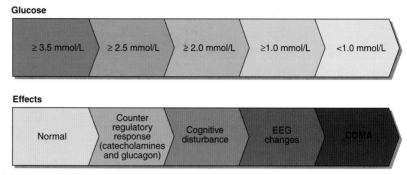

Fig. 1 **The clinical effects of hypoglycaemia.**

Clinical effects

Hypoglycaemia normally leads to suppression of insulin secretion, an increase in catecholamine secretion and stimulation of glucagon, cortisol and growth hormone. The catecholamine surge accounts for the signs and symptoms most commonly seen in hypoglycaemia, i.e. sweating, shaking, tachycardia as well as feeling weak, jittery and nauseated. Hypoglycaemia decreases the glucose fuel supply to the brain and symptoms of cognitive impairment must always be sought since they reflect neuroglycopenia. They include confusion, poor concentration, detachment and, in more severe instances, convulsions and coma. The clinical effects of hypo-glycaemia are summarized in Figure 1.

Assessment

The diagnosis of hypoglycaemia is established when three criteria ('Whipple's triad') are satisfied.

- There must be symptoms consistent with hypoglycaemia.
- There must be laboratory confirmation of hypoglycaemia.
- Symptoms must be relieved by the administration of glucose.

As a preliminary step to formal assessment, patients may be supplied with blood spot strips and asked to take fingerprick blood samples during symptomatic episodes. It may be necessary to try to precipitate symptoms, e.g. by prolonged fasting. If a blood sample is being collected for glucose analysis during a symptomatic episode, *an additional sample should be collected*

simultaneously for insulin. This need not be analysed at the time, or indeed at all unless hypoglycaemia is confirmed, but the insulin level critically alters the differential diagnosis of hypoglycaemia (Figs 2 and 3).

Specific causes of hypoglycaemia

Causes of hypoglycaemia may be divided into two groups: those which usually produce hypoglycaemia in the *fasting* patient, and those in which the low glucose is a response to a stimulus (*reactive* hypoglycaemia).

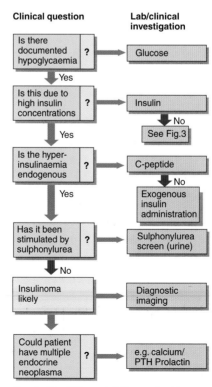

Fig. 2 **The differential diagnosis of hypo-glycaemia in the presence of high insulin levels.**

Fasting hypoglycaemia

Causes of fasting hypoglycaemia include:

- *Insulinoma.* These insulin-producing β-cell tumours of the pancreas may be isolated or part of the wider multiple endocrine neoplasia (MEN) syndrome (see pp. 140–141). Insulin-induced weight gain is a characteristic feature. Localization of the tumour may be difficult.
- *Malignancy.* Hypoglycaemia may be found with any advanced malignancy. Some tumours, e.g. retroperitoneal sarcomas, cause hypoglycaemia by producing insulin-like growth factors.

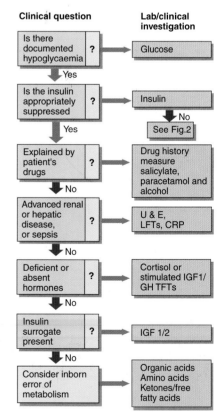

Fig. 3 **The differential diagnosis of hypo-glycaemia in the absence of high insulin levels.**

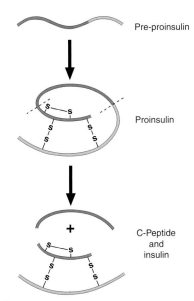

Pre-proinsulin

Proinsulin

C-Peptide and insulin

Fig. 4 **Insulin and C-peptide.**

- *Hepatic and renal disease.* Both the liver and kidneys are capable of gluconeogenesis. Hypoglycaemia is occasionally a feature of advanced hepatic or renal impairment, but this is not usually a diagnostic dilemma.
- *Addison's disease.* Given the fact that glucocorticoids antagonize the actions of insulin, it should not be surprising that hypoglycaemia is occasionally a feature of adrenal insufficiency.
- *Sepsis.* Overwhelming sepsis may be associated with hypoglycaemia; the mechanism is unclear.

Reactive hypoglycaemia

- *Insulin-induced.* Inappropriate or excessive insulin predictably produces hypoglycaemia. Occasionally it is important to distinguish between exogenous insulin (administered by the patient or someone else) and endogenous insulin. Standard assays for insulin cannot distinguish between the two kinds. However, insulin and its associated connecting peptide (or C-peptide) are secreted by the islet cells in equimolar amounts, and thus measurement of C-peptide along with insulin can differentiate between hypoglycaemia due, for example, to an insulinoma (high C-peptide) and that due to exogenous insulin (low C-peptide) (Fig. 4).
- *Drug-induced.* Oral hypoglycaemics, e.g. sulphonylureas, can produce hypoglycaemia. Urinary screens for sulphonylureas exist. Other drugs that occasionally give rise to hypoglycaemia less predictably include salicylate, paracetamol and β-blockers.

- *Alcohol.* Hypoglycaemia is not uncommon in alcoholic patients. Mechanisms include inhibition of gluconeogenesis, malnutrition and liver disease.
- *'Dumping syndrome'.* Accelerated gastric emptying following gastric resection may result in the rapid absorption of large amounts of glucose with a resultant surge of insulin release. Smaller, more frequent meals may help to minimize this phenomenon.

Diabetic patients

In diabetic patients, hypoglycaemia is rarely a diagnostic dilemma. Precipitating factors include:

- insufficient carbohydrate intake
- excess of insulin or sulphonylurea
- strenuous exercise
- excessive alcohol intake.

Neonatal hypoglycaemia

Certain groups of neonates are especially vulnerable to hypoglycaemia:

- *Small for gestational age infants.* Depleted glycogen stores and impaired gluconeogenesis contribute.
- *Babies of diabetic mothers.* A fetus that is exposed to maternal hyperglycaemia will develop hyperplasia of the islet cells and associated hyperinsulinaemia. After delivery, the neonate is unable to suppress its high insulin levels that are now inappropriate, and hypoglycaemia results.
- *Nesidioblastosis.* Hyperplasia of the islet cells may develop even when the mother is not diabetic; the reasons are unclear.
- *Inborn errors of metabolism.* Many inborn errors are associated with hypoglycaemia. Glycogen storage diseases and galactosaemia are the best examples.

> ### Clinical note
> The use of 50% dextrose as an intravenous bolus has remarkable effects in reversing the signs and symptoms of hypoglycaemia. This solution is like syrup and may cause thrombophlebitis. Care must also be taken not to cause extravasation.

Case history 26

A 25-year-old woman with IDDM complained of repeated episodes of sleep disturbances, night sweats and vivid, unpleasant dreams.

- What is the most likely cause of this woman's symptoms and how might the diagnosis be confirmed?

Comment on page 165.

Hypoglycaemia

- Hypoglycaemia is not a diagnosis but is a biochemical sign associated with a diverse group of diseases.
- Management is by glucose therapy irrespective of the underlying cause.
- Excess insulin, excess alcohol or low calorie intake in a diabetic patient are the most common causes of hypoglycaemia.
- Insulinoma is characterized by hypoglycaemia in the face of inappropriately high plasma insulin.
- Hypoglycaemia in the neonate may result in brain damage.

Calcium regulation and hypocalcaemia

Calcium homeostasis

The amount of calcium present in the extracellular fluid is very small in comparison to that stored in bone. Even in the adult, calcium in bone is not static; some bone is resorbed each day and the calcium returned to the ECF. To maintain calcium balance, an equal amount of bone formation must take place. Figure 1 shows how much calcium is exchanged between one compartment and another daily.

Calcium homeostasis is modulated by hormones (Fig. 2). Parathyroid hormone (PTH), which consists of 84 amino acids, is secreted from the parathyroid glands in response to a low unbound plasma calcium. PTH causes bone resorption and promotes calcium reabsorption in the renal tubules, preventing loss in the urine. 1,25-Dihydroxycholecalciferol (1,25 DHCC) maintains intestinal calcium absorption. This sterol hormone is formed from vitamin D (cholecalciferol), following hydroxylation in the liver (at carbon-25) and kidney (at carbon-1). However, hydroxylation in the kidney is PTH dependent, and so even the absorption of calcium from the gut relies (albeit indirectly) on PTH.

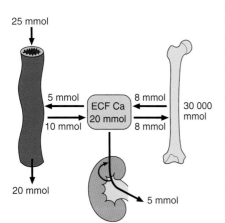

Fig. 1 **Normal calcium balance.** Calcium is exchanged each day, in the amounts shown, between the extracellular fluid and the gut, bone and kidney.

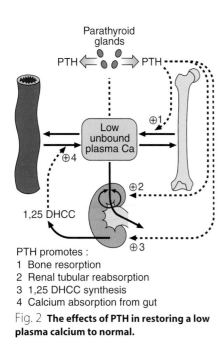

Parathyroid glands

PTH promotes :
1 Bone resorption
2 Renal tubular reabsorption
3 1,25 DHCC synthesis
4 Calcium absorption from gut

Fig. 2 **The effects of PTH in restoring a low plasma calcium to normal.**

Serum calcium

A healthy person has a total serum calcium of around 2.4 mmol/L. About half is bound to protein, mostly to albumin. Binding is pH dependent and is decreased in acidosis, because the amino acid side chains on albumin become more positively charged. Conversely, binding is increased if an alkalosis is present. Hence, the percentage of unbound calcium increases in acidosis and decreases if there is an alkalosis.

Unbound calcium is the biologically active fraction of the total calcium in plasma and maintenance of its concentration within tight limits is required for nerve function, membrane permeability, muscle contraction and glandular secretion. It is the unbound calcium concentration that is recognized by the parathyroid glands, and PTH acts to keep this concentration constant.

Laboratories routinely measure total calcium concentration (that is both the bound and unbound fractions) in a serum sample. However, this may give rise to problems in the interpretation of results because changes in serum albumin concentration cause changes in total calcium concentration. If albumin concentration falls, total serum calcium is low because the bound fraction is decreased (Fig. 3). Remember that the homeostatic mechanisms for regulating plasma calcium respond to the unbound fraction, not to the total calcium. Patients with a low albumin have total serum calcium lower than the reference values, yet have normal unbound calcium. *These patients should not be thought of as hypocalcaemic.*

In order to circumvent this problem and to ensure that patients with a low albumin are not mistakenly labelled as hypocalcaemic, clinical biochemists use the convention of the 'adjusted calcium'. Most laboratories measure both total calcium and albumin, and, if the albumin is abnormal, calculate what the total calcium would have been if the albumin had been normal. One such calculation is:

Adjusted calcium (mmol/L) = Total measured calcium + 0.02(47 − albumin)

Hypocalcaemia

Aetiology

The causes of hypocalcaemia include:

- *Hypoparathyroidism.*
- *Magnesium deficiency.* This is the commonest cause in hospital patients.
- *Vitamin D deficiency.* This may be due to malabsorption, or an inadequate diet with little exposure to sunlight. It may lead to the bone disorders, osteomalacia in adults and rickets in children (see pp. 74–75).
- *Renal disease.* The diseased kidneys fail to synthesize 1,25 DHCC (see pp. 28–29). Increased PTH secretion in response to the hypocalcaemia may lead to bone disease if untreated.
- *Pseudohypoparathyroidism.* PTH is secreted but there is failure of target tissue receptors to respond to the hormone.
- *Rarer causes* such as malignancy, acute rhabdomyolysis, acute pancratitis, ethylene glycol poisoning or bone marrow transplantation.

Clinical features

The clinical features of hypocalcaemia include: neurological features such as tingling, tetany, and mental changes; cardiovascular signs such as an abnormal ECG and cataracts.

A strategy for the investigation and differential diagnosis of hypocalcaemia is shown in Figure 4.

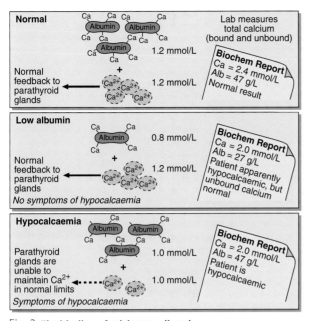

Fig. 3 **The binding of calcium to albumin.**

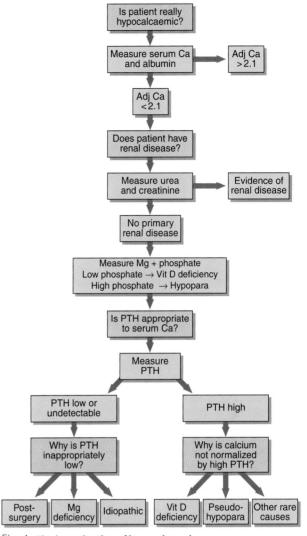

Fig. 4 **The investigation of hypocalcaemia.**

Treatment

The management calls for the treatment of the cause of the hypocalcaemia, if this is possible. Oral calcium supplements are commonly prescribed in mild disorders. 1,25 DHCC, or the synthetic vitamin D metabolite 1α-hydroxycholecalciferol, can be given.

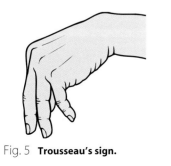

Clinical note

Trousseau's sign is the most reliable indication of latent tetany. A sphygmomanometer cuff is inflated to above systolic pressure for at least 2 minutes while observing the hand. A positive response will be the appearance of typical carpal spasm, which relaxes some 5 seconds or so after the cuff is released.

Fig. 5 **Trousseau's sign.**

Case history 27

A 70-year-old woman attended her GP complaining of generalized bone pain. Biochemistry results on a serum specimen taken at the surgery showed the following:

Calcium	Phosphate	Albumin	Ca (adj)
	— mmol/L —	g/L	mmol/L
1.80	1.1	39	1.96

■ What further investigations would be appropriate?

Comment on page 165.

Calcium regulation and hypocalcaemia

■ 'Adjusted calcium' should be used to avoid the problems of interpreting the total calcium concentration in patients who have abnormal serum albumin concentrations.

■ If a hypocalcaemic patient has low or undetectable PTH in serum, he/she is hypoparathyroid.

■ If PTH concentrations are appropriately elevated to the low calcium, then the reason for the hypocalcaemia is most likely to be vitamin D deficiency.

■ Patients with chronic renal failure often have hypocalcaemia due to the inability of renal cells to synthesize 1,25-dihydroxycholecalciferol. Secondary hyperparathyroidism and bone disease may result.

Hypercalcaemia

Patients today are unlikely to present with gross bone disease or severe renal calculi as a consequence of untreated primary hyperparathyroidism. General practitioners who are aware of the telltale signs and symptoms of hypercalcaemia can identify this disorder before gross bone abnormalities or renal problems have had time to develop. The widespread use of multichannel analysers in clinical biochemistry laboratories can detect unsuspected hypercalcaemia even before symptoms become apparent. A high serum calcium concentration may be an unexpected finding in a patient in any clinic or hospital ward, as the symptoms of hypercalcaemia are non-specific. All such findings should be followed up.

Clinical features

Symptoms of hypercalcaemia include:

- neurological and psychiatric features such as lethargy, confusion, irritability and depression
- gastrointestinal problems such as anorexia, abdominal pain, nausea and vomiting, and constipation
- renal features such as thirst and polyuria, and renal calculi
- cardiac arrhythmias.

Diagnosis

The commonest causes of hypercalcaemia are primary hyperparathyroidism and hypercalcaemia of malignancy.

A diagnostic decision chart is shown in Figure 1. *Primary hyperparathyroidism* is most often due to a single parathyroid adenoma, which secretes PTH independently of feedback control by plasma calcium. *Hypercalcaemia associated with malignancy* is the commonest cause of a high calcium in a hospital population. Some tumours secrete a protein called PTHrP (parathyroid hormone-related protein), which has PTH-like properties.

Rarer causes of hypercalcaemia include:

- *Inappropriate dosage of vitamin D or metabolites*, e.g. in the treatment of hypoparathyroidism or renal disease or due to self-medication.
- *Granulomatous diseases* (such as sarcoidosis or tuberculosis) or certain tumours (such as lymphomas) synthesize 1,25-dihydroxycholecalciferol.
- *Thyrotoxicosis* very occasionally leads to increased bone turnover and hypercalcaemia.
- *Diuretic therapy*: the hypercalcaemia is usually mild.
- *Immobilization*: especially in young people and patients with Paget's disease.
- *Renal disease.* Long-standing secondary hyperparathyroidism may lead to PTH secretion becoming independent of calcium feedback. This is termed tertiary hyperparathyroidism.
- *Calcium therapy.* Patients are routinely given calcium-containing solutions during cardiac surgery, and may have transient hypercalcaemia afterwards.
- *Diuretic phase of acute renal failure or in the recovery from severe rhabdomyolysis.*
- *Milk alkali syndrome*: the combination of an increased calcium intake together with bicarbonate, as in a patient self-medicating with proprietary antacid, may cause severe hypercalcaemia, but the condition is very rare.

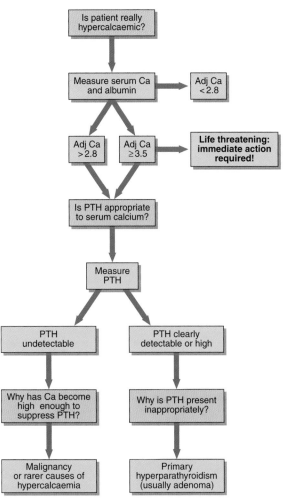

Fig. 1 **Investigation of hypercalcaemia.**

Treatment

Treatment is **urgent** if the adjusted serum calcium is greater than 3.5 mmol/L; the priority is to reduce it to a safe level. Intravenous saline is administered first to restore the glomerular filtration rate and promote a diuresis. Although steroids, mithramycin, calcitonin and intravenous phosphate have been used, compounds known as the bisphosphonates have been found to have the best calcium-lowering effects. Bisphosphonates such as pamidronate have become the treatment of choice in patients with hypercalcaemia of malignancy (Fig. 2). It acts by inhibiting bone resorption.

The cause of the hypercalcaemia should be treated if possible. Surgical removal of a parathyroid adenoma usually provides a complete cure for a patient with primary hyperparathyoidism. Immediately after successful surgery, transient hypocalcaemia may have to be treated with vitamin D metabolites, until the remaining parathyroids begin to operate normally.

Familial hypocalciuric hypercalcaemia

Although a definitive differential diagnosis of hypercalcaemia can often be made, there is one rare condition where a wrong diagnosis can lead to unnecessary surgery. In familial

Serum calcium
(mmol/L)

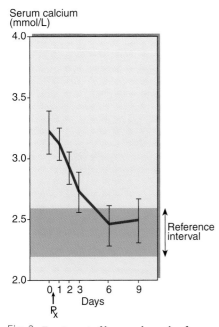

Fig. 2 Treatment of hypercalcaemia of malignancy with pamidronate.
The graph shows the response of serum calcium in 12 patients treated with a single dose of the bisphosphonate pamidronate in 0.9% saline infused over 6 hours, after initial rehydration.

hypocalciuric hypercalcaemia (FHH), a high plasma calcium is sensed by the parathyroids as normal; the patient has normal detectable levels of PTH, despite having hypercalcaemia. There are usually no symptoms of hypercalcaemia, but the patient may be labelled as primary hyperparathyroid, because of the detectable PTH in the face of a high serum calcium. On neck exploration, no parathyroid adenoma is found and it may be discovered subsequently that family members also have asymptomatic hypercalcaemia. Patients with the condition require no treatment; indeed, many would be better off remaining undiagnosed, such is the likelihood of unnecessary surgery.

The hypercalcaemia in FHH may be mild and without symptoms. It is sometimes possible to distinguish this condition from primary hyperparathyroidism on the basis of a urinary calcium excretion, which is inappropriately low for the serum calcium concentration in the patient with FHH. However, in practice, the urinary calcium excretion reference values in both conditions overlap. The possibility of FHH must always be considered when investigating the cause of asymptomatic hypercalcaemia in a relatively young patient.

Case history 28

A 48-year-old woman came to her GP with a 12-month history of increasing tiredness and muscle fatigue. In recent weeks she had been increasingly thirsty and had polyuria. Her GP tested a urine sample for glucose, which he found to be negative, and then arranged that her urea and electrolytes be measured. He decided to request a calcium profile on the serum sample as well.

Biochemistry results in a serum specimen were:

Na$^+$	K$^+$	Cl$^-$	HCO$_3^-$	Urea	Creatinine
		mmol/L			μmol/L
149	3.5	109	20	7.5	160

Calcium	Phosphate		Albumin	Ca (adj)
mmol/L	mmol/L		g/L	mmol/L
3.30	0.51		35	3.54

- What are the most likely diagnoses in this patient?
- What other investigations would be appropriate?

Comment on page 165.

Clinical note

If hypercalcaemia is not detected early, the high circulating PTH causes a characteristic pattern of bone resorption, known as osteitis fibrosa cystica (shown in Figure 3). As awareness of hypercalcaemia has grown and detection methods have improved, such severe bone abnormalities are seen much less frequently.

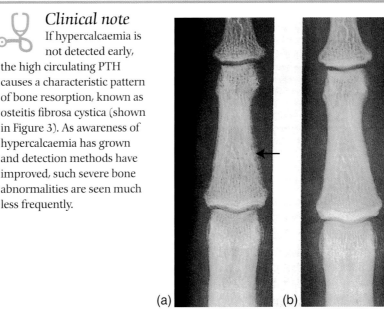

(a) (b)

Fig. 3 Classic subperiosteal resorption in a patient with severe primary hyperparathyroidism.
(a) Radiograph shows resorption in the phalanges. **(b)** Same finger 5 months after removal of parathyroid adenoma.

Hypercalcaemia

- Consideration of both serum calcium and albumin concentrations, as an 'adjusted' calcium, will give a correct assessment of the severity of the hypercalcaemia.

- Hypercalcaemia will most likely be due to the presence of a parathyroid adenoma, or will be associated with a malignancy. In the former, serum PTH will be high or inappropriately detectable, whereas in hypercalcaemia of malignancy the high calcium suppresses parathyroid function and serum PTH is undetectable.

- Serum calcium in excess of 3.5 mmol/L is life-threatening.

- Bisphosphonates such as pamidronate have the ability to reduce serum calcium rapidly by inhibiting bone resorption.

Phosphate and magnesium

Phosphate

Phosphate is abundant in the body and is an important intracellular and extracellular anion. Much of the phosphate inside cells is covalently attached to lipids and proteins. Phosphorylation and dephosphorylation of enzymes are important mechanisms in the regulation of metabolic activity. Most of the body's phosphate is in bone (Fig. 1). Phosphate changes accompany calcium deposition or resorption of bone. Control of ECF phosphate concentration is achieved by the kidney, where tubular reabsorption is reduced by PTH. The phosphate that is not reabsorbed in the renal tubule acts as an important urinary buffer.

Plasma inorganic phosphate

At physiological hydrogen ion concentrations, phosphate exists in the ECF both as monohydrogen phosphate and as dihydrogen phosphate. Both forms are together termed 'phosphate', and the total is normally maintained within the limits 0.80–1.40 mmol/L. Sometimes the term 'inorganic phosphate' is used to distinguish these forms from organically bound phosphate such as in ATP. Approximately 20% of plasma phosphate is attached to protein, although in contrast to the binding of calcium, this is of little significance.

In plasma, calcium and phosphate often have a reciprocal relationship. In particular, if phosphate rises, calcium falls.

Hyperphosphataemia

Persistent hyperphosphataemia may result in calcium phosphate deposition in soft tissues. Causes of a high serum phosphate concentration include:

- *Renal failure.* Phosphate excretion is impaired. This is the commonest cause of hyperphosphataemia.
- *Hypoparathyroidism.* The effect of a low circulating PTH decreases phosphate excretion by the kidneys, and this contributes to a high serum concentration.
- *Redistribution.* Cell damage (lysis), e.g. haemolysis, tumour damage and rhabdomyolysis.
- *Pseudohypoparathyroidism.* There is tissue resistance to PTH.

Hypophosphataemia

Severe hypophosphataemia (<0.3 mmol/L) is rare and causes muscle weakness, which may lead to respiratory impairment. The symptomatic disorder requires immediate intravenous infusion of phosphate. Modest hypophosphataemia is much more common. Alcoholic patients are especially prone to hypophosphataemia.

Causes of a low serum phosphate include:

- *Hyperparathyroidism.* The effect of a high PTH is to increase phosphate excretion by the kidneys and this contributes to a low serum concentration.
- *Treatment of diabetic ketoacidosis.* The effect of insulin in causing the shift of glucose into cells may cause similar shifts of phosphate, which may result in hypophosphataemia.

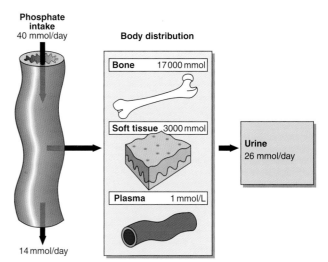

Fig. 1 **Normal phosphate balance.**

- *Alkalosis, especially respiratory due to movement of phosphate into cells.*
- *Refeeding syndrome.* Hypophosphataemia is frequently encountered when malnourished patients are first fed, due to movement of phosphate into cells.
- *Oncogenic hypophosphataemia (hungry bone syndrome).* This is a rare cause of severe hypophosphataemia, and the causative factor produced by the tumour remains to be identified.
- *Ingestion of non-absorbable antacids, such as aluminium hydroxide.* These prevent phosphate absorption.
- *Congenital defects of tubular phosphate reabsorption.* In these conditions phosphate is lost from the body.

Magnesium

Although the biological and biochemical importance of magnesium ions (Mg^{2+}) is well understood, the role of this cation in clinical medicine is sometimes overlooked. Magnesium ions are the second most abundant intracellular cations, after potassium. Some 300 enzyme systems are magnesium activated, and most aspects of intracellular biochemistry are magnesium dependent, including glycolysis, oxidative metabolism and transmembrane transport of potassium and calcium.

As well as these intracellular functions, the electrical properties of cell membranes are affected by any reduction in the *extracellular* magnesium concentration. Any detailed consideration of magnesium biochemistry has to take into account the interactions between Mg^{2+}, K^+ and Ca^{2+} ions.

Magnesium influences the secretion of PTH by the parathyroid glands, and severe hypomagnesaemia may cause hypoparathyroidism.

Magnesium homeostasis

Since magnesium is an integral part of chlorophyll, green vegetables are an important dietary source, as are cereals and animal meats. An average dietary intake is around 15 mmol per day which generally meets the recommended dietary

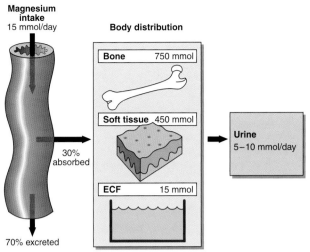

Magnesium
intake
15 mmol/day

Body distribution

Bone 750 mmol

Soft tissue 450 mmol

ECF 15 mmol

Urine
5–10 mmol/day

30% absorbed

70% excreted

Fig. 2 **Normal magnesium balance.**

intake. Children and pregnant or lactating women have higher requirements. About 30% of the dietary magnesium is absorbed from the small intestine and widely distributed to all metabolically active tissue (Fig. 2).

Serum magnesium

Hypermagnesaemia is uncommon but is occasionally seen in renal failure. Hypomagnesaemia is usually associated with magnesium deficiency. The symptoms of hypomagnesaemia are very similar to those of hypocalcaemia: impaired neuromuscular function such as tetany, hyperirritability, tremor convulsions and muscle weakness.

Magnesium deficiency

Since magnesium is present in most common foodstuffs, low dietary intakes of magnesium are associated with general nutritional insufficiency. Symptomatic magnesium deficiency can be expected as a result of:

- dietary insufficiency accompanied by intestinal malabsorption, severe vomiting, diarrhoea or other causes of intestinal loss
- osmotic diuresis such as occurs in diabetes mellitus
- prolonged use of diuretic therapy especially when dietary intake has been marginal
- prolonged nasogastric suction
- cytotoxic drug therapy such as cisplatin, which impairs renal tubular reabsorption of magnesium
- treatment with the immunosuppressant drug ciclosporin.

Laboratory diagnosis

The repeated demonstration of a magnesium concentration of less than 0.7 mmol/L in a serum specimen is evidence of marked intracellular depletion and of a clinical condition that may benefit from magnesium therapy. However, intracellular magnesium depletion may exist where the serum magnesium concentration is within the reference interval. Research procedures are required to detect these marginal states. These include the use of NMR spectroscopy to detect 'free' Mg^{2+} inside cells, and direct determination of Mg^{2+} in peripheral white blood cells, or in muscle biopsy samples.

Management

The provision of magnesium supplements in oral diets is complicated by the fact that they often cause diarrhoea. Indeed oral magnesium salts are often given as laxatives for this reason. A variety of oral, intramuscular and intravenous regimens have been proposed. Administration of magnesium salts, by whatever route, is contraindicated when there is a significant degree of renal impairment. In these circumstances any supplementation must be monitored carefully to avoid toxic effects associated with hypermagnesaemia.

Clinical note
Intravenous magnesium is the treatment of choice in severe pre-eclampsia to prevent convulsion and lower the blood pressure.

Case history 29

A 46-year-old woman, known to have radiation enteritis with chronic diarrhoea and associated malabsorption syndrome, presented to the outpatient department complaining of severe tingling of recent onset in her hands and feet. The patient had a past history of hypocalcaemic tetany 18 months previously, but serum calcium had since remained normal on therapy with 1α-hydroxycholecalciferol, 0.75 µg daily, plus oral calcium supplements.

Calcium	Phosphate	Albumin	Calcium (adj)	Alk phos	Magnesium
——— mmol/L ———		g/L	mmol/L	U/L	mmol/L
1.30	1.1	39	1.46	110	0.25

The patient did not respond to treatment with increased calcium supplements and continued 1α-hydroxycholecalciferol.

- What would you predict the patient's PTH status to be?
- What treatment is appropriate and why?

Comment on page 165.

Phosphate and magnesium

- Hyperphosphataemia is commonly a consequence of renal impairment.
- Hypophosphataemia may be due to the effects of a high circulating parathyroid hormone concentration, or to redistribution into cells.
- Magnesium deficiency results from a combination of poor dietary intake and increased urinary or intestinal losses.
- Magnesium deficiency may occur as a complication of intestinal disease or surgery, renal damage by nephrotoxins, diuretics or in diabetes.
- The demonstration of a low serum magnesium suggests severe deficiency, whereas marginal magnesium deficiency states may be present even when magnesium is within reference limits.

Bone disease

The finding that a patient has hypercalcaemia or hypocalcaemia does not imply that there will be marked bone changes. Conversely, severe bone disease can occur whilst serum calcium levels appear quite normal. The main bone diseases are:

- osteoporosis
- osteomalacia and rickets
- Paget's disease.

Bone metabolism

Bone is constantly being broken down and reformed in the process of bone remodelling (Fig. 1). The clinician looking after patients with bone disease will certainly need to know to what extent bone is being broken down, and, indeed, if new bone is being made. Biochemical markers of bone resorption and bone formation can be useful in assessing the extent of disease, as well as monitoring treatment.

Hydroxyproline, from the breakdown of collagen, can be used to monitor bone resorption. However, urinary hydroxyproline is markedly influenced by dietary gelatin. Better markers of resorption are required. One candidate would seem to be another collagen degradation product: the fragments of the molecule containing the pyridinium cross-links. Deoxypyridinoline is one such cross-link that is specific for bone, and not metabolized or influenced by diet.

The activity of the enzyme alkaline phosphatase has traditionally been used as an indicator of bone turnover. The osteoblasts that lay down the collagen framework and the mineral matrix of bone have high activity of this enzyme. Increased osteoblastic activity is indicated by an elevated alkaline phosphatase activity in a serum specimen. Indeed, children who have active bone growth compared with adults have higher 'normal' alkaline phosphatase activity in serum. However, alkaline phosphatase is also produced by the cells lining the bile canaliculi and is a marker for cholestasis. The bone isoenzyme of alkaline phosphatase may be measured, but there is need for a more specific and more sensitive marker.

Osteocalcin meets some of these requirements. It is synthesized by osteoblasts and is an important non-collagenous constituent of bone. Not all of the osteocalcin that an osteoblast makes is incorporated into the bone matrix. Some is released into plasma, and provides a

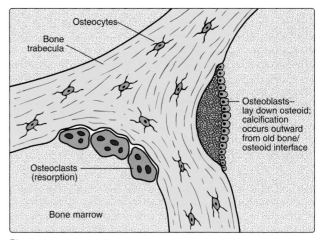

Fig. 1 **Bone remodelling.**

sensitive indicator of osteoblast activity. The test is available in specialized laboratories.

Common bone disorders

Osteoporosis

Osteoporosis is the commonest of bone disorders and is discussed separately on page 76.

Osteomalacia and rickets

Osteomalacia is the name given to defective bone mineralization in adults (Fig. 2). Rickets is characterized by defects of bone and cartilage mineralization in children. Vitamin D deficiency was once the most common reason for rickets and osteomalacia, but the addition of vitamin D to foodstuffs has almost eliminated the condition except in the elderly or house-bound, the institutionalized, and in certain ethnic groups. Elderly Asian women with a predominantly vegetarian diet are particularly at risk. Vitamin D status can be assessed by measurement of the main circulating metabolite, 25-hydroxycholecalciferol, in a serum specimen. The metabolism of vitamin D is shown in Figure 3.

In severe osteomalacia due to vitamin D deficiency, serum calcium will fall, and there will be an appropriate increase in PTH secretion. Serum alkaline phosphatase activity will also be elevated.

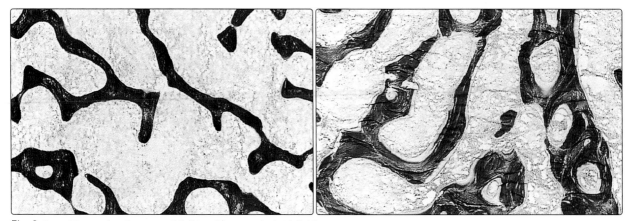

Fig. 2 **Bone biopsy showing normal (left) and osteomalacic (right) bone.**

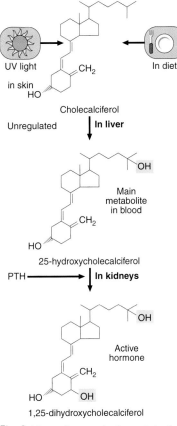

Fig. 3 **The main steps in the metabolism of vitamin D.**

The bony features of osteomalacia and rickets are also shared by other bone diseases (see later).

Paget's disease

Paget's disease is common and characterized by increased osteoclastic activity, which leads to increased bone resorption. Increased osteoblastic activity repairs resorbed bone, but the new bone is laid down in a disorganized way. The clinical presentation is almost always bone pain, which can be particularly severe. Serum alkaline phosphatase is high, and urinary hydroxyproline excretion is elevated. These provide a way of monitoring the progress of the disease. Although a viral cause for Paget's disease has been proposed, the aetiology remains obscure.

Other bone diseases

Examples include:

- *Vitamin-D-dependent rickets, types 1 and 2.* These are rare bone diseases resulting from genetic disorders leading to the inability to make the active vitamin D metabolite, or from receptor defects that do not allow the hormone to act.

- *Tumoral calcinosis.* This is characterized by ectopic calcification around the joints.
- *Hypophosphatasia.* This is a form of rickets or osteomalacia that results from a deficiency of alkaline phosphatase.
- *Hypophosphataemic rickets.* This is believed to be a consequence of a renal tubular defect in phosphate handling.
- *Osteopetrosis.* This condition is characterized by defective bone resorption.
- *Osteogenesis imperfecta.* Brittle bone syndrome is an inherited disorder which occurs around once in every 20 000 births.

Diagnosis of these and other rare conditions may require help from specialized laboratories.

Biochemistry testing in calcium disorders or bone disease

The role of the routine biochemistry laboratory in diagnosis and treatment of patients with calcium disorders and bone disease is to provide measurements of calcium, albumin, phosphate and alkaline phosphate in a serum specimen as first line tests. Follow-up tests that may be requested include:

- PTH
- magnesium
- urine calcium excretion
- 25-hydroxycholecalciferol
- urine hydroxyproline excretion
- osteocalcin.

Characteristic biochemistry profiles in some common bone diseases are shown in Table 1.

Case history 30

A 66-year-old man presented to the bone clinic with severe pains in his right leg and pelvis. Radiological examination revealed pagetic lesions in his legs, pelvis and also his skull. Biochemical results in a serum sample were unremarkable except for alkaline phosphatase which was grossly elevated at 2700 U/L. It was decided to treat him with a bisphosphonate drug.

- How would you monitor this patient's response?

Comment on page 165.

Table 1 **Biochemical profiles in bone diseases**

Disease	Profile
Bone metastases	Calcium may be high, low or normal
	Phosphate may be high, low or normal
	PTH is usually low
	Alkaline phosphatase may be elevated or normal
Osteomalacia/Rickets	Calcium will tend to be low, or may be clearly decreased
	PTH will be elevated
	25-hydroxycholecalciferol will be decreased if the disease is due to vitamin D deficiency
Paget's disease	Calcium is normal
	Alkaline phosphatase is grossly elevated
Osteoporosis	Biochemistry is unremarkable
Renal osteodystrophy	Calcium is decreased
	PTH is very high
Osteitis fibrosa cystica (primary hyperparathyroidism)	Calcium is elevated
	Phosphate is low or normal
	PTH is increased, or clearly detectable and thus 'inappropriate' to the hypercalcaemia

---

Bone disease

- Alkaline phosphatase is a marker for bone formation. Urinary hydroxyproline is a marker for bone resorption. Better markers for bone turnover are being evaluated.

- Osteomalacia due to vitamin D deficiency can be confirmed by finding a low 25-hydroxycholecalciferol concentration. In severe disease, alkaline phosphatase will be increased. Calcium may well fall and there will be an appropriate rise in PTH.

- The characteristic biochemical marker of Paget's disease is a grossly increased alkaline phosphatase activity, as a consequence of increased bone turnover.

Osteoporosis

Osteoporosis is a major public health problem. One in four women and one in twenty men over the age of 60 in Britain will have an osteoporosis-related fracture. It is a major cause of morbidity and mortality in the elderly.

Osteoporosis is characterized by a reduction in bone mass per unit volume. The composition of the matrix is essentially normal, but there is just less of it. The cortical areas of bones are thinner than normal and the trabeculae are smaller and less extensive (Fig. 1). Both sexes show a gradual bone loss throughout life but women lose bone rapidly in the postmenopausal years. This is called primary osteoporosis and is of unknown aetiology.

Accelerated bone loss leading to secondary osteoporosis may be caused by:

- certain drugs, especially long-term use of corticosteroids or heparin
- immobilization
- smoking
- alcohol
- Cushing's syndrome
- gonadal failure
- hyperthyroidism
- gastrointestinal disease.

Diagnosis

Serial measurements of bone density are required to demonstrate bone loss but frequently on presentation the diagnosis

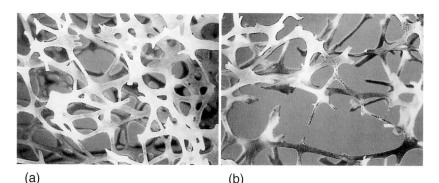

(a)   (b)

Fig. 1 **Bone showing (a) normal trabeculae and (b) bone loss in osteoporosis.**

can be made from a single measurement. It may take months or years to quantify the rate of bone loss with confidence.

For many patients the first indication of the disease is when they suffer a vertebral compression fracture, a fracture of the distal radius or a fractured neck of femur. Crush fractures of vertebrae may occur slowly and relatively painlessly over a period of time (Figs 2 and 3).

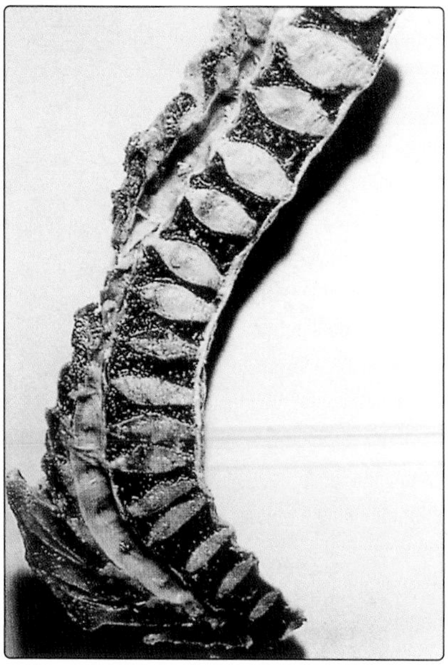

The role of the clinical biochemistry laboratory

Biochemical tests cannot be used to diagnose primary osteoporosis or monitor accelerated bone loss because the results of the common biochemical analyses overlap in healthy subjects and patients with the disorder. However, biochemical tests are of value in the diagnosis of hyperthyroidism, gonadal failure or

Cushing's syndrome, which cause secondary osteoporosis.

Markers of bone turnover are increasingly being evaluated for their role in the diagnosis and management of osteoporosis.

Treatment

Prevention, rather than cure, is the current goal. This should start in childhood with a good diet and exercise. The most powerful predictor of osteoporosis is the skeletal mass at 16 years of age.

Once skeletal maturity has been attained, it is the magnitude of the subsequent bone loss that may lead to osteoporosis. Stopping smoking is important. At the menopause, hormone replacement therapy is of benefit, not only for the relief of menopausal symptoms but also to prevent rapid bone loss.

When osteoporosis is established, the treatment options are as yet unsatisfactory. Oral calcium supplements, oestrogens and fluoride have all been advocated. Bisphosphonates may be beneficial.

Osteoporosis

- Osteoporosis is a major cause of morbidity and mortality in the elderly.

- It is characterized by a reduction in bone mass per unit volume.

- Although both sexes show a gradual bone loss throughout life, women lose bone rapidly in the postmenopausal years. This 'primary osteoporosis' is of unknown aetiology.

- Bone loss causing secondary osteoporosis may be accelerated by a number of factors such as the use of corticosteroids, smoking and immobilization.

Fig. 2 **Crush fractures of vertebral bodies in a patient with osteoporosis.**

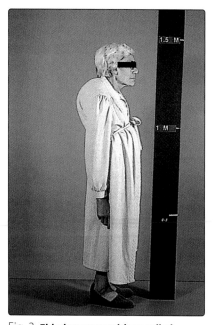

Fig. 3 **Elderly woman with so-called 'Dowager's hump' from collapsed vertebrae due to osteoporosis.**

Endocrinology

Endocrine control

Biochemical regulators

Homeostasis, the tendency to maintain stability, is essential to survival. It is achieved by a system of control mechanisms. Endocrine control is achieved by biochemical regulators. Some of these are hormones, i.e. they are released from specialized glands into the blood to influence the activity of cells and tissues at distant sites. Others are paracrine factors, which are not released into the circulation, but which act on adjacent cells, e.g. in the regulation of the immune system. Finally, autocrine factors act on the very cells responsible for their synthesis. These different kinds of regulation are illustrated in Figure 1.

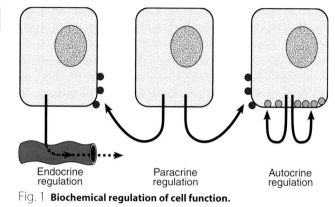

Endocrine regulation   Paracrine regulation   Autocrine regulation

Fig. 1 **Biochemical regulation of cell function.**

Hormone structure

The diverse biological effects of different hormones are reflected in different molecular structures.

Three broad classes are recognized:

- *Peptides or proteins.* Most hormones fall into this class, although they vary enormously in size. For example, the hypothalamic factor thyrotrophin-releasing hormone has just three amino acids, whilst the pituitary gonadotrophins are large glycoproteins with subunits.
- *Amino acid derivatives.* Examples include the thyroid hormones and adrenaline (epinephrine).
- *Steroid hormones.* This large class of hormones includes glucocorticoids and sex steroid hormones, all of which are derived structurally from cholesterol.

Assessment of endocrine control

Many endocrine diseases arise from failure of control mechanisms (Table 1). Assessment of endocrine control presents particular difficulties.

- *Low concentrations.* Hormone concentrations in blood are some-times so low that they are at or below the lower limit of analytical detection. In the past, it was often the biological response to hormones that formed the basis of relatively crude bioassays of hormone activity. The advent of immunoassays in the 1960s revolutionized endocrinology by permitting the measurement of hormones that had previously been well below the limits of detection. However, despite the refinement of

immunoassay technology by, for example, the introduction of monoclonal antibodies, measurement of structurally related hormones continues to be a problem for the clinical biochemistry laboratory, as is immunoassay interference (see below).
- *Variability.* Even where it is possible to measure the concentration of a hormone accurately, the result of a single measurement may be difficult to interpret. This is because the concentration may vary substantially for various reasons, some of which are illustrated in Figure 2. For example, because growth hormone is released in a pulsatile fashion, an undetectable level is largely meaningless. The marked circadian rhythm of cortisol likewise makes interpretation of a random cortisol measurement on an untimed sample difficult or impossible.
- *Hormone binding.* Steroid and thyroid hormones bind to specific hormone-binding glycoproteins in plasma. It is the unbound or 'free' fraction of the hormone that is biologically active. Failure to measure the binding protein may lead to misinterpretation of hormone results. For example, accurate assessment of androgen status requires measurement of sex hormone-binding globulin (SHBG) in addition to testosterone; from both measurements the free androgen index is calculated.

Types of endocrine control

Negative feedback

The basic operation of a negative feedback loop is shown in Figure 3. It is perhaps easier to understand the

features of such a loop with reference to a particular axis, e.g. thyroid. Hormone A in this axis is thyrotrophin-releasing hormone (TRH), hormone B is thyroid-stimulating hormone (TSH) and hormone C is thyroid hormone (T_4). Like a dial on a thermostat, the hypothalamus sets the point of optimal control for the system by secreting TRH at a certain level; this will correspond to a certain intended concentration of T_4. By means of negative feedback from T_4, the hypothalamus senses any difference between the actual concentration of T_4 and the intended concentration, and readjusts the TRH level (set point) accordingly. This stimulates TSH release from the pituitary in a log-linear fashion, i.e. TSH rises exponentially with increasing TRH, thus permitting an extremely precise degree of control.

Positive feedback

Negative feedback control is ubiquitous in endocrinology, but there is one notable example of positive feedback. During the follicular phase of the menstrual cycle, the release by the hypothalamus of gonadotrophin-releasing hormone (GnRH) fluctuates. Both follicle-stimulating hormone (FSH) and luteinizing hormone (LH) are released in response by the pituitary; the FSH stimulates the developing follicles to produce increasing amounts of oestrogen. At a particular point in the cycle the feedback from oestrogen on LH production switches from being negative to being positive, and the resulting LH surge triggers ovulation. The reasons for this switch are not entirely clear (after all, the hypothalamic-pituitary-ovarian axis normally operates as a negative feedback loop), but positive feedback requires a threshold concentration of

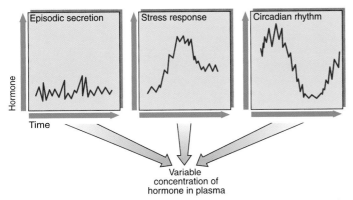

Fig. 2 **Reasons why a single blood hormone measurement may have little clinical value.**

oestradiol (thought to be in the region of 700 pmol/L) to persist for at least 48 hours. The hormonal changes during a normal menstrual cycle are illustrated on page 99.

Pitfalls in interpretation

- *Immunoassay interference.* Up to 40% of the population may have unsuspected antibodies that can interfere with immunoassays, by interacting either with the analyte being measured or with the antibody being used in the immunoassay mixture. These antibodies can produce falsely lowered or falsely raised results, with potentially serious consequences. Crucially, these interferences are specific to the patient's serum, so quality control will not detect the problem. If there is a discrepancy between the clinical and biochemical pictures, or if a result is totally unexpected, this possibility should always be considered. This kind of problem is well recognized for some assays, e.g. thyroglobulin, prolactin.
- *Log-linear responses.* In response to alterations in TRH TSH may rise exponentially. This kind of relationship means that the biological significance of a rise in TSH from 1 to 5 mU/L is the same as a rise from 10 to 50 mU/L. Moreover, this kind of relationship applies to all trophins released by the anterior pituitary, including growth hormone, the trophic hormone for insulin-like growth factors. Interestingly, the (skewed) distribution of serum prolactin behaves in a similar way, as if it too was a trophin like TSH or ACTH, even though, as yet, no prolactin-controlled hormone has been identified.

Dynamic function tests

Where the results of clinical assessment and baseline biochemical investigations fail to rule in or rule out a serious endocrine diagnosis, dynamic function tests may be required.

Table 1 **Examples of endocrine disease**
Oversecretion
Cushing's disease where a pituitary adenoma secretes ACTH
Undersecretion
Primary hypothyroidism where the thyroid gland is unable to make sufficient thyroid hormone despite continued stimulation by TSH
Failure of hormone responsiveness
Pseudohypoparathyroidism where patients become hypocalcaemic despite elevated plasma PTH concentration because target organs lack a functioning receptor signalling mechanism

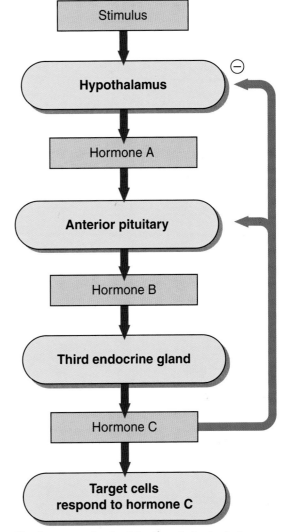

Fig. 3 **Negative feedback in a hypothalamic pituitary endocrine gland system.**

Indeed, these are routine in the investigation of some disorders like acromegaly. They are dealt with in detail on page 80.

Clinical note

The overriding influence of stress on the endocrine system makes the diagnosis of endocrine disorders in the critically ill patient very difficult. Ill patients may have hyperglycaemia, high serum cortisol or abnormal thyroid hormone results. These could be misinterpreted as diabetes mellitus, Cushing's syndrome or thyroid disease.

Endocrine control

- Endocrinology is the study of hormones, a class of biochemical regulators that are secreted into blood to act at distant sites in the body.
- Hormone concentrations in plasma are very variable.
- For a clear demonstration of abnormalities of hormone secretion or regulation, dynamic tests are often necessary.

Dynamic function tests

Much of clinical endocrinology is concerned with diseases that involve either a deficiency or an excess of hormones. It is not always possible to diagnose these diseases on the basis of clinical assessment and baseline laboratory investigations. Dynamic function tests (DFTs) involve either stimulating or suppressing a particular hormonal axis, and observing the appropriate hormonal response. In general, if a deficiency is suspected, a stimulation test should be used; if excess is suspected, a suppression test is used. Often, the stimulus is an exogenous analogue of a trophic hormone; in other cases it is provided by biochemical or physiological stress, e.g. hypoglycaemia or exercise.

On subsequent pages, individual DFT procedures are discussed in the context of specific hormonal axes. Here, we describe the principles that underpin some of these DFTs, and look at aspects of interpretation. The abbreviations used for the various hormones and the tests are listed in Tables 1 and 2 respectively.

Insulin stress test

This test is carried out when hypopituitarism is suspected. It is also known as the insulin tolerance test. Enough insulin is administered to produce hypoglycaemic stress (blood glucose <2.2 mmol/L). This tests the ability of the anterior pituitary to produce ACTH and GH in response. Cortisol is measured instead of ACTH; this assumes that the adrenals can respond normally to ACTH. A peak GH in excess of 20 mU/L is regarded as evidence of adequate reserve. For cortisol there is less consensus about what should be regarded as an adequate response; however, anything less than 500 nmol/L is inadequate, and many endocrinologists use cut-offs substantially in excess of this, e.g. 550 nmol/L. An example of the results of an insulin stress test is shown in Figure 1.

TRH test

TRH is given as an intravenous bolus; blood sampling is at 0, 20 and 60 minutes (Fig. 2). In normal

Table 1 **Acronyms for some hormones**	
Adrenocorticotrophic hormone	ACTH
Arginine vasopressin	AVP
Corticotrophin releasing hormone	CRH
Follicle stimulating hormone	FSH
Gonadotrophin releasing hormone	GnRH
Growth hormone	GH (or HGH)
Growth hormone releasing hormone	GHRH
Luteinizing hormone	LH
Parathyroid hormone	PTH
Thyroid stimulating hormone	TSH
Thyrotrophin releasing hormone	TRH
Thyroxine	T_4
Triiodothyronine	T_3

Table 2 **Commonly used abbreviations for various dynamic function tests**	
IST	Insulin stress test
OGTT	Oral glucose tolerance test
SST	Short Synacthen test
DST	Dexamethasone suppression test
CAPFT	Combined anterior pituitary function test

subjects TRH elicits a brisk release of both TSH and prolactin. This test may be used to assess the adequacy of anterior pituitary reserve, or to evaluate suspected hypothalamic disease, in which the TSH response to TRH is characteristically delayed (TSH higher at 60 minutes than at 20 minutes). Much less frequently it may be indicated in suspected hyper- or hypothyroidism. Where there has been prolonged negative feedback due to hyperthyroidism, the pituitary response to TRH is flat (TSH rises by <2 mU/L); conversely, an exaggerated TSH response (>25 mU/L) is seen in hypothyroidism.

GnRH test

In normal adults, GnRH produces a marked rise in LH and a smaller rise in FSH; typical expected increments in adults are >15 U/L for LH and >2 U/L for FSH. In children the FSH response is greater than the LH response. This test is indicated where there is clinical or biochemical evidence of hypogonadism, particularly in the absence of the expected compensatory rises in LH and FSH. It may be performed alone or as part of a combined anterior pituitary function test (see p. 83). The latter simply consists of the three separate DFTs described above (IST, TRH test and GnRH test) performed simultaneously. Collectively they provide a comprehensive assessment of anterior pituitary reserve.

Biochemical Medicine

Clinical Laboratory Services

Name:	Sex: F	PID: 2702601234	DoB: 27 Feb 1960
			Lab No: C03000033
N/W Biochemical Medicine	Clinician: Dr M.J. MURPHY		NBIOC MURM2H

INSULIN STRESS TEST

Time	GLUCOSE mmol/L	CORTISOL nmol/L	GH mU/L	TSH mU/L	FREE T4 pmol/L	FSH U/L	LH U/L	OESTRADIOL pmol/L
0 min	4.1	295	0.1	1.3	4.2	0.8	0.5	<70
30	0.5	374	0.4					
60	0.8	354	0.2					
90	2.1	261	10.0					
120	3.9	182	3.5					

Lab. comments: (1) Adequate hypoglycaemia achieved
(2) Inadequate cortisol response
(3) Inadequate GH response
(4) TSH clearly not compensating for low free T4 - TRH test not required
(5) Gonadal axis results consistent with secondary hypogonadism

Sample Date/Time
27 Feb

Request entered: 27 Feb 12.30   Report printed: 5 Mar

REPORT RECEIVED

DOCTOR'S INITIALS

Fig. 1 **Results of an insulin stress test.**

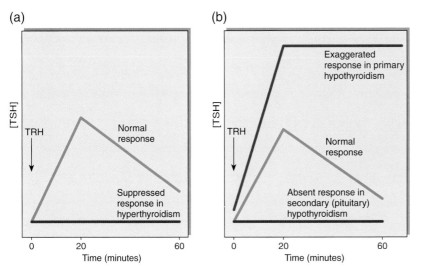

Fig. 2 **Pituitary responses to TRH. (a)** Used in the investigation of hyperthyroidism. **(b)** Used in the investigation of pituitary or hypothalamic hypothyroidism.

Oral glucose tolerance test with GH measurement

Just as hypoglycaemia stimulates GH secretion, so hyperglycaemia suppresses it. This forms the basis for performing an oral glucose tolerance test (OGTT) with GH measurement. Normal adults suppress GH to <2 mU/L, but acromegalic patients do not; failure to suppress is therefore highly suggestive of acromegaly. Following treatment, patients who fail to suppress GH below 5 mU/L have a higher prevalence of diabetes, heart disease and hypertension.

Synacthen tests

Short Synacthen test

The short Synacthen test (SST) is one of the most commonly performed DFTs. The procedure is described on page 95. Of the three criteria that are used to define a normal response (see Fig. 3 on p. 95), the final cortisol is the most important, and the increment the least important. As with the IST, there is lack of agreement on what constitutes an adequate cortisol response to Synacthen; cut-offs for the final level vary between 500 and 580 nmol/L.

Long Synacthen test

Where the response to an SST is inadequate or equivocal, it may not be clear whether the adrenal insufficiency is primary, or secondary to pituitary or hypothalamic disease. Secondary adrenal insufficiency is most frequently seen following the use of long-term steroid therapy, which causes central suppression of the axis. If the SST is repeated after the administration of a much larger dose of Synacthen (1 mg) a normal response may be observed, confirming the diagnosis.

Dexamethasone suppression tests

Dexamethasone is an exogenous steroid that mimics the negative feedback of endogenous glucocorticoids. Dexamethasone suppression tests (DSTs) are important in the investigation of suspected overactivity of the hypothalamic-pituitary-adrenal axis.

Low dose dexamethasone suppression test

In its simplest form, the low dose DST – usually performed on an outpatient basis – involves the patient taking 1 mg dexamethasone orally at 23:00 and attending for a cortisol blood test the following morning at 08:00 or 09:00. If the cortisol has suppressed to <50 nmol/L, cortisol overproduction is unlikely and no further action is normally required.

High dose dexamethasone suppression test

Failure to suppress in response to low dose dexamethasone may occur because of autonomous ACTH production by the pituitary (Cushing's disease), or ectopic ACTH production (usually malignant), or adrenal production of cortisol (see p. 96). The high dose DST (8 mg) is used to distinguish the first two of these options. ACTH production in Cushing's disease does usually suppress in response to high dose dexamethasone, whereas malignant production of ACTH usually does not.

Dynamic function tests – protocol variation

Protocols for individual DFTs vary from one centre to another. For example, an additional cortisol specimen is collected at 60 minutes in some SST protocols, although this rarely alters the interpretation of the SST. Likewise, the long Synacthen test may be performed as a day-long procedure, with 1 mg Synacthen administered in the morning and cortisol samples collected for up to 24 hours; others perform this test as outlined on p. 95. The reasons for the different protocols are often practical rather than evidence-based but it is always wise to check with the local laboratory before proceeding with any DFT.

> *Clinical note*
> Insulin-induced hypoglycaemia is designed to induce stress. If a patient requires intravenous glucose therapy to correct severe hypoglycaemia the test should not be abandoned. Obviously in such cases adequate stress has been induced, and useful information may still be obtained.

> **Dynamic function tests**
> - Dynamic function tests are often required for the diagnosis of endocrine disorders.
> - These tests involve either stimulating or suppressing a particular hormonal axis.
> - Many of these tests are complex and require careful attention to appropriate timing of samples for their results to be meaningful.

Pituitary function

The pituitary gland

Pituitary function is regulated by the hypothalamus, to which it is connected via the pituitary stalk, which comprises portal blood capillaries and nerve fibres. The anterior pituitary is influenced by a variety of stimulatory and inhibitory hormones through these capillaries. The posterior pituitary is a collection of specialized nerve endings that derive from the hypothalamus.

Anterior pituitary hormones

- *TSH (thyroid-stimulating hormone)*, acts specifically on the thyroid gland to elicit secretion of thyroid hormones.
- *ACTH (adrenocorticotrophic hormone)* acts specifically on the adrenal cortex to elicit secretion of cortisol.
- *LH (luteinizing hormone) and FSH (follicle-stimulating hormone)*, known jointly as the gonadotrophins, act cooperatively on the ovaries in women and the testes in men to stimulate sex hormone secretion and reproductive processes.
- *GH (growth hormone)* acts directly on many tissues to modulate metabolism. Metabolic fuels (e.g. glucose, free fatty acids) in turn modify GH secretion.
- *Prolactin* acts directly on the mammary glands to control lactation. Gonadal function is impaired by elevated circulating prolactin concentrations.

The hypothalamic factors that control anterior pituitary hormone secretion are shown in Figure 1.

Hyperprolactinaemia

Hyperprolactinaemia is common and can cause infertility in both sexes. An early indication in women is amenorrhoea and galactorrhoea, whereas in men there may be no early signs and the first indication of the presence of a prolactinoma may be when a large growing tumour begins to interfere with the optic nerves. Causes of hyperprolactinaemia include:

- stress (venepuncture is sufficient to raise plasma prolactin in some patients)
- drugs (e.g. oestrogens, phenothiazines, metoclopramide, α-methyl dopa)
- seizures (acutely)
- primary hypothyroidism (prolactin is stimulated by the raised TRH)
- other pituitary disease.

If these causes are excluded, the differential diagnosis is between:

- a prolactinoma (a prolactin-secreting pituitary tumour, commonly a microadenoma)
- idiopathic hypersecretion, which may be due to impaired secretion of dopamine, the hypothalamic factor that inhibits prolactin release.

Differentiating between these, after exclusion of stress, drugs and other disease, is by detailed pituitary imaging together with dynamic tests of prolactin secretion. A rise in serum prolactin following administration of TRH or metoclopramide is observed in idiopathic hyperprolactinaemia but not in the presence of a pituitary tumour.

In a small portion of cases a raised prolactin is due to the presence of macroprolactin, an immune complex.

Posterior pituitary hormones

Hypothalamic neurons synthesize arginine vasopressin (AVP) and oxytocin, which pass along axonal nerve fibres in the pituitary stalk to the posterior pituitary where they are stored in granules in the terminal bulbs of nerves in close proximity to systemic veins.

Secretion of AVP, also known as antidiuretic hormone (ADH), is stimulated by:

- increased plasma osmolality via hypothalamic osmoreceptors
- severe blood volume depletion via cardiac baroreceptors
- stress and nausea.

The role of AVP in fluid and electrolyte regulation is discussed on pages 14–15. A pituitary tumour arising in the anterior gland may cause impaired secretion of this posterior pituitary hormone, with consequent diabetes insipidus.

Oxytocin is released in response to suckling of the breast and uterine contraction at the onset of labour.

Pituitary tumours

Diagnosis

Pituitary tumours may be either functional (that is they secrete hormones) or non-functional. The incidence of different tumour types is shown in Figure 2. Local effects include headaches, papilloedema and visual field defects. There may be specific signs of hormone excess particularly in acromegaly, Cushing's syndrome and prolactinoma. There may be signs of hypopituitarism in skin, hair and musculature.

The impact of the tumour on pituitary function requires formal assessment by dynamic function tests. GH and ACTH-secreting cells are most vulnerable, and an insulin stress test (see p. 80) may suffice. However, comprehensive assessment of anterior pituitary reserve requires a combined anterior pituitary function test (Fig. 3). TRH, GnRH and insulin are administered. All hormones are assessed at 0, 30 and 60 minutes, and GH additionally at 90 and 120 minutes. It is usual also to assess basal thyroid (thyroxine) and gonadal (testosterone or oestradiol) function.

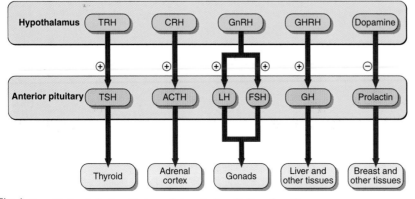

Fig. 1 **Hypothalamic factors that regulate anterior pituitary functions.**

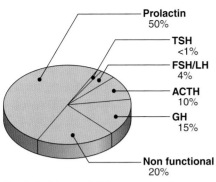

Prolactin 50%

TSH <1%

FSH/LH 4%

ACTH 10%

GH 15%

Non functional 20%

Fig. 2 **Incidence of different types of pituitary tumours.**

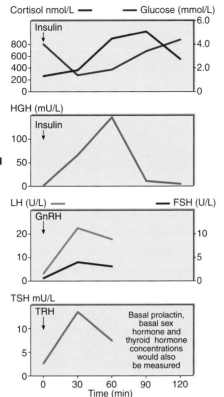

Fig. 3 **Normal responses in a combined anterior pituitary function test.**

The administration of insulin is contraindicated if there is established coronary disease or epilepsy. A clinician must be on hand throughout the test, and intravenous dextrose and hydrocortisone must be readily available in the event of severe or prolonged hypoglycaemia resulting in neuroglycopenia, e.g. loss of consciousness or fits.

Because of its associated dangers, insulin-induced hypoglycaemia is being replaced by administration of GHRH and CRH to investigate GH and cortisol secretion.

Treatment

- *Medical.* Dopamine agonist drugs like bromocriptine and cabergoline are widely used to treat hyperprolactinaemia, especially when due to microprolactinomas. They may also be used to shrink large suprasellar prolactinomas before surgery.
- *Surgery.* Trans-sphenoidal hypophysectomy is the standard procedure. Patients undergoing this are routinely given steroid cover (usually hydrocortisone), in case they cannot mount an adequate cortisol response to the stress of the operation. For the same reason, postoperative assessment of pituitary reserve should be deferred for several days.
- *Radiation.* The impact of radiation on pituitary function is cumulative, and irradiated patients require annual dynamic function testing of their anterior pituitary reserve thereafter.

Hypopituitarism

There are many causes of hypopituitarism, a relatively uncommon condition in which there is failure of one or more pituitary functions. These causes include tumour, infarction, trauma, congenital malformation, infection and hypothalamic disorder.

The clinical presentation of hypopituitarism depends on the age of the patient. In infancy, short stature or impaired development may point to the condition. In the reproductive years, women may present with amenorrhoea or infertility. Men may present with decreased libido or a lack of male secondary sex characteristics. Elderly patients may complain of symptoms relating to ACTH or TSH deficiency such as hypoglycaemia or hypothermia.

> **Clinical note**
> Imaging techniques are very important in the diagnosis of pituitary tumours in conjunction with the biochemical findings.

Case history 31

A 36-year-old man complained of impaired vision while driving, particularly at night. After clinical and initial biochemical assessment, a combined anterior pituitary stimulation test was performed (IV insulin 0.1 U/kg, TRH 200 µg, GnRH 100 µg).

Time (min)	Glucose mmol/L	Cortisol nmol/L	GH mU/L	PRL mU/L	FSH U/L	LH U/L	TSH mU/L	Free T₄ nmol/L	Testosterone nmol/L
0	3.6	320	1.5	17 000	<0.7	<1.0	<1.0	6	6.1
30	0.9	310	1.7	16 400	0.8	3.7	2.7		
60	1.8	380	1.6	18 000	1.2	3.7	4.1		
90	2.7	370	1.4						
120	3.3	230	1.4						

- A lower than normal dose of insulin was used. Why?
- What is the most likely diagnosis?
- What precautions should be taken before surgery?

Comment on page 165.

Pituitary function

- Adenomas secreting each of the anterior pituitary hormones have been identified.
- Around 20% of pituitary tumours appear not to secrete hormone.
- It is important to establish if a pituitary tumour, whether hormone secreting or not, has interfered with the other hypothalamic–pituitary connections.
- Hyperprolactinaemia is common. Once stress, drugs or other disease have been eliminated as possible causes, dynamic tests and detailed radiology are used to differentiate between prolactinoma and idiopathic hypersecretion.
- Hypopituitarism is uncommon; the clinical presentation depends on the age of the patient.

Growth disorders and acromegaly

Normal growth

Growth in children can be divided into three stages (Fig. 1). Rapid growth occurs during the first 2 years of life; the rate is influenced by conditions in utero, as well as the adequacy of nutrition in the postnatal period. The next stage is relatively steady growth for around 9 years and is controlled mainly by growth hormone (GH). If the pituitary does not produce sufficient growth hormone, the yearly growth rate during this period may be halved and the child will be of short stature. The growth spurt at puberty is caused by the effect of the sex hormones in addition to continuing GH secretion. The regulation of GH secretion is outlined in Figure 2.

GH is only one of many hormones involved in growth. Insulin-like growth factors, thyroxine, cortisol, the sex steroids and insulin are also involved.

Growth hormone insufficiency

Any child whose height for age falls below the 3rd centile on a standard chart, or who exhibits a slow growth rate, requires further investigation. If GH deficiency is diagnosed, and treatment is required, then the earlier it is given the better the chance that the child will eventually reach normal size.

Growth hormone insufficiency is a rare cause of impaired physical growth. It is important to differentiate between children whose slow growth or growth failure is due to illness or disease and those whose short stature is a normal variant of the population. Causes of short stature are:

- having parents who are both short
- inherited diseases such as achondroplasia, the commonest cause of severe dwarfism
- poor nutrition
- systemic chronic illness, such as renal disease, gastrointestinal disorders or respiratory disease
- psychological factors such as emotional deprivation
- hormonal disorders.

Standard graphs relating age and height are available for the normal population. Accurate measurements of height should be made to establish whether a child is small for chronological age. These measurements are repeated after 6 and 12 months to assess the growth rate. The height of the parents should also be assessed. The bone age is the best predictor of final height in a child with short stature; this is determined by radiological examination of hand and wrist. In most growth disorders bone age is delayed and by itself is of little diagnostic value, but taken together with height and chronological age,

> ### Clinical note
> In the investigation of normal looking children with short stature, coeliac disease must always be considered. The diagnosis is frequently overlooked.

a prediction of final height may be obtained.

Tests of growth hormone insufficiency

Growth hormone deficiency may be present from birth or due to later pituitary failure. A variety of stimulation tests have been used to evaluate GH deficiency. Serum GH concentrations rise in response to exercise, and this may be used as a preliminary screening test. They also rise during sleep, and high concentrations in a nocturnal sample may exclude GH deficiency. The lack of GH response to the stress of exercise or clonidine, a potent stimulant of GH secretion, is diagnostic. Some centres have now abandoned the use of insulin-induced hypoglycaemia as a diagnostic test in children because of its hazards.

The GH response to stimulation requires the presence of sex steroids. Thus, prepubertal children, and hypogonadal adults, require 'priming'

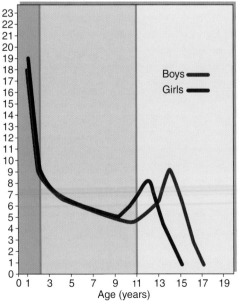

Fig. 1 **Median height velocity curve for boys and girls showing the three growth stages.**

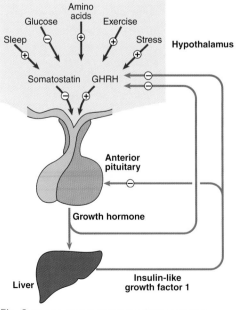

Fig. 2 **The normal regulation of GH secretion.**

by the administration of either testosterone or oestrogen before GH reserve is assessed.

Increasingly, urinary growth hormone measurements are being used to assess possible GH lack in children. Random serum IGF 1 determinations may be of value. Levels within reference limits exclude GH deficiency.

Treatment

Genetically engineered GH is available and is used in the treatment of that small group of children with proven GH deficiency.

Excessive growth

Growth hormone excess in children is characterized by extremely rapid linear growth (gigantism). The condition is uncommon and is most often due to a GH secreting pituitary tumour. Other causes of tall stature in children are rare and include:

- *Hyperthyroidism.* An increased growth rate, with advanced bone age, is a feature of hyperthroidism in children, or hypothyroid children over-replaced with thyroxine.
- *Inherited disorders* such as Klinefelter's syndrome (a 47 XXY karyotype). The relative deficiency of testosterone is associated with delayed epiphyseal closure.
- *Congenital adrenal hyperplasia.* (CAH may also be associated with short stature, due to premature epiphyseal closure, due to androgen excess.)

Acromegaly

Increased GH secretion later in life, after fusion of bony epiphyses, causes acromegaly (Fig. 3). The most likely cause is a pituitary adenoma. Clinical features include:

- coarse facial features
- soft tissue thickening, e.g. the lips
- characteristic 'spade-like' hands
- protruding jaw (prognathism)
- sweating
- impaired glucose tolerance or diabetes mellitus.

Diagnosis

Formal diagnosis of acromegaly requires an oral glucose tolerance test with GH measurement (see p. 81). Acromegalic patients do not suppress fully in response to hyperglycaemia (Fig. 4), and

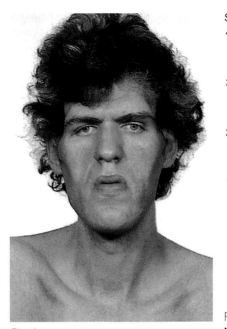

Fig. 3 **Clinical picture of an acromegalic patient.**

indeed in some patients a paradoxical rise in GH may be observed.

IGF 1 is produced in response to GH and provides useful additional biochemical information. It is now routinely measured in the diagnosis and especially monitoring of treated acromegaly, with an elevated level suggestive of active disease. Other measurements, e.g. IGF binding protein 3 (IFGBP3), have not yet attained widespread clinical use.

Treatment

- *Surgery.* Trans-sphenoidal hypophysectomy is the first-line treatment for most acromegalic patients. Its success depends on the size of the tumour.
- *Radiation.* This is usually reserved for patients whose disease remains active despite surgery. It may take years after pituitary irradiation before safe levels of GH are achieved. Medical treatment is required in the interim.
- *Medical.* Dopamine agonists like bromocriptine were widely used in the past, but response rates were low.

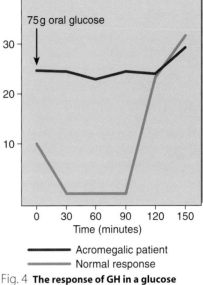

Fig. 4 **The response of GH in a glucose tolerance test in a normal and acromegalic patient.**

The advent of long-acting synthetic analogues of somatostatin, such as octreotide, has transformed the medical management of acromegaly. These are expensive drugs with side effects, and it is sensible to screen patients for responsiveness by measuring GH after administering octreotide (octreotide suppression test).

Case history 32

James is 5 years old and is much smaller than his classmates at school. His growth rate has been monitored and has clearly dropped off markedly in the past year. He is an active child, and on examination has normal body proportions. His mother and father are of average height. His bone age is that of a 3-year-old child.

- What biochemical tests would be appropriate in the investigation of this boy?

Comment on page 165.

Growth disorders and acromegaly

- GH deficiency is a rare cause of short stature in children, and is investigated only after other causes of short stature have been eliminated.
- Diagnosis of GH deficiency is made on the failure of serum GH to rise in response to stimuli.
- Gigantism in children is caused by increased GH secretion, usually from a pituitary tumour. Acromegaly is the consequence of increased GH secretion in adults.
- Lack of suppression of serum GH levels in response to a glucose tolerance test is the diagnostic test for acromegaly.
- Serum IGF 1 concentrations are of value in the diagnosis of acromegaly and the monitoring of treatment.

Thyroid pathophysiology

Introduction

Thyroxine (T_4) and tri-iodothyronine (T_3) are together known as the 'thyroid hormones'. They are synthesized in the thyroid gland by iodination and coupling of two tyrosine molecules whilst attached to a complex protein called thyroglobulin. T_4 has four iodine atoms while T_3 has three (Fig. 1).

The thyroid gland secretes mostly T_4 whose concentration in plasma is around 100 nmol/L. The peripheral tissues, especially the liver and kidney, deiodinate T_4 to produce approximately two-thirds of the circulating T_3, present at a lower concentration of around 2 nmol/L. Most cells are capable of taking up T_4 and deiodinating it to the more biologically active T_3. It is T_3 that binds to receptors and triggers the end-organ effects of the thyroid hormones. Alternatively, T_4 can be metabolized to reverse T_3 (rT_3), which is biologically inactive. By modulating the relative production of T_3 and rT_3, tissues can 'fine tune' their local thyroid status. Exactly how this is accomplished is not yet fully understood.

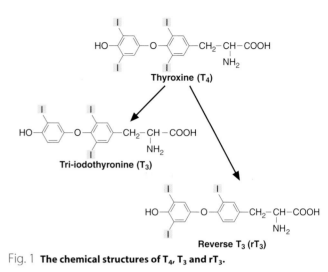

Fig. 1 **The chemical structures of T_4, T_3 and rT_3.**

Thyroid hormone action

Thyroid hormones are essential for the normal maturation and metabolism of all the tissues in the body. Their effects on tissue maturation are most dramatically seen in congenital hypothyroidism, a condition which, unless treated within 3 months of birth, results in permanent brain damage. Hypothyroid children have delayed skeletal maturation, short stature and delayed puberty.

Thyroid hormone effects on metabolism are diverse. The rates of protein and carbohydrate synthesis and catabolism are influenced. An example of the effect of thyroid hormones on lipid metabolism is the observation of a high serum cholesterol in some hypothyroid patients. This is a consequence of a reduction in cholesterol metabolism due to down regulation of low-density lipoprotein (LDL) receptors on liver cell membranes, with a subsequent failure of sterol excretion via the gut.

Binding plasma

In plasma, over 99.95% of T_4 is transported bound to proteins. Thyroxine binding globulin (TBG) carries 70% of T_4, albumin approximately 25% and transthyretin (formerly called prealbumin) around 5%. Over 99.5% of T_3 is transported by the same proteins. It is the unbound, or 'free', T_4 and T_3 concentrations that are important for the biological effects of the hormones, including the feedback to the pituitary and hypothalamus. Changes in binding protein concentration complicate the interpretation of thyroid hormone results, e.g. in pregnancy.

Regulation of thyroid hormone secretion

The components of the hypothalamic–pituitary–thyroid axis are TRH, TSH and the thyroid hormones. TRH, a tripeptide, is secreted by the hypothalamus and in turn causes the synthesis of a large glycoprotein hormone, TSH, from the anterior pituitary. This drives the synthesis of thyroid hormones by the thyroid. Production of TSH is regulated by feedback from circulating unbound thyroid hormones. A knowledge of these basics is essential for the correct interpretation of results in the investigation of thyroid disease. Remember:

- If a patient's thyroid is producing too much thyroid hormone, then the circulating TSH will be suppressed.
- If the thyroid is not secreting enough thyroid hormone, the TSH levels will be very high in an attempt to stimulate the gland to secrete more.

Thyroid function tests

Biochemical measurements in the diagnosis of thyroid disease have traditionally been known as 'thyroid function tests'. TSH and some estimate of T_4 status (either total T_4 or free T_4) are the first-line tests.

- *TSH.* Measurement of TSH is a good example of how better technology has helped in the diagnosis and monitoring of disease. Early assays for TSH were unable to measure low concentrations of the hormone – the detection limits of the radioimmunoassays overlapped significantly with concentrations of the low end of the reference interval in healthy subjects. Now, very sensitive TSH assays can detect much lower concentrations and it is possible to tell with a greater degree of certainty whether TSH secretion really is lower than normal.

  Because of its log-linear relationship with TRH, TSH is very sensitive to derangements in thyroid control, and many laboratories use TSH alone as the first-line thyroid function test. There is, however, one situation in which TSH cannot be used to diagnose primary thyroid disease, or to monitor replacement, namely hypopituitarism. For example, TSH is undetectable post hypophysectomy and an estimate of T_4 status must be used instead to monitor the adequacy of replacement.

- *Total T_4 or free T_4.* Following the introduction of replacement thyroxine or of anti-thyroid treatment, e.g. carbimazole, or indeed following any alteration in dosage, TSH may take up to 8 weeks to adjust to its new level. During this time, it is essential to have some estimate of T_4 status. This applies particularly to the monitoring of anti-thyroid treatment; patients can become profoundly hypothyroid quite quickly.

- *Total T_3 or free T_3.* Occasionally it may be useful to have an estimate of T_3 status in addition to T_4. In hyperthyroidism, the rise in T_3 is almost always disproportionate to the rise in T_4; an estimate of T_3 status may permit earlier identification of thyrotoxicosis. In some patients only the T_3 rises – the T_4 remains within the reference interval (T_3 toxicosis).

- *Antibodies.* The titre of autoantibodies to thyroid tissue antigens may be helpful in the diagnosis and monitoring of autoimmune thyroid disease. Anti-thyroid peroxidase (anti-TPO) may be useful in hypothyroidism and stimulating anti-TSH receptor antibodies in thyrotoxicosis.

Drugs and the thyroid

Various drugs affect thyroid function tests. The effects of some of these are summarized in Table 1.

Goitre

A goitre is an enlarged thyroid gland (Fig. 2). This may be associated with hypofunction, hyperfunction or, indeed, normal concentrations of thyroid hormones in blood. With such a clinical presentation, the biochemistry laboratory can confirm if a patient is hypothyroid, hyperthyroid or euthyroid.

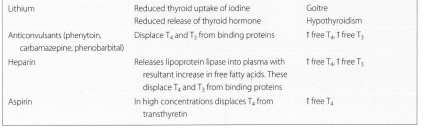

Table 1 **Drugs affecting thyroid function tests**

Drug	Mechanism	Major effects
Amiodarone	Reduced peripheral deiodination	↑T_4,↓T_3, transient ↑ in TSH
	Amiodarone can also stimulate or inhibit release of thyroid hormones from thyroid	Hyperthyroidism Hypothyroidism
Lithium	Reduced thyroid uptake of iodine	Goitre
	Reduced release of thyroid hormone	Hypothyroidism
Anticonvulsants (phenytoin, carbamazepine, phenobarbital)	Displace T_4 and T_3 from binding proteins	↑ free T_4, ↑ free T_3
Heparin	Releases lipoprotein lipase into plasma with resultant increase in free fatty acids. These displace T_4 and T_3 from binding proteins	↑ free T_4, ↑ free T_3
Aspirin	In high concentrations displaces T_4 from transthyretin	↑ free T_4

Clinical note

Autoimmune thyroid disorders are relatively common. Their presence should alert the clinician to the possibility that other autoimmune disorders, some of which are uncommon, may have been overlooked. Examples are:

- insulin-dependent diabetes mellitus
- autoimmune hypoparathyroidism
- primary gonadal failure
- autoimmune destruction of the adrenal cortex causing Addison's disease
- pernicious anaemia
- vitiligo.

Case history 33

A 49-year-old woman receiving hormone replacement therapy was found to have a thyroid nodule. No lymphadenopathy was detectable and clinically she appeared to be euthyroid. A technetium scan revealed a 'cold' nodule and an ultrasound scan indicated it was cystic.

Biochemistry results in a serum specimen:

T_4	TSH
(nmol/L)	*(mU/L)*
172	0.40

- Explain why the T_4 is elevated.
- What other investigations should be performed in this patient?

Comment on page 165.

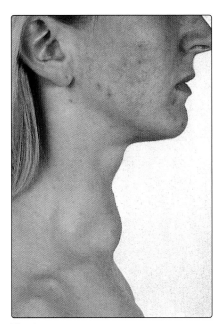

Fig. 2 **A patient with a goitre.**

Thyroid pathophysiology

- The thyroid gland synthesizes, stores, and secretes the thyroid hormones T_4 and T_3, which are important for normal development and metabolism.
- The secretion of thyroid hormones is controlled primarily by TSH from the anterior pituitary.
- Most T_4 and T_3 circulates in plasma bound to protein. Only a small proportion is not bound, yet it is this 'free' fraction that is biologically important.
- Knowledge of TSH, thyroid hormone and binding protein concentrations in serum may all be needed in the assessment of a patient's thyroid status.
- A patient may have severe thyroid disease, such as a large goitre or thyroid cancer, yet have normal concentrations of thyroid hormones in blood.

Hypothyroidism

Hypothyroidism usually develops slowly. It is therefore easily missed clinically and clinical biochemistry has an important role to play in diagnosis.

Clinical features

The clinical features of hypothyroidism include:

- lethargy and tiredness
- cold intolerance
- weight gain
- dryness and coarsening of skin and hair
- hoarseness
- slow relaxation of muscles and tendon reflexes
- many other associated signs including anaemia, dementia, constipation, bradycardia, muscle stiffness, carpal tunnel syndrome, subfertility and galactorrhoea.

Causes

Over 90% of cases of hypothyroidism occur as a consequence of:

- autoimmune destruction of the thyroid gland (Hashimoto's disease)
- radioiodine or surgical treatment of hyperthyroidism.

   Rarer causes include:

- transient hypothyroidism due to treatment with drugs such as lithium carbonate
- TSH deficiency, which may be a component of panhypopituitarism
- congenital defects such as blocks in the biosynthesis of T_4 and T_3, or end-organ resistance to their action
- severe iodine deficiency.

Diagnosis

Hypothyroidism is caused by a deficiency of thyroid hormones. Primary hypothyroidism is failure of the thyroid gland itself and is one of the most commonly encountered endocrine problems. The demonstration of an elevated TSH concentration is usually diagnostic. Secondary hypothyroidism, failure of the pituitary to secrete TSH, is much less common. Isolated pituitary deficiency of TSH is rare, but impairment of the hypothalamic–pituitary–thyroid axis may happen

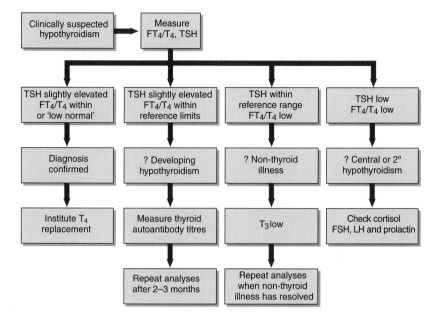

Fig. 1 **Strategy for the biochemical investigation of suspected hypothyroidism**.

as a result of any pituitary disease or damage.

   Clinical features other than those of hypothyroidism may indicate the need for investigation of pituitary function (see pp. 82–83), and the TRH test will be included in such a protocol.

   A strategy for the biochemical investigation of clinically suspected hypothyroidism is shown in Figure 1.

Treatment

Replacement therapy with T_4 is the treatment of choice since the hormone is readily available in a pure stable form, and is inexpensive. Monitoring TSH concentrations can be helpful in assessing the adequacy of treatment. Once the dosage is established, the patient will be required to continue treatment for life (Fig. 2).

   Figure 3 shows the need for careful monitoring of treatment. This graph shows the changes in thyroid hormone results as a hyperthyroid woman patient became hypothyroid after radioiodine treatment, and it subsequently proved difficult to stabilize her on a replacement dose of thyroxine.

Screening for neonatal hypothyroidism

Congenital hypothyroid disorders occur with a frequency of one in every 4000 live births (pp. 154–155).

If they are diagnosed at an early age, replacement thyroid hormone can be given and normal development can occur. Delays in treatment result in cretinism (see p. 154). Elevated TSH, measured in blood spots, is diagnostic of disorders of the thyroid itself, i.e. primary neonatal hypothyroidism. The TSH screening test does not pick up pituitary dysfunction in the newborn.

Non-thyroidal illness

In health the major factor that regulates the serum concentration of TSH is the feedback of thyroid hormone activity on the pituitary and, to a lesser extent, on the hypothalamus. Other factors also play a role. There is a diurnal rhythm with the serum TSH peaking around midday when the concentration is approximately 30% higher than at midnight, when it is at its nadir. In systemic illness the normal regulation of TSH, T_4 and T_3 secretion, and the subsequent metabolism of the thyroid hormones, is disturbed. Increased amounts of T_4 are converted to the biologically inactive reverse T_3, rather than to T_3. The resultant reduction in thyroid hormone activity does not result in an increased serum TSH concentration. TSH secretion is suppressed, and the secretion of T_4 and T_3 by the thyroid gland is therefore decreased.

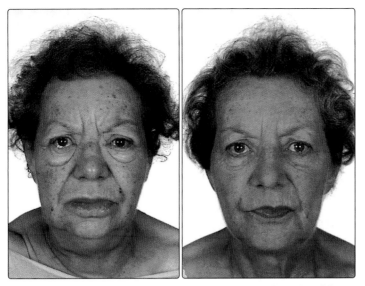

Fig. 2 **A patient before and after successful treatment of primary hypothyroidism.**

not be performed in patients during an acute illness unless there are good clinical grounds for suspecting that underlying hypothyroidism is a major feature of their illness. Thyroid function testing should be postponed until after the acute phase has passed. Patients with non-thyroidal illness results should not be given T_4 since there is no evidence that this would benefit them.

The concentrations of the transport proteins also decrease. A low serum albumin and transthyretin (pre-albumin) are classic features of the metabolic response to illness, and increased free fatty acid concentrations compete with T_4 and T_3 for their binding sites.

These changes result in sick patients having low serum T_4, T_3 and TSH, and if thyroid function tests are requested the results may well be misinterpreted. A typical non-thyroidal illness pattern might be:

Free T_4	T_3	TSH
pmol/L	nmol/L	mU/L
6.0	0.6	5.1

These results were obtained in a man with acute pancreatitis. In developing hypothyroidism the T_3 would be maintained within the reference range. In decreased TBG states the T_4 and T_3 would fall in parallel. A low T_3 is almost invariably due to the presence of non-thyroidal illness.

This condition is also known as the 'low T_3 syndrome'. The message is simple: thyroid function tests should

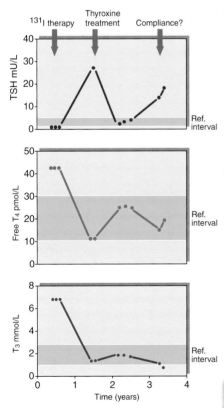

Fig. 3 **Biochemical monitoring of a patient during treatment for thyroid disease.**
This 55-year-old woman was first diagnosed as hyperthyroid, and received radioiodine therapy. She became profoundly hypothyroid, and was treated with thyroxine. Her thyroid hormone results at first indicated good replacement, but recently they indicate that she is under-replaced. It is possible that she is not taking her thyroxine tablets regularly.

Case history 34

Investigation of a 63-year-old woman with effort angina revealed a serum TSH of 96 mU/L and a serum free T_4 of 3.7 pmol/L. An ECG showed some evidence of ischaemia but was not diagnostic of myocardial infarction. Further biochemical investigation revealed:

Cholesterol (mmol/L)	Creatine kinase	AST
	—— (U/L) ——	
9.3	290	35

■ How should these results be interpreted?

Comment on page 165.

Clinical note

Patients with severe hypothyroidism should be initially treated with very small doses of thyroxine – 25 μg (i.e. 0.025 mg) daily. At higher doses, patients are at an increased risk of developing angina or suffering a myocardial infarction. The dose should be slowly increased over a number of months until the patient is rendered euthyroid.

Hypothyroidism

■ Hypothyroidism is common and is most often due to the destruction of the thyroid gland by autoimmune disease, surgery or radioiodine therapy.

■ Primary hypothyroidism is confirmed by an elevated TSH in a serum specimen.

■ A TRH test is used to investigate secondary hypothyroidism due to pituitary or hypothalamic causes.

■ Hypothyroidism is managed by thyroxine replacement, and therapy is monitored by measuring the serum TSH concentration.

■ Patients with severe non-thyroidal illness may show apparent abnormalities in thyroid hormone results, known as the 'low T_3 syndrome' or non-thyroidal illness pattern of results.

Hyperthyroidism

Thyrotoxicosis occurs when tissues are exposed to high levels of the thyroid hormones. Used correctly, the term 'hyperthyroidism' refers to the over-activity of the thyroid gland, but thyrotoxicosis can also occur from ingestion of too much T_4 or, rarely, from increased pituitary stimulation of the thyroid.

Clinical features

The clinical features of hyperthyroidism may be dramatic and include:

- weight loss despite normal appetite
- sweating and heat intolerance
- fatigue
- palpitation – sinus tachycardia or atrial fibrillation
- agitation and tremor
- generalized muscle weakness; proximal myopathy
- angina and heart failure
- diarrhoea
- oligomenorrhoea and subfertility
- goitre
- eyelid retraction and lid lag.

Causes

Hyperthyroidism can result from:

- Graves' disease (diffuse toxic goitre)
- toxic multinodular goitre
- solitary toxic adenoma
- thyroiditis
- exogenously administered iodine and iodine-containing drugs, e.g. amiodarone
- excessive T_4 and T_3 ingestion.

Graves' disease is the most common cause of hyperthyroidism, and is an autoimmune disease in which antibodies to the TSH receptor on the surface of thyroid cells appear to mimic the action of the pituitary hormone. The normal regulatory controls on T_4 synthesis and secretion are lacking. Pituitary secretion of TSH is completely inhibited by the high concentrations of thyroid hormones in the blood. Although the eyelid retraction commonly seen in the patient with Graves' disease (Fig. 3) is due to the effects of high thyroid hormone concentration, not all of the eye

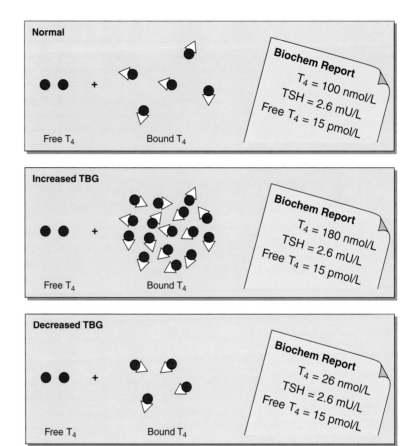

Fig. 1 **The interpretation of thyroid hormone results when TBG concentration changes.**

signs are caused this way. Rather, the thyroid and orbital muscle may have a common antigen that is recognized by the circulating autoantibodies. The inflammatory process in the eye may lead to severe exophthalmos. This may even occur in the euthyroid patient.

Diagnosis

The demonstration of a suppressed TSH concentration and raised thyroid hormone concentration will confirm the diagnosis of primary hyperthyroidism. In particular, the finding that TSH is undetectable in one of the modern sensitive assays for this hormone strongly suggests that

the symptomatic patient has primary hyperthyroidism.

Occasionally, biochemical confirmation of suspected hyperthyroidism will prove more difficult. The total T_4 concentration in a serum sample does not always reflect metabolic status, because of changes in binding protein concentration. In pregnancy, high circulating oestrogens cause stimulation of thyroid binding globulin (TBG) synthesis in the liver. Total T_4 concentrations will be above the reference interval although free T_4 will be normal (Fig. 1). Congenital TBG deficiency can also cause confusion if a specimen is screened for thyroid hormones, even if thyroid disease is not suspected (Fig. 1). TBG deficiency is encountered much less frequently than increased TBG.

Table 1 Thyroid hormone and binding protein results in pregnancy

Patient	T_4 nmol/L (55–144)	T_3 nmol/L (0.9–2.8)	TSH mU/L (0.35–5.0)	TBG mg/L (12–30)	Free T_4 pmol/L (9–24)	Comment
1	130	2.0	3.4	25	18	Euthyroid
2	175	3.6	1.1	35	14	Euthyroid, pregnant
3	190	5.0	<0.05	36	30	Hyperthyroid, pregnant

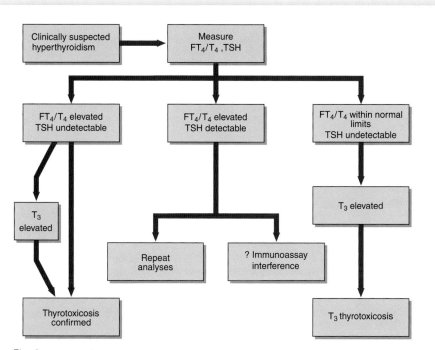

Fig. 2 **Strategy for the biochemical investigation of suspected hyperthyroidism.**

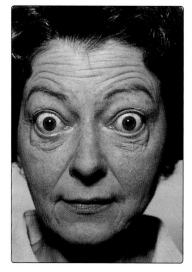

Fig. 3 **Lid retraction and exophthalmos in a patient with Graves' disease.**

Free T_4 assays are routinely used as first-line tests of thyroid dysfunction. TSH secretion is very sensitive to changes in free T_4, and many laboratories use TSH on its own to screen for thyroid disease. Free T_4 analyses are invaluable in diagnoses where binding proteins are altered, e.g. in pregnancy, in women on the oral contraceptive pill and in patients with the nephrotic syndrome (Table 1).

In a few patients with clinical features of hyperthyroidism, total T_4 concentration is found to be within the reference interval. Subsequent investigations reveal an elevated T_3 concentration. This is referred to as 'T_3 toxicosis'. TSH is undetectable in these patients.

A strategy for the biochemical investigation of clinically suspected hyperthyroidism is shown in Figure 2.

Treatment

There are three methods for the treatment of Graves' disease:

- *Antithyroid drugs* (such as carbimazole and propylthiouracil). These are of most use in the younger patient.
- *Radioiodine.* Therapy with sodium ^{131}I is commonly used in older patients. Most will eventually require replacement thyroxine. Thus 'thyroid function tests' should be checked regularly to detect developing hypothyroidism.
- *Surgery.* Many patients who have subtotal thyroidectomy may later require thyroxine replacement. Occasionally the parathyroids may be damaged and the patient may become hypocalcaemic post-operatively due to lack of PTH.

Thyroid function tests are important in the monitoring of all three treatments. In these circumstances it must be remembered that it takes a number of weeks before the tissue effects of thyroid hormones accurately reflect the concentration in the serum.

In particular, TSH may take 6–8 weeks to adjust to its new level.

Thyroid eye disease

Clinically, thyroid eye disease can be a prominent feature of Graves' disease (Fig. 3). It may pursue a separate or similar course to the thyroid disease; typically it takes longer to resolve. It may be exacerbated by the administration of radioiodine, and steroid treatment may be required.

Case history 35

A 28-year-old woman with thyrotoxicosis has had two courses of carbimazole. Results from her recent visit to the thyroid clinic now show:

TSH	Free T_4
mU/L	pmol/L
<0.05	66

- What has happened?
- What other biochemistry might be useful here?

Comment on page 166.

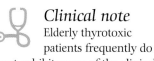

Clinical note

Elderly thyrotoxic patients frequently do not exhibit many of the clinical features of hyperthyroidism. This is called 'apathetic hyperthyroidism'. Isolated idiopathic atrial fibrillation may be the only manifestation in some patients. Others may present with weight loss that may lead to anxiety and a futile search for malignant disease.

Hyperthyroidism

- Autoimmune disease is the commonest cause of hyperthyroidism.
- Diagnosis is confirmed by suppressed TSH and elevated T_4 in a serum specimen, although T_3 concentration, free hormone levels and binding protein status may all be needed in difficult situations.
- The management of hyperthyroidism is by antithyroid drugs, radioiodine therapy or partial thyroidectomy. TSH and T_4 are used to monitor thyroid function after all of these treatments.

Adrenocortical pathophysiology

The hormones of the adrenal (suprarenal) glands are essential for survival. The adrenal cortex is the source of the two important steroid hormones, aldosterone and cortisol (Fig. 1). The adrenal medulla is embryologically and histologically distinct from the cortex and is part of the sympathetic nervous system. Medullary cells synthesize, store and secrete adrenaline, along with noradrenaline and dopamine. The adrenal medullary hormones are discussed further on pages 134–135.

Cortisol

Cortisol is produced in the zona fasciculata and zona reticularis of the adrenal cortex, the end product of a cascade of hormones that make up the hypothalamic–pituitary–adrenocortical axis (Fig. 2). Corticotrophin releasing hormone (CRH) is secreted by the hypothalamus under the influence of cerebral factors. Adrenocorticotrophic hormone (corticotrophin, or simply ACTH) is secreted by the anterior pituitary under the control of CRH to maintain the fascicular and reticular zones of the adrenal cortex and to stimulate the secretion of cortisol. Hypothalamic secretion of CRH and pituitary secretion of ACTH are modulated by cortisol in negative feedback loops.

Adrenal cortex cells have many low-density lipoprotein receptors on their surface. This enables them to take up cholesterol rapidly, from which the adrenal steroid hormones are synthesized (Fig. 3).

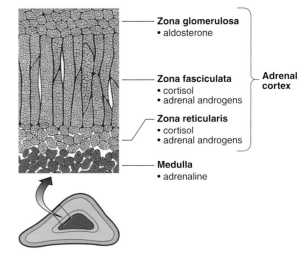

Fig. 1 **The histology of an adrenal gland.**

Zona glomerulosa
• aldosterone

Zona fasciculata
• cortisol
• adrenal androgens

Zona reticularis
• cortisol
• adrenal androgens

Adrenal cortex

Medulla
• adrenaline

The conversion of cholesterol to pregnenolone is the rate-limiting step in the biosynthesis of cortisol; this conversion is stimulated by ACTH. Cortisol biosynthesis from pregnenolone involves the action of a specific reductase/isomerase and three separate hydroxylase enzymes. Inherited defects of all of these enzymes have been characterized.

Cortisol is an important hormone with effects on many tissues in the body. It plays a major role in metabolism by promoting protein breakdown in muscle and connective tissue and the release of glycerol and free fatty acids from adipose tissue. Thus, cortisol provides the substrates necessary for gluconeogenesis, which it promotes in the liver.

Natural or synthetic steroids with cortisol-like effects are called glucocorticoids. Such compounds can act as anti-inflammatory or immunosuppressive agents. Synthetic glucocorticoids have found therapeutic applications in a wide range of clinical situations, e.g. asthma and connective tissue disorders.

Adrenal androgens

The fascicular and reticular zones of the adrenal cortex also produce androgens – androstenedione, DHA (dehydroepiandrosterone) and DHA sulphate. These compounds probably owe their androgenic activity to peripheral conversion to testosterone. In females the adrenal cortex is an important source of androgens, but in

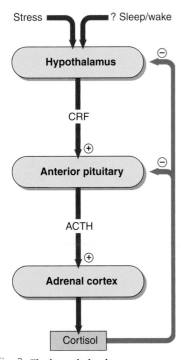

Fig. 2 **The hypothalamic–pituitary–adrenocortical axis.**

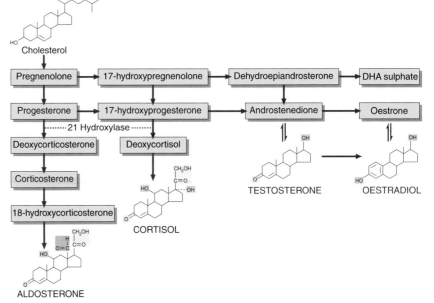

Fig. 3 **Pathways of steroid metabolism.**

adult males this source is insignificant compared with testosterone made by the testes.

Assessing the function of the hypothalamic–pituitary–adrenocortical axis

Cortisol secretion fluctuates widely throughout the day, and single serum measurements are of limited value in clinical practice. There is a marked diurnal rhythm. Dynamic tests of cortisol production involving stimulation of the adrenal cortex by synthetic ACTH, or of stimulation or suppression of the whole HPA axis, form an important part of investigations of adrenocortical hyper- or hypofunction and are discussed on the following pages.

Aldosterone

Aldosterone is produced exclusively by the zona glomerulosa and is primarily controlled by the renin–angiotensin system (p. 15). The metabolic pathway for the synthesis of aldosterone utilizes many of the same enzymes involved in cortisol biosynthesis. The glomerular zone lacks the 17-hydroxylase enzyme and has the additional 18-hydroxylase and 18-hydroxysteroid dehydrogenase enzymes necessary for aldosterone synthesis.

Other factors, including ACTH, are also involved in the regulation of aldosterone synthesis. Aldosterone is responsible for promoting sodium reabsorption and potassium excretion in the kidney.

A natural or synthetic steroid with aldosterone-like activity is called a mineralocorticoid. All of the 21-hydroxylated steroids have mineralocorticoid effects to varying degrees.

Congenital adrenal hyperplasia (CAH)

CAH is the result of an inherited enzyme defect in corticosteroid biosynthesis. The adrenals cannot secrete cortisol and electrolyte disturbances may involve severe hyponatraemia and hyperkalaemia if aldosterone biosynthesis is also affected. If the condition is not diagnosed quickly the afflicted infant may die.

Because of the lack of cortisol, negative feedback to the pituitary is absent and ACTH secretion continues to drive steroid biosynthesis (Fig. 3). Cortisol precursors are secreted in large amounts, their nature depending on which enzyme is lacking. The 21-hydroxylase is the deficient enzyme in 95% of cases of CAH. Here, large amounts of 17-hydroxyprogesterone are secreted. Elevated plasma concentrations are diagnostic as early as 2 days after birth. Increased stimulation of adrenal androgen production can cause virilization in baby girls, and precocious puberty in boys.

One variant of the condition, the late onset form, presents as menstrual irregularity and hirsutism in young women. This is presumably the result of a partial enzyme defect.

Relationship of adrenal cortex and medulla

For a multicellular organism to survive it is essential that the extracellular fluid bathing the tissues is continually circulating so that nutrients may be supplied to the cells and waste products removed from their environment. The adrenal medulla and the two separate hormone systems of the adrenal cortex act in harmony to ensure that this occurs. Adrenaline (epinephrine) and noradrenaline (norepinephrine) through their inotropic effects on the heart and their vasoconstrictor actions on the arterioles maintain the blood pressure and facilitate tissue perfusion. Cortisol facilitates the synthesis of adrenaline and potentiates its vasopressor effects. Cortisol is also required for the efficient excretion of water in the kidney. Aldosterone, through its action in promoting sodium reabsorption, maintains the extracellular volume.

Case history 36

A 40-year-old man was investigated for severe skeletal muscle pains. The following biochemical results in a serum sample were unexpected:

Na⁺	K⁺	Cl⁻	HCO₃⁻	Urea	Creatinine
		mmol/L			*μmol/L*
130	6.1	90	17	7.6	150

- Suggest a likely diagnosis.
- What other biochemistry tests might be helpful in the investigation of this patient?

Comment on page 166.

Clinical note

Stress is the most important stimulus for ACTH secretion and it, along with the sleep/wake-induced ACTH rhythm, will override the negative feedback control mechanisms. As a result, when investigating disturbances in ACTH/cortisol secretion, it is essential to eliminate stress (e.g. due to illness or trauma) and to ensure that a normal sleep/wake cycle has been established.

Adrenocortical pathophysiology

- The adrenal glands comprise three separate hormone systems:
  - the zona glomerulosa, which secretes aldosterone
  - the zona fasciculata and reticularis, which secrete cortisol and the adrenal androgens
  - the adrenal medulla, which secretes adrenaline.

- Steroids with cortisol-like activity are known as glucocorticoids; they are potent metabolic regulators and immunosuppressants.

- Steroids with aldosterone-like activity are called mineralocorticoids; they promote renal sodium retention.

- Adrenal steroid concentrations in serum fluctuate widely. Single measurements are, therefore, of limited value in clinical investigations, and dynamic tests are widely used in diagnosis.

- Congenital adrenal hyperplasia is an inherited enzyme defect in corticosteroid biosynthesis that can prove fatal unless diagnosed early.

- 21-Hydroxylase deficiency is the most commonly encountered form of CAH. The finding of a raised plasma 17-hydroxyprogesterone confirms the diagnosis.

Hypofunction of the adrenal cortex

Adrenal insufficiency

Acute adrenal insufficiency is a rare condition that if unrecognized is potentially fatal. Because of its low incidence it is often overlooked as a possible diagnosis. It is relatively simple to treat once the diagnosis has been made, and patients can lead a normal life. The clinical features of adrenal insufficiency are shown in Figure 1.

In areas where tuberculosis is endemic, adrenal gland destruction may be due to TB; in developed countries autoimmune disease is now the main cause of primary adrenal failure. Both cortisol and aldosterone production may be affected. Secondary failure to produce cortisol is more common. Frequently, this is due to long-standing suppression and subsequent impairment of the hypothalamic–pituitary–adrenocortical axis from therapeutic administration of corticosteroids. The causes of adrenal insufficiency are summarized in Figure 2.

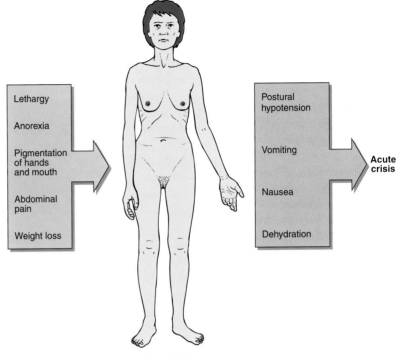

Fig. 1 **Features of adrenocortical insufficiency.**

Biochemical features

In addition to the clinical observations, a number of biochemical results may point towards adrenocortical insufficiency. These are hyponatraemia, hyperkalaemia and elevated serum urea, and may be seen in many patients with Addison's disease.

In primary adrenal insufficiency, patients become hyponatraemic for two reasons. The lack of aldosterone leads to pathological sodium loss by the kidney that results in a contraction of the extracellular fluid volume, causing hypotension and pre-renal uraemia. Patients may develop life-threatening sodium depletion and potassium retention due to aldosterone deficiency.

The hypovolaemia and hypotension stimulate AVP secretion, thus causing water retention. In the absence of cortisol, the kidneys' ability to excrete a water load is impaired, thus exacerbating hyponatraemia. Overall, however, the total body water is reduced and this is reflected by the increase in the serum urea.

Lack of negative feedback of cortisol on the anterior pituitary results in an excessive secretion of ACTH. The structure of this hormone contains part of the amino acid sequence of melanocyte-stimulating hormone. Where excessive ACTH secretion occurs, patients may show darkening of the skin and mucous membranes.

Diagnosis

If a patient is suspected to be suffering from adrenal insufficiency, it is essential to ensure that they have an adequate sodium intake whilst investigations proceed. It is important to remember that patients with adrenal insufficiency are not able to retain sodium effectively, so sodium requirements may be higher than normal.

Random cortisol

Random cortisol measurements are not wholly without value in the initial evaluation of suspected adrenal insufficiency, but caution must be exercised in interpreting the results, and the sample should always be timed.

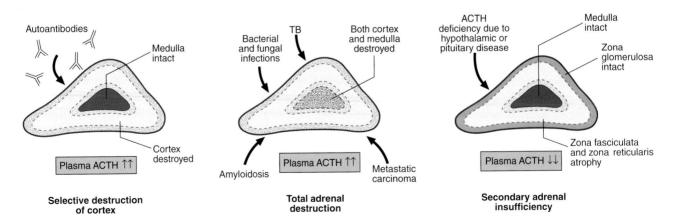

Fig. 2 **Causes of adrenocortical insufficiency.**

A very low or a very high random cortisol result is most useful.

Synacthen tests

Formal diagnosis or exclusion of adrenal insufficiency requires a short Synacthen test (SST) (see below and p. 81). Synacthen is a synthetic 1-24 analogue of ACTH and is administered intravenously at a dose of 250 µg. Cortisol is measured at 0, 30 and sometimes 60 minutes. The criteria for a normal response are shown in Figure 3.

Equivocal or inadequate responses to a SST may require a long Synacthen test (LST) to be performed (see p. 81) in order to establish whether adrenal insufficiency is primary, or secondary to pituitary or hypothalamic disease. Here, depot Synacthen (1 mg) is given intramuscularly daily for 3 days and the SST repeated on the fourth; a normal response makes primary adrenal insufficiency unlikely. Measurement of ACTH may obviate the need for a LST – unequivocally elevated ACTH in the presence of an impaired response to Synacthen confirms the diagnosis of primary adrenal failure.

Relative adrenal insufficiency

Inability to mount an adequate cortisol response is well-recognized in acutely ill patients. Such 'relative adrenal insufficiency' carries a poor prognosis; it may be identified by cortisol levels that are high in absolute terms but by a flat response to Synacthen. This is the only context in which the increment in cortisol is as useful as the other criteria for a normal response.

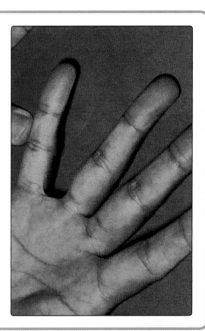

Fig. 4 **Pigmented skin creases in patient with primary adrenal insufficiency.**

Clinical note

Primary adrenal insufficiency may have an insidious onset. Pallor is a characteristic feature, as is dry flaky skin with pigmentation especially in palmar creases and pressure points (Fig. 4). Patients may present asymptomatically with apparently isolated hyperkalaemia or hyponatraemia. Addison's disease must always be considered as a possible diagnosis in patients with raised serum potassium, especially if they do not have renal failure.

Isolated aldosterone deficiency

This is rare and may be due to an adrenal lesion, such as an 18-hydroxylase defect, or to primary renin deficiency, as in the anephric patient.

Case history 37

A 31-year-old woman was admitted to a surgical ward with a 2-day history of abdominal pain and vomiting. Her blood pressure was 110/65 mmHg and her pulse 88 beats per minute and regular. A provisional diagnosis of intestinal obstruction was made. On admission, tests showed:

Na+	K+	Cl⁻	HCO₃⁻	Urea	Creatinine
		—mmol/L———			µmol/L
128	6.1	92	18	10.8	180

She was given 1.5 L of 0.9% saline intravenously, overnight, and the following morning her symptoms had resolved. Her serum sodium had increased to 134 mmol/L and her serum potassium had fallen to 4.8 mmol/L. On reviewing her history, it was found she had been unwell for a number of months with weight loss and anorexia. She was noted to be pigmented.

A short Synacthen test was performed and the serum cortisol was less than 60 mmol/L both before and after an intravenous injection of 0.25 mg of Synacthen.

■ Suggest the diagnosis.
■ How could the changes in her sodium and potassium be explained?

Comment on page 166.

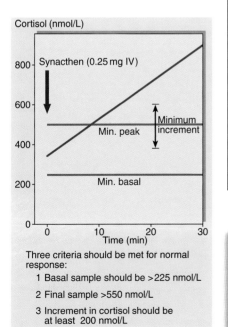

Three criteria should be met for normal response:

1 Basal sample should be >225 nmol/L

2 Final sample >550 nmol/L

3 Increment in cortisol should be at least 200 nmol/L

Fig. 3 **Synacthen test responses.**
Synacthen is given iv after basal blood samples have been taken.

Hypofunction of the adrenal cortex

■ Adrenocortical insufficiency is rare, but life-threatening.

■ Failure of the adrenal cortex to produce cortisol and aldosterone may be due to autoimmune or infiltrative diseases.

■ The Synacthen test is used in diagnosis of primary adrenocortical failure.

■ The insulin stress test is used in diagnosis of pituitary insufficiency that may lead to secondary failure of the adrenal cortex.

■ The mainstay of therapy is maintenance of sodium intake and appropriate hormone replacement.

Hyperfunction of the adrenal cortex

Hyperfunction of the adrenal cortex can be conveniently discussed in terms of the overproduction of the three main products:

- cortisol
- adrenal androgens
- aldosterone.

Cortisol excess

Prolonged exposure of body tissues to cortisol or other glucocorticoids gives rise to the clinical features that collectively are known as Cushing's syndrome (Fig. 1), after the American neurosurgeon Harvey Cushing. It most often results from prolonged use of steroid medications (iatrogenic). Much less frequently, it is caused by tumours that secrete either cortisol or ACTH (see below); these can sometimes be very difficult to diagnose.

In any investigation of Cushing's syndrome the clinician should ask two questions:

- 'Does the patient actually have Cushing's syndrome?' The possibility that a patient may have Cushing's syndrome frequently arises because they are obese or hypertensive, conditions frequently encountered in the population at large. Initial investigations will in most cases exclude the diagnosis of Cushing's syndrome.
- Once the diagnosis of Cushing's syndrome is established, then a second question may be asked: 'What is the cause of the excess cortisol secretion?' Tests used in the differential diagnosis are different from those used to confirm the presence of cortisol overproduction.

Confirming the diagnosis

Iatrogenic Cushing's syndrome is usually obvious – the patient is on steroid medications. The steroid may have been taken orally, inhaled or applied topically. Iatrogenic Cushing's syndrome is not usually a diagnostic dilemma and will not be considered further here.

Cortisol, secreted in excess by the adrenal cortex, will rapidly exceed the available capacity of the plasma binding protein, cortisol binding globulin. Unbound cortisol is filtered readily into the urine. 'Urinary free cortisol' in a 24-hour collection, or assessed as a cortisol:creatinine ratio in an early morning urine sample, is one of the initial screening tests in a patient with suspected adrenocortical hyperfunction. The latter measurement can be made on a small aliquot of urine. Repeatedly high early morning urine cortisol:

creatinine ratios are evidence enough to proceed with further investigations of the patient. If the test is negative on three occasions, Cushing's syndrome may be excluded from the differential diagnosis.

Cortisol concentrations measured at 08:00 and 22:00 normally show a circadian rhythm with the evening sample having a lower value than that in the morning. This difference is usually not apparent in the patient with Cushing's syndrome. It is essential that the patients are not stressed when such measurements are made.

Failure of 1 mg of dexamethasone taken at 23:00 to suppress the serum cortisol level at 08:00 the following morning, or failure to suppress urinary cortisol secretion overnight (as measured by an early morning urine cortisol:creatinine ratio), is another pointer towards the presence of Cushing's syndrome.

Failure of the serum cortisol to rise after insulin-induced hypoglycaemia is also a characteristic feature of Cushing's syndrome. Since patients with cortisol overproduction will be insulin-resistant, adequate hypoglycaemia may not be achieved with 0.15 units of insulin/kg body weight. A higher dose may have to be used. In normal individuals a fall of blood glucose concentration to less than 2.2 mmol/L is accompanied by a rise in serum cortisol of more than 200 nmol/L. A patient who shows such a response in the IST is unlikely to have a pathological excess of cortisol production.

Determining the cause

The possible causes of Cushing's syndrome are illustrated in Figure 2. These include:

- pituitary adenoma
- ectopic ACTH
- adrenal adenoma
- adrenal carcinoma.

Classically, ACTH is not detectable in the plasma of patients with adrenal tumours. In patients with pituitary-dependent Cushing's syndrome (known somewhat confusingly as *Cushing's disease*) the plasma ACTH may be within the reference range or modestly elevated. The plasma ACTH level is often very high in patients with ectopic ACTH production.

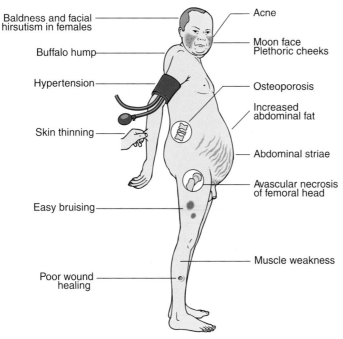

Baldness and facial hirsutism in females

Buffalo hump

Hypertension

Skin thinning

Easy bruising

Poor wound healing

Acne

Moon face
Plethoric cheeks

Osteoporosis

Increased abdominal fat

Abdominal striae

Avascular necrosis of femoral head

Muscle weakness

Fig. 1 **Some clinical features of Cushing's syndrome.**

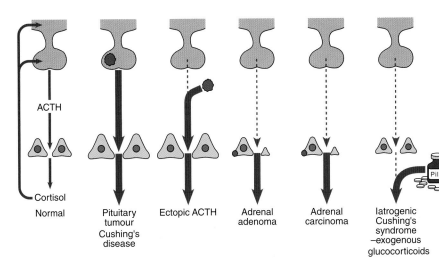

Fig. 2 **The possible causes of Cushing's syndrome.**

In patients with pituitary-dependent Cushing's disease the serum or urinary cortisol will be partially suppressed after 2 days of dexamethasone, 2.0 mg q.i.d. (Fig. 3). Failure to suppress suggests either ectopic ACTH production or the autonomous secretion of cortisol by an adrenal tumour.

The cause of Cushing's syndrome will determine the therapeutic options, and it is therefore essential that a definitive diagnosis is made. CT scans or magnetic resonance imaging of the pituitary may be helpful in detecting a pituitary adenoma in patients with Cushing's disease. Selective venous sampling with ACTH measurement is sometimes carried out to locate the ACTH source in difficult cases.

Androgen excess

Adrenocortical tumours, particularly adrenal carcinomas, may produce excess androgens (DHA, androstenedione and testosterone) causing hirsutism and/or virilization in females (see pp. 98–99). This may not necessarily be accompanied by cortisol excess, and signs of Cushing's syndrome may be absent. Patients with congenital adrenal hyperplasia (p. 93) may also present with signs of increased androgen production.

Aldosterone excess

Primary hyperaldosteronism (Conn's syndrome) is rare. In most cases, the disease is due to a single adrenocortical adenoma. Patients may present with polydipsia and polyuria, symptoms of neuromuscular abnormalities such as weakness, paraesthesiae and tetany, and hypertension. All symptoms other than hypertension are attributable to potassium depletion.

Preliminary investigations must include determination of serum and urine electrolytes over several days, with adequate sodium intake. Serum potassium will be low, and urinary potassium excretion will be elevated. Documented, careful collection of specimens for assay of aldosterone, renin or 'plasma renin activity', may be made on 2 consecutive days after 8 hours recumbency, and again with the patient ambulatory, to confirm the diagnosis.

The diagnosis of hyperaldosteronism may be made in the hypokalaemic patient if the serum aldosterone level exceeds the upper limit of normal or if the level is persistently inappropriate to the serum potassium. In primary hyperaldosteronism, where the excess aldosterone arises from an adrenal adenoma, the levels of plasma renin will be low.

Secondary hyperaldosteronism is common and is associated with renal, heart or liver disease.

Case history 38

A 31-year-old woman presented with a 3-month history of weight gain, hirsutism, amenorrhoea and hypertension. Her urine cortisol:creatinine ratio was increased, and serum cortisol diurnal rhythm was absent. Treatment with 0.5 mg of dexamethasone q.i.d. did not suppress her cortisol, and insulin-induced hypoglycaemia did not cause her serum cortisol to rise.

■ What investigations should now be carried out?

Comment on page 166.

Clinical note
Excessive alcohol intake can cause *pseudo-Cushing's syndrome* when patients may present with hypertension, truncal obesity, plethora or acne. Preliminary investigations may demonstrate hypercortisolism, which may fail to suppress with dexamethasone. The biochemical features of Cushing's syndrome will resolve after 2 or 3 weeks of abstinence.

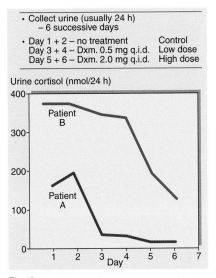

- Collect urine (usually 24 h)
  – 6 successive days
- Day 1 + 2 – no treatment   Control
  Day 3 + 4 – Dxm. 0.5 mg q.i.d.   Low dose
  Day 5 + 6 – Dxm. 2.0 mg q.i.d.   High dose

Fig. 3 **The dexamethasone suppression test.** Patient A showed a >75% fall in urinary cortisol excretion on the low dose. This is a **normal response.** Patient B showed some suppression of cortisol secretion on the high dose. This is typical of **pituitary-dependent Cushing's syndrome.**

Hyperfunction of the adrenal cortex

■ Cushing's syndrome can be a difficult diagnosis to make.

■ To confirm hypercortisolism, early morning urinary cortisol:creatinine ratios will be elevated, diurnal rhythm of serum cortisol will be absent, there will be no cortisol rise during an insulin-stress test, and serum cortisol will not suppress with a low dose of dexamethasone.

■ Once the diagnosis of Cushing's syndrome has been made, the cause can be established by the high-dose dexamethasone suppression test and by measuring ACTH.

■ Clinical and biochemical evidence of increased adrenal androgens may be present.

■ Primary excess of aldosterone is rare and due usually to an adenoma (Conn's syndrome).

Gonadal function

Sex steroid hormones

Testosterone is the principal androgen and is synthesized by the testes in the male. Oestradiol, which is secreted by the ovaries, varies widely in concentration in plasma throughout the female menstrual cycle. Steroids with oestradiol-like action are called oestrogens. Progesterone is also a product of the ovary and is secreted when a corpus luteum forms after ovulation. Normal female plasma also contains a low concentration of testosterone, about half of which comes from the ovary and half from peripheral conversion of androstenedione and dehydroepiandrosterone (DHA) sulphate, which are secreted by the adrenal cortex. Some oestradiol is present in low concentration in normal male plasma.

Testosterone and oestradiol circulate in plasma mostly bound to plasma proteins, particularly sex hormone-binding globulin (SHBG). The plasma concentration of SHBG in females is twice that in males. In both sexes the effect of an increase in SHBG is to increase oestradiol-like effects, whereas a decrease in SHBG increases androgen effects.

Testosterone and SHBG concentrations are sometimes reported by the laboratory as a ratio (the free androgen index), which gives a clearer indication of androgen status than does serum testosterone alone.

Hypothalamic–pituitary–gonadal axis

The episodic secretion of the hypothalamic hormone, gonadotrophin-releasing hormone (GnRH), stimulates synthesis and release of the gonadotrophins, LH (luteinizing hormone) and FSH (follicle-stimulating hormone), from the anterior pituitary. Despite the names, both gonadotrophins act cooperatively on the ovaries in the woman and the testes in the man to stimulate sex hormone secretion and reproductive processes.

Male gonadal function

The testes secrete testosterone and manufacture spermatozoa. Before puberty, gonadotrophin and testosterone concentrations in plasma are very low. The development of the Leydig cells and their secretion of testosterone is influenced by LH, whereas Sertoli cell function is influenced by FSH (Fig. 1). Testosterone is responsible for the development of the male secondary sex characteristics such as hair growth, deep voice and characteristic musculature.

Disorders of male sex hormones

Hypogonadism may result in deficient sperm production and decreased testosterone secretion. This may be due to a testicular deficiency (primary disorders or hypergonadotrophic hypogonadism) or to a defect in the hypothalamus or pituitary (secondary disorders or hypogonadotrophic hypogonadism). In hypogonadotrophic hypogonadism both gonadotrophins, or only LH, may be absent. There may be a generalized failure of pituitary function.

Causes of primary hypogonadism include:

- congenital defects such as Klinefelter's syndrome or testicular agenesis
- acquired defects due to testicular infections (e.g. mumps), trauma, irradiation, or cytotoxic drugs.

Causes of secondary hypogonadism include:

- pituitary tumours
- hypothalamic disorders such as Kallmann's syndrome.

Dynamic tests such as stimulation with GnRH may help to establish the cause of the hypogonadism in some patients.

Disorders of male sexual differentiation

Disorders of male sexual differentiation are rare. Testosterone production may be impaired. In the testicular feminization syndrome, androgen receptors are inactive and target tissues

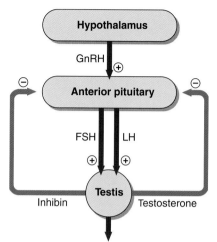

Fig. 1 **Control of testicular function by the gonadotrophins.**

cannot respond to stimulation by circulating testosterone.

Female gonadal function

Oestradiol is responsible for:

- female secondary sex characteristics
- stimulation of follicular growth
- development of the endometrium.

Concentrations are low before puberty, but then rise rapidly and fluctuate cyclically during reproductive life. After the menopause, plasma oestradiol concentrations fall despite high circulating concentrations of the gonadotrophins.

The normal hormonal control of the menstrual cycle is shown in Figure 2. At the beginning of the cycle, FSH is released and initiates follicular growth. At mid-cycle a surge of LH triggers ovulation. The ruptured follicle differentiates into the corpus luteum that secretes progesterone and oestradiol whose target is the endometrium, which it prepares for implantation.

Disorders of female sex hormones

Disorders of female sex hormones include:

- *Subfertility, amenorrhoea and oligomenorrhoea* (see p. 100).

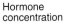
Hormone
concentration

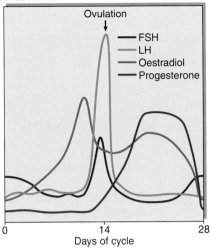

Fig. 2 **Plasma hormone concentrations throughout the female menstrual cycle.**

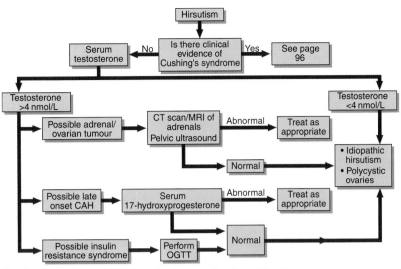

Fig. 3 **Diagnostic decision chart for the investigation of hirsutism.**

- *Hirsutism.* This is an increase in body hair with male pattern distribution. It may be idiopathic but the commonest pathological cause is obesity (insulin resistance) often in association with polycystic ovarian disease. It is essential when investigating hirsute women that serious disease is excluded. A diagnostic decision chart for the investigation of hirsutism is shown in Figure 3.

- *Virilism.* Although uncommon it is a sign of serious disease. Testosterone concentrations are markedly elevated in the virilized patient and there is evidence of excessive androgen action such as clitoral enlargement, hair growth in a male pattern, deepening of the voice and breast atrophy. Tumours of the ovary or of the adrenal are the likely cause.

The androgen screen in women

The observation of an elevated testosterone in a woman should always be investigated further. A decreased SHBG concentration is evidence of elevated androgen, as the synthesis of this protein in the liver is depressed by testosterone. By measuring the concentration of other androgens such as androstenedione and DHA sulphate (an 'androgen screen'), the source of the testosterone can be pinpointed (Fig. 4). An elevated DHA sulphate suggests that the adrenal, or an adrenal tumour, is overproducing androgens. If the ovary is the source then only androstenedione will be raised.

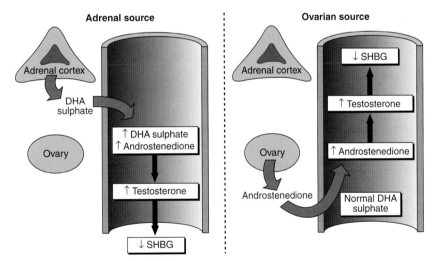

Fig. 4 **Investigation of an elevated testosterone concentration in a woman.**

Case history 39

A 29-year-old woman complained of acne and irregular periods. On examination she was overweight and moderately hirsute.

Initial investigations showed a slightly elevated testosterone of 3.7 nmol/L. LH was 15 U/L and FSH 5.6 U/L.

- What other investigations should be undertaken to make a diagnosis in this patient?

Comment on page 166.

Gonadal function

- Testosterone is the main hormone secreted by the testes in the male and is regulated by pituitary LH. Testosterone is responsible for the male secondary sex characteristics.

- Oestradiol is the main product of the ovary and is responsible for the female secondary sex characteristics, development of the ovarian follicle and proliferation of the uterine epithelium.

- Hypogonadism in the male may be primary (where the cause is a failure of testosterone synthesis or of spermatogenesis in the testes) or secondary where the problem is in the hypothalamus or pituitary.

- Gonadal dysfunction in women may present as primary or secondary amenorrhoea, infertility, hirsutism or virilism.

Subfertility

Subfertility is defined as the failure of a couple to conceive after 1 year of regular, unprotected intercourse. A full clinical history obtained prior to physical examinations should seek information about previous pregnancies, contraceptive practice, serious illnesses, past chemotherapy or radiotherapy, congenital abnormalities, smoking habits, drug usage, sexually transmitted disease and the frequency of intercourse. Physical examination should look for indications of hypothalamic–pituitary or thyroid disorders, Cushing's syndrome, galactorrhoea and hirsutism. In the male, semen analysis should detail volume, sperm density, motility and the presence of abnormal spermatozoa.

In the female, endocrine abnormalities are found in one-third of patients. Hormone dysfunction is a very rare cause of male subfertility. In some couples no cause can be identified.

Endocrine investigations in the subfertile woman

The investigation of the infertile female depends on the phase of the menstrual cycle. If there is a regular menstrual cycle, serum progesterone should be measured in the middle of the luteal phase (day 21). If progesterone is high (>30 nmol/L), the patient has ovulated and there is no need for further endocrine investigations. Other causes of subfertility should be sought. If progesterone is low (<10 nmol/L), ovulation has not occurred.

In women who present with irregular or absent menstruation (oligomenorrhoea or amenorrhoea) or who are not ovulating, hormone measurements may be diagnostic. A protocol for investigation is shown in Figure 1. Measurement of oestradiol and gonadotrophin concentrations may detect primary ovarian failure or polycystic ovarian disease. Measurement of prolactin, and androgens, may also assist.

Endocrine causes of subfertility in women include:

- *Excessive androgen secretion by the ovaries in response to insulin resistance.* This is commonly a feature of central obesity.
- *Primary ovarian failure.* This is indicated by elevated gonadotrophins and low oestradiol concentration (a postmenopausal pattern). Hormone replacement therapy assists libido and prevents osteoporosis, but does not restore fertility.
- *Hyperprolactinaemia* (pp. 82–83).
- *Polycystic ovarian disease.* This is indicated by an elevated LH and normal FSH. Oestradiol measurements are often unhelpful. Hirsutism, a feature of this condition, is associated with raised testosterone and subnormal sex hormone binding protein concentrations.
- *Cushing's syndrome* (pp. 96–97).
- *Hypogonadotrophic hypogonadism.* Rarely, subnormal gonadotrophin and oestradiol concentrations suggest the presence of a hypothalamic–pituitary

lesion such as interference from a pituitary tumour.

Endocrine investigations in the subfertile man

In the eugonadal male with normal sperm analysis, no endocrine investigations are required. In the hypogonadal male, testosterone and the gonadotrophins should be measured first (Fig. 2). Causes of subfertility in the male include:

- *Primary testicular failure.* Where both the interstitial cells and tubules are damaged, FSH and LH will be elevated and testosterone reduced. Where tubular function only is impaired, FSH is selectively increased and androgen levels may be normal.
- *Hypothalamic–pituitary disease.* Decreased testosterone with low or normal gonadotrophins suggests hypogonadotrophic hypogonadism.
- *Hyperprolactinaemia.* This is a rare cause of subfertility in the male (pp. 82–83).

> ## Subfertility
>
> - Endocrine problems are a common cause of subfertility in the female but are rare in the male.
> - An elevated serum progesterone in a specimen at day 21 of the menstrual cycle indicates that ovulation has occurred.
> - In both men and women a serum FSH concentration greater than 25 U/L indicates primary gonadal failure.
> - Hyperprolactinaemia is a common cause of female subfertility.

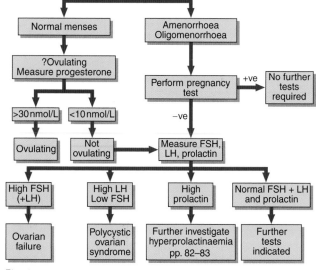

Fig. 1 **Diagnostic approach to subfertility in the woman.**

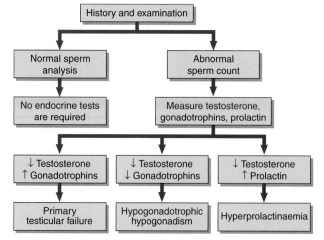

Fig. 2 **Diagnostic approach to subfertility in the man.**

Specialized Investigations

Nutritional assessment

Malnutrition is a common problem worldwide, and in developed countries it is associated particularly with poverty and alcoholism. It is also encountered among patients in hospital. Various studies have shown that patients may have evidence, not only of protein-calorie malnutrition, but also of vitamin and mineral deficiencies, especially after major surgery or chronic illness.

Malnutrition to the layman usually means starvation, but the term has a much wider meaning encompassing both the inadequacy of any nutrient in the diet as well as *excess* food intake. The pathogenesis of malnutrition is shown in Figure 1.

Malnutrition related to surgery or following severe injury occurs because of the extensive metabolic changes that accompany these events: the 'metabolic response to injury' (pp. 108–109).

The assessment of a patient suspected of suffering from malnutrition is based on:

- history
- examination
- laboratory investigations including biochemistry.

History

Past medical history may point to changes in weight, poor wound healing or increased susceptibility to infection. The ability to take a good *dietary* history is one of the most important parts of a full nutritional assessment. Taking a dietary history may involve recording in detail the food and drink intake of the patient over a 7-day period. More usually, however, a few simple questions may yield a lot of useful information about a person's diet. Depending on the background to the problem, different questions will be appropriate. For example, in the wasted patient, questions about appetite and general food intake may suggest an eating disorder such as anorexia nervosa, but in the patient presenting with a skin rash, details of the specific food groups eaten will be required to help exclude a dietary cause. In the patient at increased risk of coronary heart disease, questions on saturated fat intake may be most revealing.

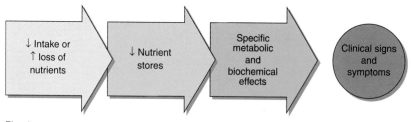

Fig. 1 **The development of malnutrition.**

Examination

Simple anthropometric measurements will include height, weight, arm circumference and skin-fold thickness.

Body mass index (weight in kg divided by the height squared in metres) is a reasonable indicator of nutritional state, except when the patient is oedematous. Arm circumference is an indicator of skeletal muscle mass, while skin-fold thickness is proportional to body fat levels. In addition, general physical examination may reveal signs of malnutrition in the skin, nails, hair, teeth and mucous membranes.

Biochemistry

A number of biochemical tests are used to complement the history and examination in assessing the general nutritional status of a patient. None are completely satisfactory and should never be used in isolation. The most common tests include:

- *Protein.* Serum albumin concentration is a widely used but insensitive indicator of protein nutritional status. It is affected by many factors other than nutrition,

e.g. hepatic and renal diseases and the hydration of the patient. Serum albumin concentration rapidly falls as part of the metabolic response to injury, and the decrease may be mistakenly attributed to malnutrition.

- *Blood glucose concentration.* This will be maintained even in the face of prolonged starvation. Ketosis develops during starvation and carbohydrate deficiency. Hyperglycaemia is frequently encountered as part of the metabolic response to injury.
- *Lipids.* Fasting plasma triglyceride levels provide some indication of fat metabolism, but are again affected by a variety of metabolic processes. Essential fatty acid levels may be measured if specific deficiencies are suspected. Faecal fat may be measured both qualitatively and quantitatively in the assessment of malabsorption (pp. 110–111).

Unlike the assessment of overall status, biochemical measurements play a key role in identifying excesses or deficiencies of specific components of the diet. Both blood and urine results may be of value. Such assays include:

Table 1 **Classification of vitamins**		
Vitamins	**Deficiency state**	**Lab assessment**
Water soluble		
C (Ascorbate)	Scurvy	Plasma or leucocyte levels
B_1 (Thiamin)	Beri-beri	Plasma levels or RBC transketolase activation
B_2 (Riboflavin)	Rarely single deficiency	Plasma levels or RBC glutathione reductase activation
B_6 (Pyridoxine)	Dermatitis/Anaemia	Plasma levels or RBC AST activation
B_{12} (Cobalamin)	Pernicious anaemia	Serum B_{12}, full blood count
Folate	Megaloblastic anaemia	Serum folate, RBC folate, full blood count
Niacin	Pellagra	Urinary niacin metabolites
Fat soluble		
A (Retinol)	Blindness	Serum vitamin A
D (Cholecalciferol)	Osteomalacia/rickets	Serum 25-hydroxycholecalciferol
E (Tocopherol)	Anaemia/neuropathy	Serum vitamin E
K (Phytomenadione)	Defective clotting	Prothrombin time

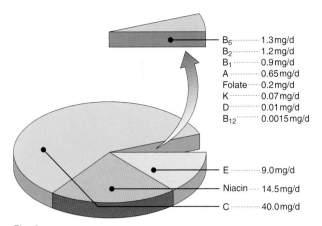

Fig. 2 **Average adult daily requirements of vitamins.**

B$_6$	1.3 mg/d
B$_2$	1.2 mg/d
B$_1$	0.9 mg/d
A	0.65 mg/d
Folate	0.2 mg/d
K	0.07 mg/d
D	0.01 mg/d
B$_{12}$	0.0015 mg/d
E	9.0 mg/d
Niacin	14.5 mg/d
C	40.0 mg/d

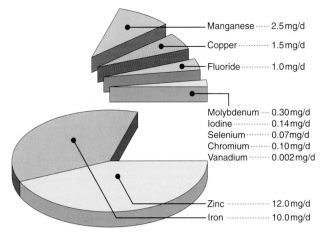

Fig. 3 **Average adult daily requirements of essential trace elements.**

Manganese	2.5 mg/d
Copper	1.5 mg/d
Fluoride	1.0 mg/d
Molybdenum	0.30 mg/d
Iodine	0.14 mg/d
Selenium	0.07 mg/d
Chromium	0.10 mg/d
Vanadium	0.002 mg/d
Zinc	12.0 mg/d
Iron	10.0 mg/d

■ *Vitamins*. These organic compounds are not synthesized by the body but are vital for normal metabolism. Usually they are classified by their solubility; they are listed in Table 1 and their average adult daily requirements shown in Figure 2. Some assays are available to measure the blood levels of vitamins directly, but often functional assays that utilize the fact that many vitamins are enzyme cofactors are used. These latter assays may help identify gross abnormalities. However, to detect subtle deficiencies and the increasing problem of excess intake, quantitative measurements are required.

■ *Major minerals*. These inorganic elements are present in the body in quantities greater than 5 g. The main nutrients in this category are sodium, potassium, chloride, calcium, phosphorus and magnesium. All of these are readily measurable in blood and their levels in part reflect dietary intake.

■ *Trace elements*. Inorganic elements present in the body in quantities less than 5 g are often found in complexes with proteins. The essential trace elements are shown in Figure 3.

Preoperative nutritional assessment

Nutritional assessment is not only necessary following surgical procedures. Patients need to be in good nutritional condition before an operation and the assessment should be done well in advance to allow build-up of reserves before surgery (Fig. 4).

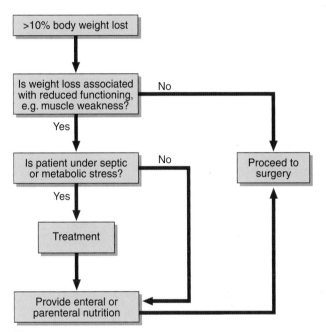

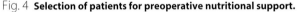

Fig. 4 **Selection of patients for preoperative nutritional support.**

Flowchart:
- >10% body weight lost
- Is weight loss associated with reduced functioning, e.g. muscle weakness? — No → Proceed to surgery
- Yes
- Is patient under septic or metabolic stress? — No → Proceed to surgery
- Yes
- Treatment
- Provide enteral or parenteral nutrition

Clinical note

Accurate measurement of height and weight are the most important features of global nutritional assessment at all stages of life – from the neonatal period to old age. These are also often very poorly recorded in patient notes.

Case history 40

A 68-year-old man with motor neuron disease is admitted because of severe anorexia and weight loss. Suspecting malnutrition, the house officer requests a battery of biochemical tests including serum vitamin E and selenium.

■ How useful will these be in the management of this patient?

Comment on page 166.

Nutritional assessment

■ Nutritional assessment is important in every patient.

■ Malnutrition is common and usually reflects the inadequacy of any nutrient or nutrients in the diet.

■ History, examination and laboratory investigations are complementary.

■ A variety of biochemical investigations may assist in the diagnosis of nutritional deficiencies and in the monitoring of patients undergoing nutritional support.

Nutritional support

Nutritional support may range from simple dietary advice to long-term total parenteral nutrition (TPN). In between is a whole spectrum of clinical conditions and appropriate forms of nutritional support (Fig. 1). As we move to the right, climbing the scale of severity of disease, we increase the level of support and in so doing increase the need for laboratory back-up. The clinical biochemistry laboratory plays an important role in the diagnosis of some disorders that require specific nutritional intervention, e.g. diabetes mellitus, iron deficiency anaemia and hyperlipidaemia, but a much greater role is played in the monitoring of patients receiving the different forms of nutritional support.

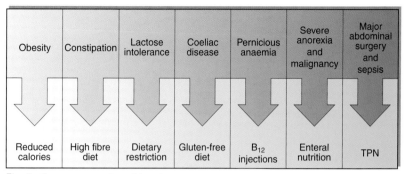

Fig. 1 **The spectrum of nutritional support.**

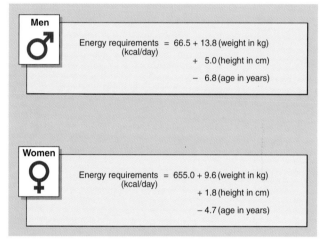

Fig. 2 **The Harris–Benedict equation.**

What do patients need?

Assessing the dietary needs of some patients is a highly specialized task, but some general guidelines can be considered. A balanced mix of nutrients must contain adequate provision for growth, healing and pathological losses, e.g. a draining fistula. Where patients are able to eat a mixed diet, the detailed consideration of their specific dietary intakes is seldom an issue. However, for those patients where the clinical team has to assume the responsibility of providing the balance of nutrients, much greater care must be taken.

Energy

Patients require energy, the amount of which can be roughly calculated from the Harris–Benedict equation (Fig. 2). This formula provides the basal energy requirements of an individual, and these must be adjusted to take account of increased requirements or losses as described above.

The principal energy sources in the diet are carbohydrates and fats. Glucose provides 4 kcal/g while fat provides 9 kcal/g. The entire calorie load may be administered using carbohydrates, but prescribing a mixture of carbohydrates and lipids is more physiological and serves to reduce the volume of the diet. This is important in tube feeding as well as in parenteral nutrition.

Nitrogen

Proteins and the amino acids provide nitrogen and also yield energy at 4 kcal/g. Amino acids are essential both for protein synthesis and for the synthesis of other nitrogen-containing compounds. Usually it is recommended that protein intake should constitute 10–15% of the total calorie requirement. Positive nitrogen balance can only be achieved if the energy intake is at least adequate to cover the resting energy expenditure. The protein needs can be calculated from knowledge of urinary urea excretion (Fig. 3). This dictates amino acid needs as well as the energy requirements to ensure that protein synthesis takes place.

Vitamins and trace elements

Vitamins and trace elements are collectively described as 'micronutrients', not because they are of limited importance, but because they are required in relatively small amounts. Recommended dietary allowances (RDAs) have been

defined for most nutrients and these are used in the make-up of artificial diets.

How should they receive it?

Patients may be fed in the following ways:

- oral feeding
- tube feeding into the gut
- parenteral feeding.

Oral feeding should be used whenever possible. Tube feeding (Fig. 4) involves the use of small bore nasogastric, nasoduodenal and gastrostomy tubes. Defined diets of homogeneous composition can be continually administered. Tube feeding in this way bypasses problems with oral pathology, swallowing difficulties (e.g. after a stroke) and anorexia. Even patients who have had gastric surgery can be tube fed postoperatively if a feeding

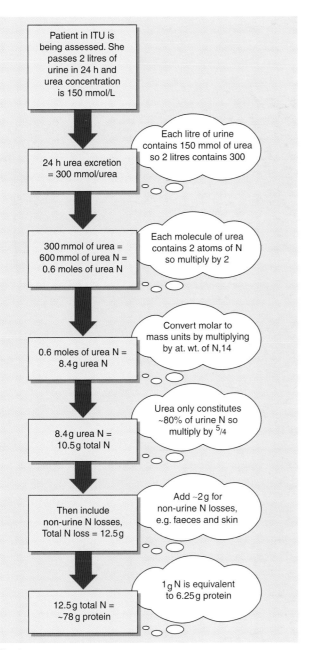

Fig. 3 **Urine urea measurements over 24 hours may be used to assess nitrogen balance.**

jejunostomy is fashioned during the operation distal to the lesion. However, tube feeding also presents mechanical problems in terms of blockage or oesophageal erosion. Gastrointestinal problems such as vomiting and diarrhoea, and metabolic problems can be minimized by the gradual introduction of the feeds and are rarely contraindications to enteral feeding. The problems associated with parenteral nutrition are even more severe and are discussed on pages 106–107. It should be noted, however, that the vast majority of patients can be fed very successfully either orally or with enteral tube feeds.

Monitoring patients

Clinical and biochemical monitoring should always go hand in hand in the assessment of any form of nutritional support. In some circumstances the contribution of the laboratory may be the simple measurement of blood glucose, while in other situations the measurements and advice provided by the lab may dictate the regimen in a patient receiving parenteral nutrition.

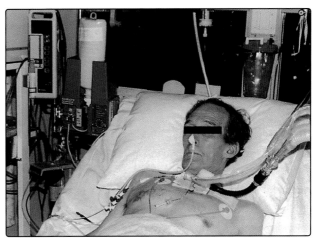

Fig. 4 **Patient on tube feeding in ITU.** Note this patient is also being ventilated via a tracheostomy and has a central line in place.

Case history 41

A patient with pernicious anaemia is being treated with parenteral vitamin B_{12}. Because she has recently been feeling tired and 'run down', her physician sends a sample to the clinical biochemistry lab requesting a serum B_{12} level.

■ Is this the most appropriate way to monitor the patient?

Comment on page 166.

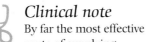
Clinical note
By far the most effective route of supplying nutrients to a patient is via the gut. By using nasogastric tubes and electively inserted stoma tubes to the stomach or small intestine, only a small minority of patients will require to be fed parenterally.

Nutritional support

■ Nutritional support is required in a wide spectrum of conditions.

■ It consists of a variety of approaches, from simple dietary advice to total parenteral nutrition.

■ The route of first choice for nutritional support is oral followed by enteral followed by parenteral.

■ Careful clinical and laboratory monitoring is required to some extent in all forms of nutritional support.

■ Most laboratory support is needed for those patients receiving parenteral nutrition.

Parenteral nutrition

The provision of nutrients to the body's cells is a highly complex physiological process involving many endocrine, exocrine and other metabolic functions. Total parenteral nutrition (TPN) completely bypasses the gastrointestinal tract, delivering processed nutrients directly into the venous blood. It is more physiological to feed patients enterally and parenteral nutrition should only be considered once other possibilities have been deemed unsuitable. The institution of TPN is never an emergency and there should always be time for consultation and for baseline measurements to be performed. A team approach is desirable (Fig. 1).

Indications for parenteral nutrition

Patients who are unable to eat or absorb food adequately from the gastrointestinal tract should be considered for parenteral nutrition. The circumstances where this occurs include:

- inflammatory bowel disease, e.g Crohn's disease
- short bowel syndrome, e.g. mesenteric artery infarction.

Route of administration

Parenteral nutrition may be given in the following ways:

- *Via peripheral veins.* This route may be successfully used for a short period of 1–2 weeks.
- *Via a central venous catheter.* This route is used where long-term IV. feeding is anticipated. Central vein catheters may remain patent for years if cared for properly.

Although most recipients of TPN are inpatients, many individuals who require long-term TPN have successfully managed to administer TPN in the home. These patients have permanent central catheters through which prepackaged nutrition fluids are administered, usually at night.

Components of TPN

TPN should, as its name suggests, provide complete artificial nutrition. An appropriate volume of fluid will

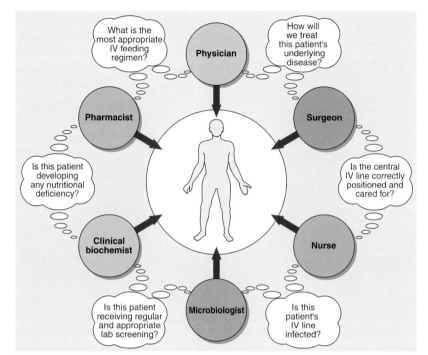

Fig. 1 **Team approach to TPN.**

contain a source of calories, amino acids, vitamins and trace elements (Fig. 2). The calorie source is a mixture of glucose and lipid. Many patients who receive TPN are given standard proprietary regimens and prepackaged solutions. These have made TPN much easier, but as with any such approach in medicine there are some patients who require more tailored regimens.

Complications

Total parenteral nutrition is the most extreme form of nutritional support and can give rise to considerable difficulties. In order to pre-empt these,

consistent careful nursing care and biochemical monitoring are required.

Catheter site sepsis is a constant fear in these patients. The nutrient-containing infusion fluids are, of course, also excellent bacterial and fungal growth media, and risk of infection is further heightened by the presence of a foreign body, the catheter. Strict attention to aseptic technique both in the siting of a catheter and in its maintenance will serve to avoid many of these problems.

Misplacement of a catheter and infusion of nutrient solutions extravascularly can be very serious. Central catheters should be placed under X-ray control. The possibility of embolism, either thrombotic or air,

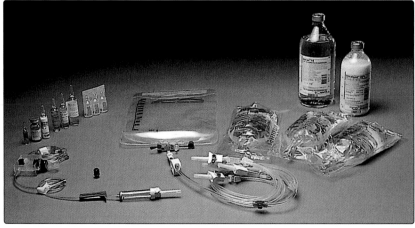

Fig. 2 **TPN preparations.**

should be easily avoided as long as their potential is recognized.

The most common metabolic complication is that of hyperglycaemia. Against a background of increased stress hormones, especially if there is infection, there may be marked insulin resistance and consequently an increased glucose level. The use of insulin to correct these metabolic effects is best avoided. The composition of the IV regimen should be adjusted if metabolic disorders occur. Many other biochemical abnormalities have been reported in association with TPN. These include:

- hypokalaemia
- hypomagnesaemia
- hypophosphataemia
- hypercalcaemia
- acid–base disorders
- hyperlipidaemia.

If patients are properly monitored both clinically and biochemically during their TPN these potential disorders should be avoided.

Monitoring patients on TPN

In addition to baseline assessment of patients receiving TPN, there should also be a strict policy for careful clinical and biochemical monitoring of these patients (Fig. 3). This is especially important if the TPN is medium to long term. The tests described on pages 102–103 have particular relevance here.

Special attention must be paid to the micronutrients in long-term TPN patients as any imbalance here may result in a single nutrient deficiency state. Such situations are increasingly rare except in those patients relying solely on artificial diets for their nutrients.

Because biochemical changes may precede the development of any clinical manifestation of a nutritional deficiency, careful laboratory monitoring should be instituted.

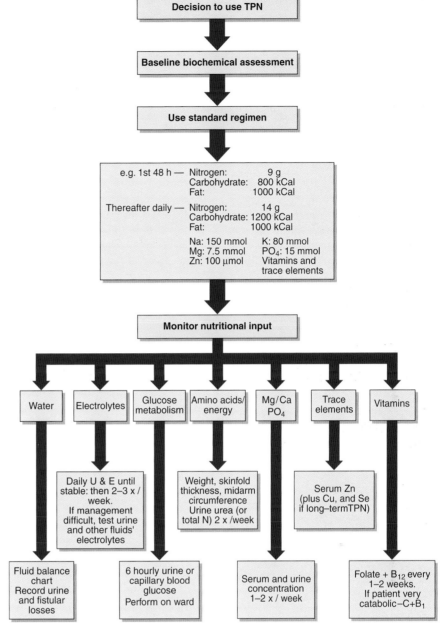

Fig. 3 **Intravenous nutrition and its monitoring**.

However, measurement of trace elements and vitamins is often affected by the acute phase response and care needs to be taken in interpretation.

Clinical note

Patients often receive lipid emulsions as part of their IV regimen. Visible lipaemia in a blood sample usually suggests that the patient is unable to clear the lipid from the plasma.

Case history 42

A 54-year-old man was admitted with a superior mesenteric artery thrombosis. He had gross bowel ischaemia and necrosis. Subsequently he had only 15 cm of viable small bowel.

- What form of feeding would be appropriate in this man?
- What assessment should be made before commencing treatment?

Comment on page 166.

Parenteral nutrition

- TPN is never an emergency procedure and should be carefully planned.
- A multidisciplinary team approach to TPN is the most effective.
- The main problems are due to sepsis, and mechanical and metabolic complications.
- The use of commercial preparations has made the incidence of deficiency states much less common.
- Patients receiving TPN require careful clinical and biochemical monitoring.

The metabolic response to injury

The body reacts to all forms of noxious stimuli with an inflammatory response. This is a complex series of events that varies from mild hyperaemia due to a superficial scratch to major haemodynamic and metabolic responses to a severe injury.

The problems faced by the traumatized individual are listed in Table 1. The metabolic response to injury (Fig. 1) can be thought of as a protective physiological response designed to keep the individual alive until healing processes repair the damage that has been done. It is mediated by a complex series of neuroendocrine and cellular processes, all of which contribute to the overall goal – survival. The metabolic response to injury becomes clinically important only when the degree of injury is severe.

The phases of the metabolic response to injury

The metabolic response to injury has two phases, the *ebb* and the *flow* (Fig. 2). The ebb phase is usually short and may correspond to clinical shock, resulting from reduced tissue perfusion. The physiological changes that occur here are designed to restore adequate vascular volume and maintain essential tissue perfusion. The severity of the ebb phase determines clinical outcome. If the ebb phase is mild or moderate, patients will have an uncomplicated transition to the flow phase. However, if severe, patients may develop the systemic inflammatory response syndrome (SIRS). The features of this are shown in Table 2. This is a complex pathophysiological state involving a vast array of inflammatory mediators and hormonal regulators, but the underlying mechanisms have yet to be clarified. No therapeutic strategies have been found to be helpful, perhaps because of our incomplete understanding of the SIRS. However, a proportion of patients will recover with intensive life support, including ventilation and dialysis.

A number of biochemical parameters are deranged in this syndrome, because the normal homeostatic mechanisms are overridden by the stress response. A low level of albumin, zinc, iron and selenium are characteristic along with disordered hormonal regulation, e.g low T_4, TSH and T_3, and nearly all of these patients will develop SIAD (see p. 16).

The flow phase may last for days to weeks depending on the extent of the injury. In this phase, metabolism is altered to ensure that energy is available for dependent tissues at the expense of muscle and fat stores (Table 3).

The acute phase protein response

The acute phase protein response leads to greatly increased de novo synthesis (principally by the liver) of a number of plasma proteins along with a decrease in the plasma concentration of some others. This response is stimulated by the release of cytokines such as interleukin 1 and 6 and tumour necrosis factor, and raised concentrations of the hormones cortisol and glucagon. The major human acute phase proteins are listed in Table 4.

The acute phase protein response is an adaptive response to disease. Its role is not fully understood but certain aspects can

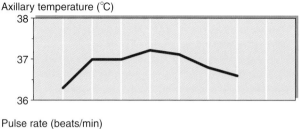
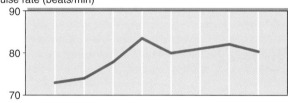
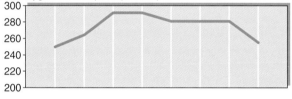
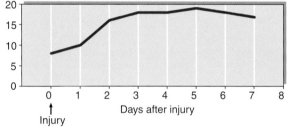

Fig. 1 **The changes in body temperature, pulse rate, oxygen consumption and urinary nitrogen excretion which accompany injury.**

Table 1 **Major problems faced by traumatized individuals**
Bleeding and circulatory collapse
Pain
Major tissue damage
Food and water deprivation
Immobilization
Infection

Table 2 **Criteria for the diagnosis of SIRS**
Temperature >38°C or <36°C
Heart rate > 90/min
Respiratory rate >20/min
PCO_2 <32 mmHg or ventilated
White blood cell count > 12 000 or <4000/mm³

be seen to be of benefit to the individual. The increases in C-reactive protein (CRP) and complement will contain and eliminate infection; increased coagulation factors will aid and prevent excess blood loss; protease inhibitors will prevent the spread of tissue necrosis when lysosomal enzymes are released by damaged cells at the site of injury.

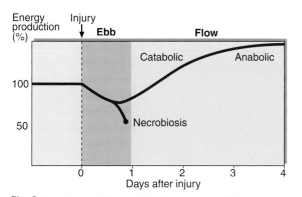

Fig. 2 **The phases of the metabolic response to injury.**

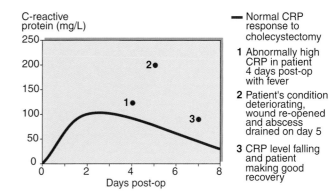

Fig. 3 **CRP concentrations in a patient who developed an occult abscess following abdominal surgery.**

Table 3 **Biochemical changes in the metabolic response to injury**

Metabolic change	Consequence
Increased glycogenolysis	Leads to increased circulating blood glucose to be used as an energy substrate
Increased gluconeogenesis	Leads to increased circulating blood glucose to be used as an energy substrate
Increased lipolysis	Leads to increased free fatty acids which are used to provide energy and increased glycerol which may be converted to glucose
Increased proteolysis	Leads to increased amino acids which may be catabolized to provide energy or used for tissue synthesis and wound healing

Table 4 **The acute phase protein response**

Protein types	Increased	Decreased
Protease inhibitors	α_1-Antitrypsin α_2-Macroglobulin	
Coagulation proteins	Fibrinogen Prothrombin Factor VIII Plasminogen	
Complement proteins	C1s C2, B C3, C4, C5 C56 C1 INH	Properdin
Miscellaneous	Haptoglobin Caeruloplasmin C-reactive protein Serum amyloid-A protein	Albumin HDL LDL

The precise role of other proteins in this response such as caeruloplasmin and serum amyloid A remains to be established.

Clinical uses

In practice the major use of the acute phase response is to monitor the course of the inflammatory process in the patient. This is done in two ways:

- *By measuring serum CRP.* CRP concentrations change very rapidly and can be used to monitor changes on a daily basis (Fig. 3).
- *By monitoring the erythrocyte sedimentation rate (ESR).* This reflects fibrinogen and immunoglobulin concentration. ESR changes slowly, and is used to monitor the inflammatory process over weeks rather than days.

In neonates and immunosuppressed patients, bacterial infection can be difficult to diagnose in its early stages. This includes patients with AIDS. Failure to make the diagnosis may have fatal consequences. In practice, a serum CRP concentration of >100 mg/L (normal <10 mg/L) is frequently taken to indicate the presence of infection.

Starvation and the metabolic response to injury

The metabolic responses to injury and to starvation are quite different. After injury the body is at war, defences are mobilized, metabolic activity increases and resources are directed to the site of action. In starvation, the body is in a state of famine, resources are rationed and metabolic activity is limited to the minimum for survival. Hypoalbuminaemia is often erroneously perceived as an index of nutritional status. However, in short-term starvation not associated with injury, serum albumin is characteristically within the reference interval or even increased.

Case history 43

A 28-year-old man was admitted to the intensive therapy unit after a serious road traffic accident in which he sustained multiple injuries. After initial resuscitation and surgery to his injuries he was considered stable but in coma.

- What is the role of biochemical measurements in this patient's management?

Comment on page 167.

Clinical note

Antibiotic therapy for an infection, perhaps indicated by increased CRP concentration, should be started only after appropriate specimens have been taken for bacteriological investigation.

The metabolic response to injury

- The metabolic response to injury is a protective physiological response.
- The ebb phase may progress to recovery or to the SIRS.
- The flow phase involves changes in metabolism to ensure that energy is made available to dependent tissues.
- The flow phase persists until the inflammatory response provides for tissue healing and/or eradication of infection.
- C-reactive protein (CRP) and albumin measurements are useful in monitoring day-to-day changes in the inflammatory response.

Malabsorption

Physiology of digestion and absorption

Having been initially broken down in part by cooking and mastication, food is assimilated by the body by the combined action of two processes: digestion and absorption. The major nutrients (carbohydrate, protein and fat) are broken down enzymatically to low-molecular-weight compounds. Digestive enzymes are secreted by the stomach, pancreas and small intestine.

The transport of the products of digestion into gut epithelial cells and from there to the portal blood is termed absorption. The absorption of some nutrients is passive while others require active transport.

Malabsorption

Failure of digestion is properly called maldigestion. The term 'malabsorption' describes impairment of the absorptive mechanisms, but in practice is used to encompass both disorders. Malabsorption is a condition that can occur at any stage of life from a variety of causes (Fig. 1).

The clinical effects of malabsorption result from the failure to absorb nutrients. The major consequences of generalized malabsorption arise from inadequate energy intake that results in weight loss in adults and growth failure in children.

Diagnosis

In suspected malabsorption a detailed dietary history is essential to establish eating patterns and habits. Endoscopy and biopsy are by far the most important tools available for the investigation of gastrointestinal tract disorders. They allow macro- and microscopic study of the intestinal mucosa and are the standard techniques used to diagnose major causes of malabsorption such as coeliac disease. Radiological tests are of assistance when detecting abnormal anatomy of the bowel and motility. Though not usually investigated, it is important to assess the state of teeth and gums, and the adequacy of salivary secretion, as they play an important role in initiating digestion.

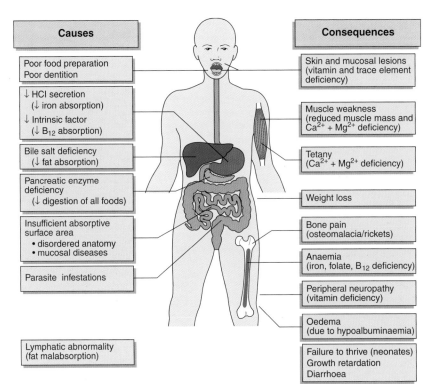

Fig. 1 **Causes and consequences of malabsorption.**

Provided that dietary input is adequate, the presence of malabsorption from the small bowel will often be indicated by changes in the faeces, in particular by diarrhoea. Diarrhoea due to malabsorption can be assumed only if other causes, such as infection and laxative abuse, have been excluded. Laxative abuse is an important diagnosis that may be missed. A laxative screen can be performed in cases of suspected abuse.

In the case of fat malabsorption, the faeces will contain fat, which can be detected by microscopic examination of the stools or by quantitative analysis. Where small molecules such as monosaccharides are not absorbed, they exert an osmotic effect that will prevent water absorption in the large intestine, giving rise to a large volume of watery stools.

Biochemical investigations

Laboratory tests in the investigation of gastrointestinal disorders fall into one of two groups: tests that identity malabsorption and tests of pancreatic function. The most frequently performed tests are outlined below. There is little agreement amongst investigators as to the best tests to use.

Tests of malabsorption

- *Faecal fat.* The presence of fatty stools is an important sign of malabsorption. Faecal specimens over a 5-day period may be collected and total fat content measured.
- *Faecal microscopy.* The presence of fat globules can be observed directly.
- *Butterfat test.* Chylomicrons detected in the plasma of patients after a standard fat load indicate that some fat digestion and absorption has occurred.
- ^{14}C-*triglyceride breath test.* An oral dose of radiolabelled triglyceride (e.g. ^{14}C-triolein in which the fatty acid contains the label) is absorbed and metabolized. The $^{14}CO_2$ in expired air is a measure of the effectiveness of digestion and absorption.
- *Xylose absorption test.* Serum measurements of this 5-carbon sugar are made after an oral dose and provide an indication of intestinal ability to absorb monosaccharides.

Tests of pancreatic function

- *Lundh test.* Duodenal contents are collected after a meal and the activity of a pancreatic enzyme, such as trypsin or amylase, is measured.

Table 1	Additional biochemical tests used in the investigation of gastrointestinal disease
Test	**Purpose**
Urea breath test	Used to identify patients with *Helicobacter pylori* infection, which is strongly associated with peptic ulcer disease
Hydrogen breath test	Assesses bacterial overgrowth in the intestine
Lactose tolerance test	Different disaccharides may be used to detect specific functional enzyme defects such as lactase or sucrase
Faecal chymotrypsin or elastase	Indirect pancreatic function tests used in the assessment of pancreatic function mainly in cystic fibrosis
Intestinal permeability	Biologically inert polymers are used to assess mucosal permeability by measuring their excretion in urine after an oral load
Schilling test	Assesses vitamin B_{12} absorption

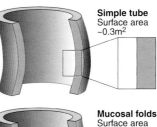

Simple tube
Surface area
~0.3m^2

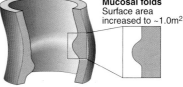

Mucosal folds
Surface area
increased to ~1.0m^2

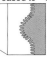

Mucosal villi
Surface area
increased to ~10m^2

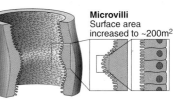

Microvilli
Surface area
increased to ~200m^2

Fig. 2 **Effects of mucosal structure on absorptive surface area of the small intestine.**

- *Secretin test.* An intravenous injection of secretin stimulates pancreatic secretion, which is assessed by aspiration of duodenal contents and measurement of trypsin or amylase activity.
- *Pancreolauryl test.* Fluorescein dilaurate is hydrolysed by cholesterol esterase in pancreatic secretions. The water-soluble fluorescein is absorbed and excreted in urine where its fluorescence gives an indirect measure of pancreatic function.

Other tests that may be employed in the investigation of malabsorption and gastrointestinal disease are shown in Table 1.

Gastrointestinal disease

There are many disorders associated with malabsorption. Generalized malabsorption occurs for a number of reasons. These include:

- Inadequate digestion, which is seen in chronic pancreatitis as a consequence of insufficient pancreatic enzyme release such as in cystic fibrosis.
- Inadequate intestinal mucosal surface (Fig. 2) as occurs in coeliac disease.
- Inflammation affecting the mucosa, submucosa and frequently the entire bowel structures as occurs in Crohn's disease.
- Infections of the bowel causing intestinal hurry. These may be acute as in salmonella, or chronic as in tropical sprue.
- Abnormal bowel anatomy or insufficient bowel. This may occur after repeated surgery for chronic disorders such as Crohn's disease or after bowel infarction and removal of the necrotic bowel.

Malignant disease is not usually associated with malabsorption unless there is abnormal bowel motility that allows bacterial flora to proliferate, or if the tumour secretes a hormone such as VIP, which causes diarrhoea (p. 140).

Inadequate bile salt secretion occurs in many forms of liver disease and gives rise to fat malabsorption. Patients may present with the clinical features of generalized malabsorption on top of the underlying liver disease. Inadequate fat absorption is associated with impaired absorption of vitamin D (a fat-soluble vitamin). In the absence of adequate sunlight exposure, patients may become vitamin D deficient and unable to absorb calcium from the gut. This may lead to the development of osteomalacia or rickets.

The malabsorption of specific substances tends to occur in certain well-defined conditions such as vitamin B_{12} malabsorption, which leads to pernicious anaemia. This occurs when intrinsic factor production is lost due to gastric mucosal atrophy. Patients may also have inherited deficiencies of intestinal saccharidases, such as lactase, which cause malabsorption when the patient drinks milk or eats milk products. This is known as lactose intolerance.

Clinical note

Many patients with malabsorption recognize that certain things in their diet – usually fatty foods – cause diarrhoea. They avoid these foods and reduce their fat intake. As a result, faecal fat excretion may be normal because of this low dietary fat intake.

Case history 44

A 69-year-old woman, who had made an excellent recovery after local excision of a breast tumour 8 years previously, presented with weight loss, bone tenderness and weakness. Her symptoms had developed over a number of months. Her family were concerned that she was not caring for herself nor eating adequately. There was no clinical evidence of recurrence of breast cancer. LFTs showed only an elevated alkaline phosphatase (430 U/L).

- What other biochemical tests would be of assistance in making a diagnosis?

Comment on page 167.

Malabsorption

- In suspected malabsorption, a detailed dietary history is essential to establish eating patterns and habits.
- Endoscopy and biopsy are the most important tools and frequently allow a specific diagnosis to be made.
- Laboratory tests in the investigation of gastrointestinal disorders fall into one of two groups: tests of malabsorption and tests of pancreatic function.

Iron

Iron is an essential element in humans, being the central ion in haem, the non-protein component of haemoglobin, myoglobin and the cytochromes (Fig. 1). Iron deficiency causes a failure in haem synthesis and since haemoglobin is required for delivery of oxygen to the tissues, this leads to anaemia and tissue hypoxia. However, free iron is highly toxic to cells and must be bound to protein at all times.

Iron physiology

Iron levels are controlled by regulating iron uptake, since there is no mechanism for controlling its excretion. Dietary intake of iron is about 0.35 mmoL (20 mg) per day and there are 50–70 mmoL (3–4 g) of iron in the body, distributed as shown in Figure 2. Iron in the tissue stores is bound to the iron storage proteins ferritin (soluble) and haemosiderin (insoluble). The 1% of body iron in the plasma is associated with the iron binding glycoprotein, transferrin, each molecule of which binds two Fe^{2+} ions.

Serum iron concentrations differ with age and sex. Normal adult concentrations are 10–40 mmo/L. There is a marked circadian rhythm in serum iron concentrations, which can vary by 50% over 24 hours.

Laboratory investigation of iron disorders

- *Serum iron determinations* are of limited routine value, being of most assistance in the diagnosis of iron overload and acute iron poisoning.
- *Transferrin* can be measured directly or indirectly as the *total iron binding capacity (TIBC)*. Normally transferrin is about 30% saturated with iron. When saturation falls to 15%, iron deficiency is likely and some degree of clinical effect can be expected. A higher percentage saturation indicates iron overload. Transferrin and, therefore, also total serum iron, is decreased as part of the acute phase response. Protein energy malnutrition also decreases transferrin synthesis and hence its serum concentration.

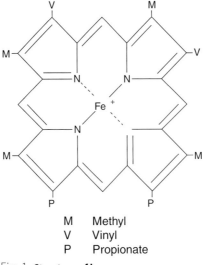

M Methyl
V Vinyl
P Propionate

Fig. 1 **Structure of haem.**

- *Serum ferritin* is the best indicator of body iron stores. The concentration is normally greater than 12 µg/L. The acute phase response can result in increases in serum ferritin, making the diagnosis of marginal iron deficiency difficult or impossible in these circumstances.
- *Red cell protoporphyrin*, a haem precursor, is markedly increased in iron deficiency. The concentration is usually less than 1 µmol/L of red cells. Levels are also increased in some forms of porphyria and by exposure to organic lead compounds. For a full investigation of iron status, the haemoglobin concentration, the appearance of the erythrocytes (deficiency), and liver biopsy (excess) may be required.

Iron deficiency

Iron deficiency anaemia is the commonest of all single-nutrient deficiencies, causing seriously impaired quality of life. The principal causes are chronic blood loss and poor dietary intake of bio-available iron. Uptake of iron can be decreased by a number of dietary constituents, such as phytic acid, and can also occur in malabsorptive conditions, such as coeliac disease. In iron deficiency anaemia it is important to diagnose the underlying condition, especially malignant disease, the presence of intestinal parasites or any other intestinal pathology that may cause chronic blood loss. In women, even when well-nourished, iron deficiency may develop during pregnancy due to the increased iron requirements of the developing fetus.

Iron deficiency anaemia develops in three stages:

1. Depletion of iron stores: confirmed by serum ferritin levels of less than 12 µg/L.
2. Deficient erythropoiesis with normal haemoglobin but increased red cell protoporphyrin. Iron concentration falls, the synthesis of transferrin is increased and the percentage saturation is decreased.
3. Iron deficiency anaemia, in which both iron and haemoglobin are low and there is a microcytic, hypochromic anaemia (Fig. 3). Low stainable iron is seen in the bone marrow.

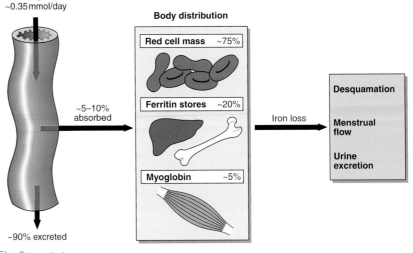

Fig. 2 **Iron balance.**

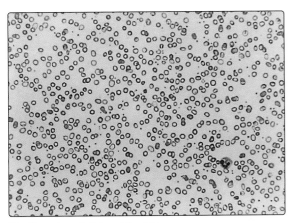

Fig. 3 **An iron-deficient blood film.**

Fig. 4   **The effect of desferrioxamine on iron excretion in overdose.**

Treatment

Oral iron salts or glycine chelates or intramuscular injection of sodium ferrate gluconate are used to treat deficiency. It can take up to 6 months to replete the body stores. With oral treatment, compliance may be a problem, due to nausea, diarrhoea and other intestinal complaints. These are all lessened if the iron salts are taken with food.

Iron overload

Iron overload may be caused by chronic blood transfusions, inappropriate total parenteral nutrition and where there is ineffective haematopoiesis, as in renal failure. Other important causes of iron overload are haemochromatosis and iron poisoning. Since there is no major mechanism for excretion of iron except by cell desquamation and occult blood loss, iron overload is also a possibility when iron therapy is prescribed. In iron overload the serum ferritin concentrations may rise to 500–5000 µg/L.

Haemochromatosis

This is a relatively common inherited disease characterized by increased iron absorption ($2–3 \times$ normal) that leads to iron deposition in various organs. Whole body iron content may be increased tenfold. The excess iron leads to free radical generation, fibrosis and organ failure. The commonest mutation (C282Y) in the HFE gene codes for a membrane-bound glycoprotein that binds β_2 microglobulin. This complex then binds the transferrin receptor (Tfr) and the whole complex controls iron uptake. African iron overload is related to a similar but separate mutation. The clinical presentation varies widely depending upon dietary iron uptake, alcohol abuse or the presence of hepatotoxins. Women are less severely affected than men, being protected by physiological iron loss during menstruation and in pregnancy.

Clinical features include chronic fatigue and, in extreme cases, skin pigmentation, diabetes mellitus, cardiomyopathy, hepatic cirrhosis and hepatoma. Serum iron is increased, with almost complete saturation of transferrin. Transferrin saturation is the test with the greatest sensitivity and specificity for haemochromatosis, but serum ferritin is also increased to greater than 500 µg/L. The best way to confirm hereditary haemochromatosis is genotyping, which is 99% sensitive. Liver biopsy is also used to confirm iron overload. Chronic iron overload is usually treated by venesection, the removal of 500 mL blood accounting for approximately 250 mg iron. In chronic treatment, ferritin levels should be maintained below 100 µg/L.

Iron poisoning

Iron poisoning in children is common and may be life-threatening. Symptoms include nausea and vomiting, abdominal pain and haematemesis. In severe cases, hypotension and coma can result. Serum iron is increased and transferrin is >70% saturated. Treatment is by chelation of the iron in the stomach and the plasma with desferrioxamine. Chelated iron is excreted in the urine as a deep orange coloured complex (Fig. 4).

Clinical note

A microcytic hypochromic anaemia, and the absence of stainable iron in a bone marrow biopsy, are the best diagnostic indices of established iron deficiency.

Case history 45

A 42-year-old woman presented with a history of increasing lethargy, dizziness and breathlessness. She had brittle hair and nails. She complained of heart palpitation on exercise and reported particularly heavy periods. Biochemical investigation revealed the following results:

Serum iron	4 µmol/L
Transferrin saturation	10%
Ferritin	<5 µg/L

- What is the diagnosis and what other investigations should have been done first?

Comment on page 167.

Iron

- Iron deficiency is commonly caused by the combination of blood loss and low dietary intake.

- Iron deficiency can be diagnosed by finding a hypochromic microcytic anaemia.

- Serum ferritin is the most reliable single biochemical test of iron deficiency.

- Iron overload may arise following repeated blood transfusions.

- Iron overload is diagnosed by finding an increased serum iron concentration and percentage transferrin saturation, and increased serum ferritin.

- Accidental iron poisoning in children is an important medical emergency.

Copper and zinc

COPPER

Copper is an essential trace metal that is a component of a wide range of intracellular metalloenzymes, including cytochrome oxidase, superoxide dismutase, tyrosinase, dopamine hydroxylase and lysyl oxidase. Most of the copper in plasma is associated with the specific copper-binding protein, caeruloplasmin.

Copper physiology

About 50% of the average daily dietary copper of around 25 μmol (1.5 mg) is absorbed from the stomach and the small intestine (Fig. 1). Although copper is present in most foodstuffs, there is evidence that not all modern diets contain sufficient copper, especially when large amounts of refined carbohydrate are consumed. Absorbed copper is transported to the liver in portal blood bound to albumin and is exported to peripheral tissues mainly bound to caeruloplasmin and, to a lesser extent, albumin.

Copper is present in all metabolically active tissue. The highest concentrations are found in liver and in kidney, with significant amounts in cardiac and skeletal muscle and in bone. The liver contains 10% of the total body content of 1200 μmol (80 mg). Excess copper is excreted in bile into the gut, and the faecal copper output (12.5 μmol/24 hours) is the sum of unabsorbed dietary copper and that re-excreted into the gut.

Laboratory assessment

A number of different investigations are needed to diagnose disorders of copper metabolism. These are:

- *Serum copper.* Normal concentrations are usually between 10 and 22 μmol/L, of which 90% is bound to caeruloplasmin. Total copper concentration may vary either due to changes in copper itself or to changes in the concentration of caeruloplasmin.
- *Serum caeruloplasmin.* The normal adult levels are 200–600 mg/L. Caeruloplasmin is increased greatly in the acute phase reaction, and in some cases may be so high as to raise

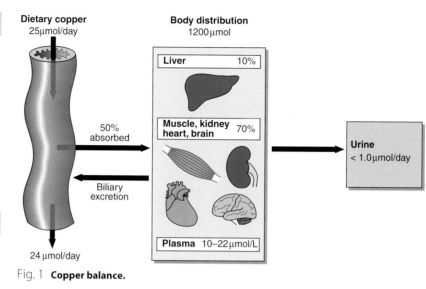

Dietary copper
25 μmol/day

Body distribution
1200 μmol

Liver 10%

50% absorbed

Muscle, kidney heart, brain 70%

Biliary excretion

Urine < 1.0 μmol/day

24 μmol/day

Plasma 10–22 μmol/L

Fig. 1 **Copper balance.**

the total copper concentration to 30–45 μmol/L. Caeruloplasmin levels may be helpful in the interpretation of serum copper concentrations.
- *Urinary copper.* Normal excretion is <1.0 μmol/24 hours.

Copper deficiency

Both children and adults can develop symptomatic copper deficiency. Premature infants are the most susceptible since copper stores in the liver are laid down in the third trimester of pregnancy. In adults, deficiency is usually found following intestinal bypass surgery or in patients on parenteral nutrition. Symptoms range from bone disease to an iron-resistant microcytic hypochromic anaemia.

Copper toxicity

Copper toxicity is uncommon and is most usually due to administration of copper sulphate solutions. Oral copper sulphate may lead to gastric perforation. Serum copper concentrations may be greatly elevated. Copper is toxic to many organs, but renal tubular damage is the major concern. Treatment is by chelation with penicillamine.

Inborn errors of copper metabolism

There are two inborn errors of copper metabolism: Menkes syndrome and Wilson's disease.

Menkes syndrome

Menkes syndrome is a very rare but fatal condition that presents in infants as growth failure and mental retardation, with lesions of the major blood vessels and bone disease. A characteristic sign is 'steely hair' (pilo torti).

Wilson's disease

All adolescents or young adults with otherwise unexplained neurological or hepatic disease should be investigated for Wilson's disease, since this condition is fatal if not diagnosed and treated. Symptoms are a result of copper deposition in liver, brain and kidney. Copper deposits in the eye can sometimes be seen as a brown pigment around the iris (the Kayser–Fleischer ring).

The inherited defect in Wilson's disease is believed to be in the gene coding for an enzyme involved in copper excretion into bile and reabsorption in the kidney. Urinary free copper excretion is high and total serum concentrations low (Table 1). Just what causes the low caeruloplasmin concentrations in these patients remains unclear. Confirmation is by measurement of copper in a liver biopsy, which is usually greater than 250 μg/g dry weight in patients with the disease.

Treatment is by administration of a chelating agent, penicillamine, to promote urinary copper excretion. Patients are maintained on oral penicillamine for life and require regular monitoring to ensure compliance and to check for side effects. Liver transplantation may also be considered, particularly in young patients with severe disease.

Table 1 **Biochemistry determinations in patients with Wilson's disease**		
Investigation	Normal adult	Wilson's disease
Serum copper µmol/L	10–22	<10
Caeruloplasmin mg/L	200–600	<200
Urinary copper µmol/24h	<1	5–15
Liver copper µg/g dry weight	20–50	>250

Case history 46

A 15-year-old girl presented with abdominal pain and diarrhoea for 3 days. She became jaundiced and a presumptive diagnosis of infective hepatitis was made, but serological tests were negative. She subsequently died of fulminant liver failure. At post mortem her liver copper concentration was found to be grossly increased.

- What investigations should be carried out on this patient's younger sister?

Comment on page 167.

Clinical note

In the general population, marginal copper deficiency may be a cardiovascular disease risk factor, since both experimental animal and human studies show that a low copper diet combined with high carbohydrate intake may lead to hypercholesterolaemia and cardiac abnormalities.

ZINC

Zinc is an essential element present in over 200 metalloproteins with a wide range of functions. Carbonic anhydrase, alcohol dehydrogenase, alkaline phosphatase and steroid hormone receptors are examples.

Zinc physiology

The average daily dietary intake of zinc is around 150 µmol (10 mg) (Fig. 2). It is present in all protein-rich foods. Around 30% is absorbed. Absorption is reduced in the presence of phytates. In the liver, zinc is incorporated into metalloenzymes, while in blood the majority of the zinc is contained in the erythrocytes. In plasma, 90% of zinc is bound to albumin and 10% to α_2-macroglobulin. Zinc reserves in the body are small and are located mainly in muscle and bone. Zinc is excreted in urine, in bile, in pancreatic fluid and in milk in lactating mothers.

Laboratory assessment

The repeated finding of a zinc concentration in a serum specimen of less than 5 µmol/L is suggestive of impending zinc deficiency and requires investigation. Unlike copper, serum zinc falls during the acute phase response to injury or infection.

Marginal zinc deficiency is best demonstrated by a positive clinical response to supplementation. Oral or intravenous zinc reverses the signs and symptoms of zinc deficiency within weeks.

Zinc deficiency

Zinc deficiency occurs in both adults and children through lack of dietary zinc. In children, the rate of growth during rehabilitation from famine has been clearly related to the dietary supply of bioavailable zinc. Zinc deficiency is known to occur in patients on intravenous nutrition and causes a characteristic skin rash (Fig. 3) and hair loss. Wound breakdown and delayed healing are other complications. Acrodermatitis enteropathica, a rare inherited disorder of zinc metabolism, manifests itself in infancy as skin rash. Untreated, the prognosis is poor, but oral zinc therapy leads to complete remission. Zinc is antagonized by cadmium, and zinc deficiency can be a consequence of chronic cadmium poisoning.

Zinc toxicity

Zinc toxicity is uncommon. It is usually due to exposure to high levels of zinc fumes. It is difficult to induce toxicity by dietary means. However, in cases of self poisoning with zinc salts, the symptoms are fever, vomiting, stomach cramps and diarrhoea.

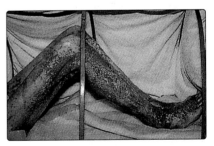

Fig. 3 **Skin lesions in zinc deficiency.**

Copper and zinc

- Diagnosis of severe copper deficiency can be made by measurement of serum copper. Values of <10 µmol/L in adults and of <5.0 µmol/L in neonates require investigation.

- The major inborn error of copper metabolism is Wilson's disease.

- Wilson's disease is treatable and requires prompt diagnosis.

- Adequate zinc is needed for growth in children.

- Symptomatic zinc deficiency in the adult causes dermatitis, hair loss and poor wound healing.

- Serum zinc concentrations persistently below 5 µmol/L warn of impending clinical deficiency.

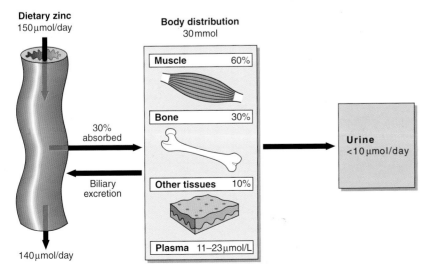

Dietary zinc 150 µmol/day

30% absorbed

Biliary excretion

140 µmol/day

Body distribution 30 mmol

Muscle	60%
Bone	30%
Other tissues	10%
Plasma	11–23 µmol/L

Urine <10 µmol/day

Fig. 2 **Zinc balance.**

Therapeutic drug monitoring

The effect of most drug therapy is assessed by observing the change in the patient's clinical state. Therapeutic drug monitoring (TDM) is the measurement of drug concentrations in blood, plasma or saliva as a means of assessing the adequacy of dosage. TDM is not necessary where there is a clear clinical effect, such as with antihypertensive or hypoglycaemic drugs, but is important with those drugs for which there is no good objective measurement of effectiveness and/or there is a serious risk of toxicity. For TDM to be of value there must be a proven relationship between the plasma drug concentration and the clinical effect.

Following the administration of a drug, the graph of plasma concentration against time, plotted on semi-logarithmic graph paper, will look like that in Figure 1. Analysis of such graphs can allow an estimate of the half-life of the drug ($t\frac{1}{2}$) and the volume of distribution, which is higher if the drug is taken up by tissues. These can be used to estimate the correct dose to give. After several similar doses have been given, the pattern reaches a steady state at which the plasma drug concentration will oscillate between a peak and a trough level. It usually takes about five half-lives for the steady state to be attained. In the steady state there is a stable relationship between the dose and the effect, and decisions can be made with confidence. For most drugs there is a linear relationship between dose and plasma concentration. However, phenytoin shows non-linear kinetics (Fig. 2).

Sampling for TDM

The concentration of drug in plasma or saliva changes constantly over the period of treatment, and in order to compare one treatment with another, some standardization must be introduced. When taking a sample for TDM it is important to:

- ask the patient about compliance
- check for interacting drugs (including complementary/herbal therapies)
- note the dose, and the time since last dose
- take the sample at an appropriate time.

Interpretation of drug levels

A great deal of information is required in order to interpret drug concentrations correctly. Where concentrations are lower than expected, the most likely cause is non-compliance. Higher than expected concentrations, in the absence of an increase in dose, indicate that a change has taken place either in other drug therapy or in hepatic or renal function. It is much easier to interpret results if cumulative reports, including dosing details, are available, since these allow comparisons between drug levels achieved. The population reference interval for each drug indicates roughly the limits within which most patients will show maximum therapeutic effect with minimum toxicity. However, a level that is therapeutic in one patient may give rise to toxicity in another (Fig. 3). The most likely reasons for the plasma drug concentration to fall above or below the reference interval are given in Table 1.

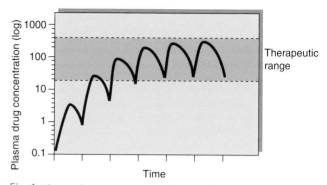

Fig. 1 **Plasma drug concentration shown after a series of identical doses equally spaced.** After approximately 5 half-lives steady state is achieved.

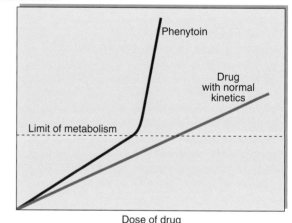

Fig. 2 **Non-linear kinetics of phenytoin.**

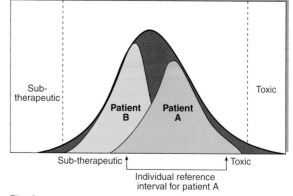

Fig. 3 **A population reference interval for a common drug.**

Table 1 **Common reasons for sub-therapeutic or toxic levels**
Sub-therapeutic levels
Non-compliance
Dose too low
Malabsorption
Rapid metabolism
Toxic levels
Overdose
Dose too high
Dose too frequent
Impaired renal function
Reduced hepatic metabolism

Table 2 **Drugs for which therapeutic drug monitoring is appropriate**	
Drug(s)	**Reason for monitoring**
Anticonvulsants	
Phenytoin	Non-linear kinetics
Carbamazepine	
Antiarrhythmics	
Digoxin	Very low therapeutic index
	Sensitive to renal dysfunction
Amiodarone	Wide variability in half-life especially in neonates
Aminoglycosides	Nephrotoxic and ototoxic
Antitubercular drugs	Drug interactions
Isoniazid	Slow and fast metabolizers exist
Immunosuppressants	
Ciclosporin A	Nephrotoxic. Measure at 2 hours
Tacrolimus	Nephrotoxic. Measure trough levels
Lithium	Very low therapeutic index
Methotrexate	If slowly metabolized folate therapy required
Theophylline	Low therapeutic index

Note Significant drug interactions between antiretroviral drugs and the antibiotics used in patients with AIDS indicate that TDM of these drugs may well become a necessary part of patient care.

Although many drugs are measured in specialist units, such as cardiology, neurology and oncology, only a few drugs are required to be measured in most laboratories. Examples of drugs for which TDM is appropriate, and the reasons why, are shown in Table 2. Many of these drugs have a low therapeutic index. This means that the concentration at which toxicity occurs is not much higher than that which is required for therapeutic effect. It should be noted that some drugs are highly bound to albumin. In patients with low albumin concentrations, the total drug concentration may be low but the effective (free) level may be adequate.

drug concentration at steady state measured, it is possible to control the plasma concentrations accurately over a long period by small dosage adjustments. The greatest benefit of TDM is obtained in those at the extremes of age.

Drug interactions

Some drugs interfere with the metabolism and excretion of others, and as a result the addition of one drug will alter the plasma concentration of another (Fig. 4). In such circumstances, rather than attempt to establish a new steady state, it may be appropriate, when a patient is receiving a short course of a drug such as an antibiotic, temporarily to change the dose of the drug it affects. Drug interactions are particularly problematical where several drugs must be co-prescribed, as in treatment of tuberculosis, AIDS and cancer.

Pharmacokinetics

Although there is considerable variation between patients and the rate at which they metabolize and excrete drugs, predictions can be made on population averages. These allow the calculation of doses that are better than the rough guidance given by the manufacturers. Once a patient with good compliance has been stabilized and the plasma

Case history 47

Mrs CG, a chronic asthmatic, well controlled on theophylline, developed a severe chest infection. She was prescribed erythromycin and later presented to her GP complaining of tachycardia and dizziness. Her plasma theophylline concentration was found to be 140 µmol/L, much higher than the therapeutic range of 55–110 µmol/L.

- Explain the theophylline result.

Comment on page 167.

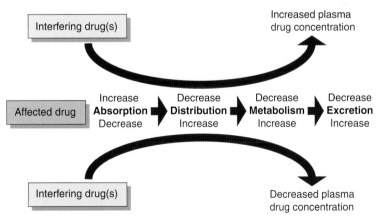

Fig. 4 **Common mechanisms of drug interactions.**

Therapeutic drug monitoring
■ TDM is only of use where the plasma concentration of a drug relates to its clinical effect.
■ TDM samples should be taken at the correct time following the dose.
■ For correct interpretation of a drug level, full details of the patient's dosing history should be obtained.
■ Poor compliance is the commonest cause of inadequate drug concentrations.
■ Used correctly, TDM can identify non-compliance and can avoid iatrogenic toxicity.

Toxicology

Clinical toxicology is the investigation of the poisoned patient. Poisoning may be due to many substances, not all of which are drugs. A diagnosis of poisoning is made more often on the basis of clinical than laboratory findings. In all cases of suspected poisoning the following biochemical tests may be requested:

- serum U & E and LFTs to assess kidney and liver function
- blood glucose to exclude hypoglycaemia
- blood gases to assess acid–base status.

In a few specific poisonings additional biochemical tests may be of value (Table 1).

Confirming poisoning

Few of the clinical signs or symptoms that may be present, including coma, are specific for any one drug or poison. A limited toxin screen in urine can be carried out in many laboratories, but a positive finding indicates only that a toxin has been taken and not the severity of the overdose.

Measurement of drug levels

Usually knowledge of the plasma concentration of a toxin will not alter the treatment of the patient. Toxins for which measurement is useful include carbon monoxide, iron, lithium, paracetamol, paraquat, phenobarbital, phenytoin, quinine, salicylate and theophylline. Quantitative analysis will give an indication of the severity of the poisoning and serial analyses provide a guide to the length of time that will elapse before the effects begin to resolve (Fig. 1).

Qualitative drug analysis simply indicates if a drug is present or not. Reasons for qualitative drug analysis include:

- differential diagnosis of coma
- confirmation of brain death
- monitoring of drug abuse
- investigation of suspected non-accidental poisoning (e.g. in children).

Treatment

Most cases of poisoning are treated conservatively, while the toxin is eliminated by normal metabolism and excretion. However, when there is hepatic or renal insufficiency, haemodialysis (for water-soluble toxins) or oral activated charcoal may be used. Such measures are usually used only for a small group of toxins including salicylate, phenobarbital, alcohols, lithium (water-soluble), carbamazepine and theophylline. When active measures are used, plasma toxin concentrations should be measured. For a few toxins there are antidotes (Table 2).

Common causes of poisoning

Poisonings in which patients may present with few clinical features are: salicylate, paracetamol, theophylline, methanol and ethylene glycol. If rapid action is not taken in such cases, the consequence can be severe or fatal illness.

Table 1 Toxins for which biochemical tests are potentially useful

Toxin	Additional biochemical tests
Amphetamine and Ecstasy	Creatine kinase, AST
Carbon monoxide	Carboxyhaemoglobin
Cocaine	Creatine kinase, potassium
Digoxin/cardiac glycosides	Potassium
Ethylene glycol	Serum osmolality, calcium
Fluoride	Calcium and magnesium
Insulin	Glucose, c-peptide
Iron	Iron, glucose
Lead (chronic)	Lead, zinc protoporphyrin
Organophosphates	Cholinesterase
Dapsone/oxidizing agents	Methaemoglobin
Paracetamol	Paracetamol
Salicylate	Salicylate
Theophylline	Glucose
Warfarin	INR (prothrombin time)

Table 2 Commonly used antidotes

Toxin	Antidote
Atropine/hyoscyamine	Physostigmine
Benzodiazepines	Flumezanil
Carbon monoxide	Oxygen
Cyanide	Dicobalt edetate
Digoxin/cardiac glycosides	Neutralizing antibodies
Ethylene glycol/methanol	Ethanol
Heavy metals	Chelating agents
Nitrates/dapsone	Methylene blue
Opiates	Naloxone
Organophosphates	Atropine/pralidoxime
Paracetamol	N-acetylcysteine
Salicylate	Sodium bicarbonate
Warfarin	Vitamin K

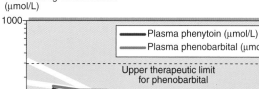
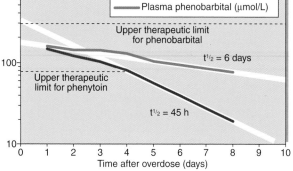

Fig. 1 **Elimination of phenytoin and phenobarbitone from plasma at different rates.**

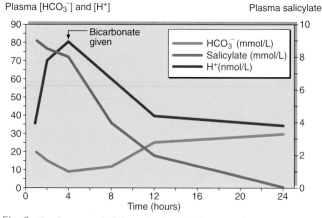

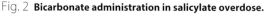
Fig. 2 **Bicarbonate administration in salicylate overdose.**

- *Salicylate* poisoning can result in severe metabolic acidosis, from which the patient may not recover. This common drug must be tested for if there is any likelihood that it has been taken. The treatment for salicylate poisoning is intravenous sodium bicarbonate, which both enhances excretion and helps correct the acidosis (Fig. 2).
- *Paracetamol (acetaminophen)* poisoning causes serious hepatocellular damage and severely affected patients may die of liver failure. In cases of poisoning, the plasma paracetamol concentration, related to time of ingestion, is prognostic (Fig. 3). A specific therapy, *N*-acetylcysteine, given intravenously, can prevent all of the hepatotoxic and nephrotoxic effects of paracetamol poisoning. Therapy should be started within 12 hours of ingestion, and hopefully before any clinical symptoms or biochemical changes develop. Patients who abuse alcohol are at particular risk from paracetamol poisoning.
- Slow release *theophylline* preparations in overdose can lead to late development of severe arrhythmias, hypokalaemia and death. In cases of suspected poisoning, the plasma theophylline concentration should be measured and its rise or fall monitored. Measures to aid elimination are of limited effect.

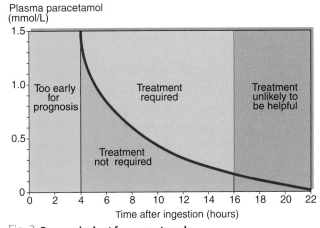

Fig. 3 **Prognosis chart for paracetamol.**

Other serious poisonings are:

- *Organophosphate and carbamate pesticides,* in which cholinergic symptoms persist for some time. Cholinesterase should be monitored.
- *Atropine,* causing anticholinergic features, e.g. hallucinations with dry mouth, dry hot skin and dilated pupils. Cases occur most often from ingestion of herbal medicines.
- *Opiates,* where overdose leads to pin-point pupils that rapidly dilate on treatment with naloxone.
- *Cardiac glycosides,* both pharmaceutical and herbal, give rise to severe bradycardia.
- *Methanol and ethylene glycol,* poisoning is not uncommon, especially in alcoholics. These toxins are metabolized to formic acid and oxalic acid respectively. Patients develop a severe metabolic acidosis and, in the case of ethylene glycol, a severe hypocalcaemia. Measuring the serum osmolality and calculating the osmolal gap can be useful here. Treatment is with intravenous ethanol to a plasma concentration of around 20 mmol/L. The ethanol is preferentially metabolized and the unchanged alcohols are gradually eliminated in the urine. An alternative is to block metabolism with fomepizole.

Chronic poisoning

Chronic poisoning occurs when there is a gradual build-up in drug concentration over a period of time, and is usually iatrogenic. Patients may present with a history only of taking their usual medication. In such cases plasma drug concentrations can be of assistance in confirming the cause of the symptoms. The drug should be withdrawn and treatment with a lower dose reinstated once the plasma levels fall.

Poisoning due to the interaction of drugs whose effect is additive is not uncommon. An example is that of alcohol and benzodiazepines, both of which may not be lethal when taken alone, but are responsible for numerous deaths when taken together in overdose. It is important to be aware that patients may also be taking over-the-counter drugs or herbal remedies that may contain pharmacologically active compounds.

Clinical note
If the plasma drug concentration is rising then drug is still being absorbed. The most likely causes are:

- the presence of a bolus of drug in the gastrointestinal tract
- correction of hypotension has led to increased absorption via the portal system.

Toxicology

- Diagnosis of poisoning is often made clinically. Symptoms may be specific or non-specific.
- Serum urea and electrolytes, blood glucose, blood gases and LFTs should be requested in every suspected poisoning.
- Analysis of specific drugs and poisons is required infrequently and only after consultation with the laboratory.
- For salicylate, paracetamol and theophylline, plasma drug concentrations are used in prognosis and should always be requested.
- Poisoning may require general supportive therapy or specific treatment.

Case history 48

A man aged 38 presented at Accident and Emergency late one afternoon, claiming to have taken 100 aspirin tablets early in the day. He was hyperventilating and complaining of ringing in his ears. He felt anxious, but his pupils were of normal size and no other abnormalities were observed. He was given gastric lavage and blood was taken for measurement of salicylate, urea and electrolytes, and blood gases. The results were as follows:

Na$^+$	K$^+$	Cl$^-$	HCO$_3^-$	Urea	Creatinine	H$^+$	PCO$_2$	PO$_2$
		─mmol/L─			μmol/L	nmol/L	kPa	kPa
140	3.7	102	20	8.1	110	35	3.7	13.3

Salicylate 4.6 mmol/L

- Comment on these results.
- What other information would be useful in determining treatment?

Comment on page 167.

Metal poisoning

Poisoning with metals is one of the oldest forms of toxicity known to man. However, it is only recently that the mechanisms of toxicity have become known. More importantly, the means of diagnosis and treatment are now available. The symptoms of poisoning are related to the amount ingested or absorbed and to the duration of exposure. In general, the elemental metals are less toxic than their salts. Organic compounds, where the metal is covalently bound to carbon, may also be toxic.

Metals associated with poisoning

The metals that give rise to clinical symptoms in man are shown in Table 1. Apart from the occasional suicide or murder attempt, most poisonings are due to environmental contamination or administration of drugs, remedies or cosmetics that contain metal salts. There are three main clinical effects of exposure to toxic metals. These are: renal tubular damage, gastrointestinal erosions and neurological damage.

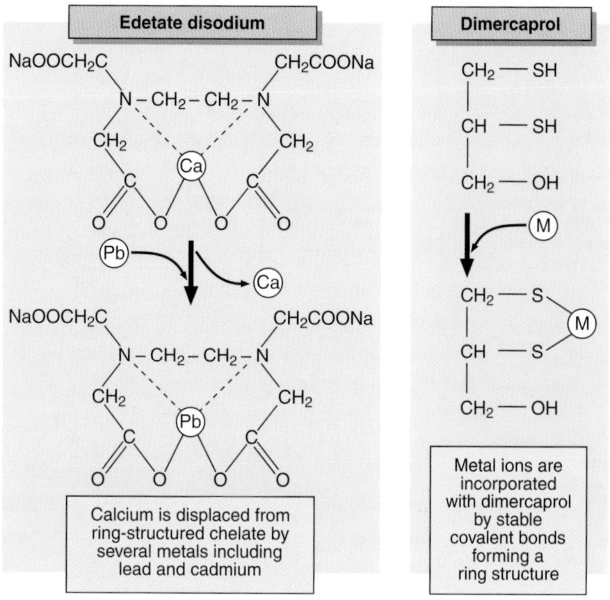

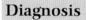

Fig. 1 **Structures and actions of chelating agents.**

Diagnosis

Metal poisoning may be suspected in cases where it is not present and missed in cases where it is the cause of the symptoms. Diagnosis may be made by measuring:

- plasma or blood levels of the metal
- urinary excretion of metals
- an associated biochemical abnormality related to the toxicity.

Blood, plasma, serum or urine can all be used for measurement, and in some cases it may also be helpful to measure the metal concentration in other tissues such as hair. The action limits for metals in plasma and urine are shown in Table 1.

Treatment

As with most poisons, treatment consists of removal of the source of the metal and increasing the elimination from the body, while correcting deranged physiological or biological mechanisms. Removal of the source may require that a person be removed from a contaminated site or workplace or that the use of a medication or cosmetic be discontinued. Elimination of heavy metals is achieved by treatment with chelating agents that bind the ions and allow their excretion in the urine (Fig. 1).

Common sources

Aluminium

Aluminium is poorly absorbed from the gastrointestinal tract, which is just as well since antacid preparations used by dyspeptic patients may contain as much as 500 mg of aluminium per tablet. Aluminium levels in water supplies are variable and may contain from less than 50 to more than 1000 µg/L. This is a potential hazard to renal dialysis patients when the aluminium can enter the body across the dialysis membrane, thus bypassing intestinal absorption. The water used in dialysis is now treated to remove contaminating metals. Acute aluminium toxicity is extremely rare. Aluminium toxicity in patients with renal dysfunction causes bone disease (aluminium osteodystrophy) and gradually failing cerebral function (dialysis dementia).

Diagnosis is by measurement of aluminium in a plasma specimen (Table 1). Aluminium content of bone biopsy material is also used, with levels greater than 100 µg/g dry weight indicating accumulation.

Treatment of aluminium toxicity is by prevention. In cases of toxicity, aluminium excretion may be enhanced by using the chelating agent desferrioxamine.

Arsenic

Arsenic never occurs as the free element, but as the ions As^{3+} and As^{5+} and may be found in some insecticides. Acute ingestion gives rise to violent gastrointestinal pain and vomiting, with shock developing. Chronic ingestion is evidenced by persistent diarrhoea, dermatitis and polyneuropathy. Arsenic is sometimes used to treat colitis and this is probably the most frequent

Table 1 **Reference and action limits for toxic metals**		
Metal	**Action limits/Indices of toxicity**	**Clinical sequelae**
Arsenic	>0.5 µg/g hair	Diarrhoea, polyneuropathy, gastrointestinal pain, vomiting, shock, coma, renal failure
Aluminium	>3 µmol/L in plasma – chronic >10 µmol/L in plasma – acute	Encephalopathy, osteodystrophy
Cadmium	>90 nmol/L in blood or >90 nmol/24 h in urine	Renal tubular damage, bone disease, hepatocellular damage
Lead	>2.0 µmol/L in blood >0.72 µmol/L in urine	Acute: colic, seizures and coma Chronic: anaemia, encephalopathy
Mercury	>120 nmol/mmol creatinine in urine	Nausea and vomiting, nephrotoxicity, neurological dysfunction
Bismuth	>5 nmol/L in blood	Acute: renal failure Chronic: encephalopathy

type of exposure. The best indicator of chronic arsenic exposure is hair analysis. The arsenic content will vary with time along the length of the hair. A level of >0.5 μg/g arsenic in hair indicates significant exposure. Urine arsenic measurements are also of value in assessing occupational exposure.

Treatment of acute and chronic arsenic poisoning is by supportive treatment and enhancement of excretion using initially a dimercaprol-type chelating agent and, once symptoms have subsided, *N*-acetyl-penicillamine. In cases of renal failure, arsenic may be removed by haemodialysis.

Cadmium

Chronic cadmium toxicity occurs in industrial workers exposed to cadmium fumes. The symptoms are those of nephrotoxicity, bone disease and, to a lesser extent, hepatotoxicity. Renal stone formation may be increased.

In diagnosis, indicators of renal damage, in particular β_2-microglobulin in urine, can be used to monitor the effects. Blood and urine cadmium estimates (Table 1) will give an objective index of the degree of exposure, and, in some cases, the cadmium content of renal biopsy tissue may be useful.

Treatment of chronic cadmium toxicity is by removal from exposure. The use of chelating agents is not recommended because mobilization of cadmium may cause renal damage.

The major source of cadmium exposure in the general population is tobacco smoke, with smokers having blood cadmium levels twice that of non-smokers.

Lead

Inorganic lead has long been known to be toxic, but acute lead poisoning is rare. Chronic toxicity is related to industrial exposure, lead leached from water pipes, or the eating of

lead-containing paints or dirt by children (pica). There is also concern over the contamination of air by organic lead constituents of petrol. Only 5–10% of lead is absorbed from the gastrointestinal tract in adults but this proportion is higher in children.

Lead poisoning causes anaemia as well as hepatic, renal and neurological sequelae. In general, the consequences of organic lead poisoning are neurological, whereas inorganic lead poisoning results in constipation, abdominal colic, anaemia and peripheral and motor neuron deficiencies. Severe cases develop encephalopathy with seizures and coma.

Biochemical evidence of lead poisoning is by the finding of raised protoporphyrin levels in the erythrocytes due to the inhibition of a number of the synthetic enzymes of the haem pathway by lead (Fig. 2). A clinical sign is the appearance of a blue line on the gums.

Lead is measured in whole blood or in urine (Table 1). Excretion can be enhanced using any of the chelating agents NaCaEDTA, dimercaprol or *N*-acetyl-penicillamine, but may require to be prolonged in order to deplete bone stores.

Mercury

Mercury poisoning may be acute or chronic and is related to exposure to elemental mercury vapour, inorganic salts or organic forms such as methyl-mercury. Metallic mercury is relatively non-toxic if ingested, but mercury vapour can give rise to acute toxicity. The symptoms are respiratory distress and a metallic taste in the mouth.

Mercurous salts, notably calomel, have been known to cause chronic toxicity following skin absorption from powders and other forms, but are less toxic than mercuric salts, notably mercuric chloride. This is highly toxic when ingested. The symptoms are nausea and vomiting, muscular

tremors, CNS symptoms and renal damage.

Diagnosis is by estimation of blood and urine mercury concentrations (Table 1). Long-term monitoring of exposure, such as may be necessary with those working with dental amalgam, may be carried out using hair or nail clippings.

Treatment of acute mercury poisoning is by use of dimercaprol, which leads to excretion via both bile and urine. Chronic exposure is best treated with *N*-acetyl-penicillamine, unless renal function is compromised.

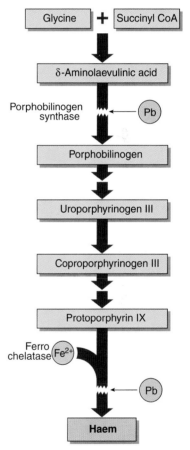

Fig. 2 **Effects of lead on haem synthesis.** Lead (Pb) inhibits porphobilinogen synthase and Fe^{2+} incorporation into haem, resulting in increased levels of δ-aminolaevulinic acid and coproporphyrin in urine and protoporphyrin in erythrocytes.

Case history 49

A 12-year-old Asian girl presents with nausea and vomiting and non-localizing neurological signs. She has been using brightly coloured facial cosmetics obtained abroad.

■ What biochemical investigations would be appropriate?

Comment on page 167.

Clinical note

Often associated in the past with murders, arsenic poisoning may still be encountered as an industrial disease. The features are abdominal pain, headache, confusion, peripheral neuropathy and coma.

Metal poisoning

■ Heavy metals are an insidious cause of gastrointestinal, renal and neurological disease.

■ Measurement of blood and urine levels is used in diagnosis of poisoning.

■ Treatment of acute exposure is with chelating agents.

Alcohol

Abuse of alcohol (ethanol) is a major contributor to morbidity and mortality, far outstripping other drugs in its effects on the individual and on society. Alcohol is a drug with no receptor. The mechanisms by which it exerts its detrimental effect on cells and organs are not well understood, but the effects are summarized in Table 1.

For clinical purposes alcohol consumption is estimated in arbitrary 'units' – one unit representing 200–300 mmol of ethanol. The ethanol content of some common drinks is shown in Figure 1. The legal limit for driving in the UK is a blood alcohol level of 17.4 mmol/L (80 mg/dL).

Table 1 **Effects of ethanol on organ systems**		
System	**Condition**	**Effect**
CNS	Acute	Disorientation → coma
	Chronic	Memory loss, psychoses
	Withdrawal	Seizures, delirium tremens
Cardiovascular	Chronic	Cardiomyopathy
Skeletal muscle	Chronic	Myopathies
Gastric mucosa	Acute	Irritation, gastritis
	Chronic	Ulceration
Liver	Chronic	Fatty liver → cirrhosis, decreased tolerance to xenobiotics
Kidney	Acute	Diuresis
Blood	Chronic	Anaemia, thrombocytopenia
Testes	Chronic	Impotence

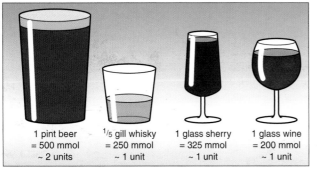

1 pint beer	1/5 gill whisky	1 glass sherry	1 glass wine
= 500 mmol	= 250 mmol	= 325 mmol	= 200 mmol
~ 2 units	~ 1 unit	~ 1 unit	~ 1 unit

Fig. 1 **Alcohol content of common drinks.**

Metabolism of ethanol

Ethanol is metabolized to acetaldehyde by two main pathways (Fig. 2). The alcohol dehydrogenase route is operational when the blood alcohol concentration is in the range 1–5 mmol/L. Above this most of the ethanol is metabolized via the microsomal P450 system. Although the end product in both cases is acetaldehyde, the side effects of induced P450 can be significant. Ethanol metabolism and excretion in a normal 70 kg man is summarized in Figure 3.

Acute alcohol poisoning

The effects of ethanol excess fall into two categories:

- those that are directly related to the blood alcohol concentration at the time, such as coma
- those that are caused by the metabolic effects of continued high ethanol concentrations.

The relative contribution of ethanol in cases of coma, especially where other drugs and/or head injury are present, may be difficult to distinguish. Blood ethanol determinations are the best guide. Where these are not available, plasma osmolality measurement and calculation of the osmolal gap may help.

Recovery from acute alcohol poisoning is usually rapid in the absence of renal or hepatic failure, and is speeded up if hepatic blood flow and oxygenation is maximized. The elimination rate of ethanol is dose-related; at a level of 100 mmol/L it is around 10–15 mmol/hour. Ethanol concentrations in a group of chronic alcoholics admitted in coma with acute alcohol poisoning are shown in Figure 4.

Alcohol inhibits gluconeogenesis and some patients are prone to develop hypoglycaemia 6–36 hours after alcohol ingestion, especially if they are malnourished or fasted. A small number of these malnourished patients develop alcoholic ketoacidosis.

Fig. 2 **The metabolism of ethanol.**

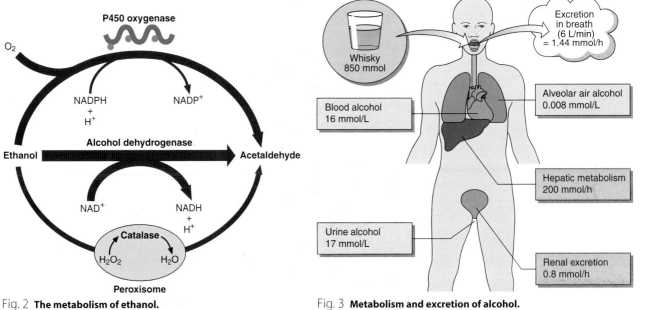

Fig. 3 **Metabolism and excretion of alcohol.**

Chronic alcohol abuse

Many of the effects of chronic alcohol abuse are due either to the toxicity of acetaldehyde and/or the failure of one or more of the many homeostatic and synthetic mechanisms in the liver. One of the earliest signs of chronic alcohol abuse is hepatomegaly. This results from the accumulation of triglyceride due to increased synthesis from the carbohydrate load and reduced protein synthesis. Continued high ethanol intake may cause the following sequelae:

- impaired glucose tolerance and diabetes mellitus
- hypertriglyceridaemia
- cirrhosis of the liver with resultant decreased serum albumin concentration
- portal hypertension with resultant oesophageal varices
- coagulation defects
- cardiomyopathy
- peripheral neuropathy.

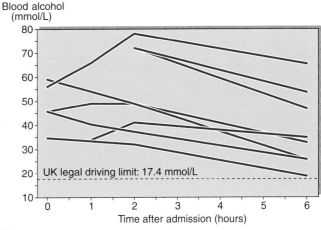

Fig. 4 **Alcohol concentrations in patients admitted in a coma.**

Diagnosis of chronic alcohol abuse

Chronic alcohol abuse can be very difficult to detect, and is usually determined from the patient's history. In order to be more objective, there has been a continued search for markers of ethanol abuse. As yet there is no highly sensitive and specific marker. However, a number of blood components are altered and these can give an indication of chronic alcohol ingestion. The most commonly used are:

- Elevated γGT. This enzyme is increased in 80% of alcohol abusers. It is not a specific indicator as it is increased in all forms of liver disease and is induced by drugs such as phenytoin and phenobarbital.
- Elevated serum triglyceride.
- Hyperuricaemia.

There are a number of other potentially useful markers, notably isoforms of transferrin that are deficient in the carbohydrate linked to the protein. This carbohydrate-deficient transferrin is present in more than 90% of patients with chronic alcohol abuse. Such assays are not yet widely available.

Once the diagnosis of chronic alcohol abuse is made, these markers are of use in monitoring behaviour, since a single 'binge' will lead to their derangement. γGT is used regularly in this manner.

Chronic alcohol abuse exposes the individual to increased risk of damage from other substances. Chronic alcoholics have higher rates of smoking-related disease, and are more susceptible to poisoning with hepatotoxic substances. They also have different rates of metabolism of therapeutic drugs and care needs to be taken in treating them with drugs that are metabolized by the cytochrome P450 system.

Admission rates to hospital with alcohol-related diseases are high, and since the diagnosis is sometimes unsuspected, it should always be considered when carrying out an initial examination (Fig. 5).

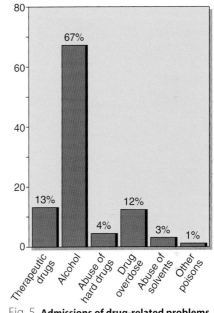

Fig. 5 **Admissions of drug-related problems to one UK hospital.**

Clinical note

Methanol and ethylene glycol (antifreeze) are both metabolized by alcohol dehydrogenase to formic and oxalic acids, which are toxic. In order to prevent this metabolism, ethanol is infused to a concentration of 20 mmol/L until the alcohols, methanol and ethylene glycol, are excreted unchanged. Alcoholics who drink ethanol as well as methanol in fact protect themselves against the worst effects of methanol poisoning.

Alcohol

- Ethanol abuse is a common clinical problem.
- An elevated serum osmolality and an increased osmolal gap can be of diagnostic value in acute ethanol poisoning.
- Chronic ethanol abuse can be difficult to detect.
- Serum γGT is of limited value for diagnosis of ethanol abuse but good for monitoring abstinence.
- The effects of chronic alcohol abuse are not limited to the liver.

Coma

The comatose patient presents a number of problems to the physician, some in relation to initial diagnosis and some later during treatment.

The depth of coma can be defined following clinical examination using a scale such as that in Figure 1. This allows clinical staff to establish the severity of the coma and to monitor changes. Obtaining the correct diagnosis is paramount. To this end the most valuable information is usually obtained from the clinical history, but frequently a reliable history is not available.

Patency of airway, blood pressure, temperature, pupillary reflex and blood glucose concentration need to be monitored repeatedly and a search should be made for evidence of trauma or needlemarks at the time of admission. A careful history and physical examination will give the correct diagnosis in over 90% of cases. Other biochemical tests can help in diagnosis or for the continued monitoring of comatose patients.

Differential diagnosis of coma

A helpful mnemonic in the diagnosis of the unconscious patient is given in Figure 2. However, within each of these categories described there are many possible causes. The first priorities in treating an unconscious patient are to ensure that airways are clear and that breathing and circulation are satisfactory.

Cerebrovascular accident

Where coma of cerebrovascular origin is suspected a CSF examination may show the presence of blood and will help to differentiate a subarachnoid haemorrhage from cerebral infarction (see p. 128). When available, imaging with a CT scan or MRI is preferable.

Infectious causes

Meningitis (bacterial and viral) and encephalitis (viral) can both lead to coma. Meningococcal meningitis has a high mortality, especially in children. Diagnosis is of great importance and CSF specimens should be obtained *before* antibiotic therapy is commenced (Fig. 3). The usual findings are:

- In *bacterial meningitis* CSF protein is increased and glucose is low or absent. There is a leucocytosis that may be visible as cloudiness in severe cases.
- In *viral meningitis* glucose is normal or only slightly depressed and protein may be normal.

Metabolic causes

The brain is acutely sensitive to failure in metabolic homeostasis, and a wide range of disorders can give rise to disorientation and later coma. Many of these cases can be corrected rapidly by treatment and thus their early diagnosis is mandatory. The most common forms are shown in Figure 2.

Hypoglycaemic and hyperglycaemic comas must always be considered. Diagnosis is by measurement of blood glucose, which should be carried out on admission. Glucose can be safely given to any diabetic in coma outside hospital, but insulin must not be administered until hyperglycaemia is confirmed. Over 99% of hypoglycaemic episodes encountered in Accident and Emergency departments will be in patients with known diabetes mellitus.

Drugs and poisons

A wide variety of drugs and poisons can give rise to coma if taken in sufficient dose. In very few cases are there specific clinical signs. Exceptions are

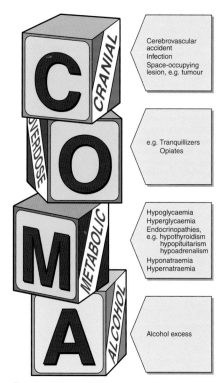

Fig. 2 **Differential diagnosis of a coma patient.**

the pinpoint pupils of opiate poisoning for which the specific antagonist naloxone is effective in restoring consciousness, and the divergent strabismus (Fig. 4) associated with tricyclic antidepressant overdose. In most cases of drug or poison-induced coma, conservative therapy is all that is required to maintain vital functions until the substance is eliminated by metabolism and excretion. The best specimen to analyse for diagnosis is urine. Where drugs such as phenytoin or theophylline are suspected, plasma levels should be measured on admission and thereafter until they fall to therapeutic levels (see pp. 118–119).

Alcohol

Alcohol is a common cause of coma in all age ranges. Coma depth and length is associated with the amount of alcohol ingested, and this shows wide interpatient variation. Alcoholic coma can be associated with head injuries, hypothermia and the presence of other drugs with which its action may be additive. In most cases, coma caused by alcohol will resolve relatively rapidly, the exception being when there is hepatic insufficiency. In cases where the blood alcohol level exceeds 80 mmol/L, haemodialysis may be required. The fact

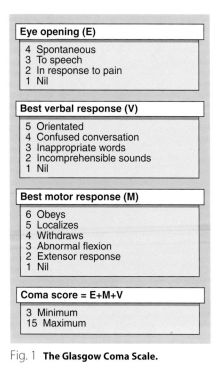

Eye opening (E)
4 Spontaneous
3 To speech
2 In response to pain
1 Nil

Best verbal response (V)
5 Orientated
4 Confused conversation
3 Inappropriate words
2 Incomprehensible sounds
1 Nil

Best motor response (M)
6 Obeys
5 Localizes
4 Withdraws
3 Abnormal flexion
2 Extensor response
1 Nil

Coma score = E+M+V
3 Minimum
15 Maximum

Fig. 1 **The Glasgow Coma Scale.**

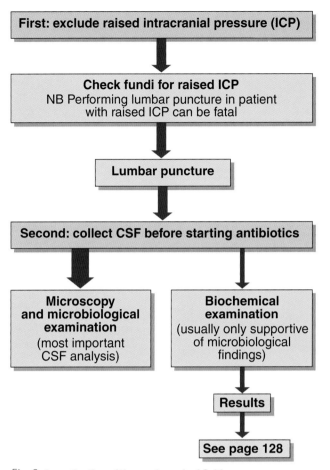

Fig. 3 **Investigation of the cerebrospinal fluid.**

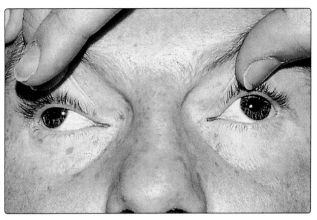

Fig. 4 **Divergent strabismus.**

Brain death

The diagnosis of brain death is made using criteria outlined in Table 1, which includes arterial blood gas analysis. Where measurable sedative drugs have been used (for example in ITU) there must be biochemical confirmation that these drugs are no longer present.

> ### Clinical note
> Coma associated with a cerebrovascular accident will have an abrupt onset and give rise (in most cases) to unilateral signs. Coma caused by metabolic or toxic causes will usually affect all parts of the body equally and will develop over a period of time.

that alcohol can be detected on the breath is not sufficient for diagnosis, and a full clinical examination should be made in all cases of alcoholic coma. If acidosis is present, methanol or ethylene glycol poisoning should also be suspected.

Carbon monoxide poisoning

Carbon monoxide poisoning accounts for a large number of deaths in the UK each year. Coma can occur with a carboxyhaemoglobin concentration above 30% of haemoglobin. Carbon monoxide poisoning may be insidious due to a faulty heater or poor ventilation and may be presaged by headaches and confusion. Treatment with oxygen restores oxyhaemoglobin. This is a dangerous form of poisoning that requires careful aftercare.

Hepatic coma

Acute or chronic hepatic failure may result in coma. This is believed to be due to the failing liver's inability to remove neurotoxins such as ammonia from the blood.

Table 1 **Criteria for confirming brain death**

ALL BRAIN-STEM REFLEXES ARE ABSENT
- The pupils are fixed and unreactive to light
- The corneal reflexes are absent
- The vestibulo-ocular reflexes are absent – there is no eye movement following the injection of 20 mL of ice-cold water into each external auditory meatus in turn
- There are no motor responses to adequate stimulation within the cranial nerve distribution
- There is no gag reflex and no reflex response to a suction catheter in the trachea
- No respiratory movement occurs when the patient is disconnected from the ventilator long enough to allow the carbon dioxide tension to rise above the threshold for stimulating respiration (PCO_2 must reach 6.7 kPa)

The diagnosis of brain death should be made by two experienced doctors, one of whom should be a consultant and the other a consultant or specialist registrar. The tests are usually repeated after an interval of 6–24 hours, depending on the clinical circumstances, before brain death is finally confirmed

Case history 51

A 20-year-old insulin-dependent diabetic was found unconscious beside his bicycle. An hour or so earlier he had left a party where he had been drinking. He was brought to the Accident and Emergency department.

- What investigations and interventions would be appropriate in this case?

Comment on page 167.

Coma

- The first priority is to ensure clear airways and satisfactory breathing and circulation.
- Lateralizing neurological signs should always be sought as evidence of a cerebrovascular accident.
- Hypoglycaemia in the known diabetic patient is the commonest metabolic cause of coma.
- A high percentage of patients in coma from all causes will have alcohol as a complicating factor.

Ascites and pleural fluid

Ascites

Diagnosis

Ascites is fluid in the peritoneal space. It can usually be detected by clinical examination (Fig. 1). Laboratory analysis of ascitic fluid may provide answers to important clinical questions, as its composition varies depending on the underlying cause.

Transudate or exudate?

Traditionally, ascites has been classified based on the protein concentration of the accumulated fluid. Transudates have less protein than exudates. Most cut-offs lie between 20 and 30 g/L. Inflammatory causes of ascites, e.g. malignancy or infection, are usually associated with exudates, whilst transudates more commonly reflect reduced plasma oncotic pressure or increased plasma hydrostatic pressure. However, total protein concentration is not always a reliable guide and comparison of serum and ascites albumin may provide better diagnostic information.

Serum-ascites albumin gradient

The serum-ascites albumin gradient (SAAG) is defined as the serum albumin concentration minus the ascitic fluid albumin concentration. The SAAG correlates directly with the portal pressure. Patients with a wide SAAG (defined as ≥11 g/L) have portal hypertension, whereas patients with a narrow SAAG (<11 g/L) do not (Table 1).

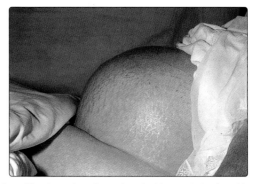

Fig. 1 **Abdominal swelling in ascites.** Reproduced with permission from Hayes PC, Simpson KJ, Gastroenterology and Liver Disease. Churchill Livingstone, Edinburgh, 1995.

Sometimes causes of ascites that are normally associated with a narrow gradient will occur in patients with portal hypertension, in which case the gradient will be wide. In these situations additional analyses may help to narrow the differential diagnosis. For example, abnormalities of pH, lactate, glucose and/or lactate dehydrogenase (LDH) may point towards an inflammatory process; increased lymphocytes in the ascitic fluid may point towards tuberculosis, lymphomas or fungal infections of the peritoneum; and malignant cells are found in nearly all patients with peritoneal carcinomatosis (where the tumour directly involves the peritoneum).

Peritonitis

Cirrhotic patients with ascites are prone to develop peritonitis, usually without an obvious focus of infection (spontaneous bacterial peritonitis or SBP). Less commonly, identifiable sources of infection, e.g. perforated viscus or intra-abdominal abscess, are responsible (secondary infection). Laboratory investigations can assist in three ways. First, they may be used to predict who is going to develop SBP. Second, they may permit rapid detection of infection. Third, they may help to differentiate SBP from secondary infection.

Prediction

A low protein concentration in ascitic fluid predisposes to SBP; the ability of macrophages to consume bacteria

disappears below a total protein concentration of 10 g/L. In addition, a high bilirubin or a low platelet count identifies individuals who are at particularly high risk.

Early detection

For early detection of peritonitis, the neutrophil count in the ascitic fluid has been found to be the best test; this is readily obtainable by doing a full blood count and differential on the ascitic fluid specimen. It has been recommended that patients with a high neutrophil count in the ascitic fluid ($>0.5 \times 10^9$/L) should be treated as if they have SBP.

SBP or secondary infection?

Secondary peritonitis tends to be more severe than SBP, probably because of the heavier bacterial load. This severity is reflected in the ascitic fluid biochemistry (Table 2). Bacteria and neutrophils consume glucose, anaerobic metabolism of which results in the production of lactate, which correlates inversely with pH. Lysis of stimulated neutrophils results in the release of LDH and other cellular proteins, with a consequent rise in the ascitic fluid total protein concentration.

Malignant ascites

Finding malignant cells in the ascitic fluid indicates the presence of malignancy, although not all patients with malignant ascites will have positive cytology. Nearly all patients with peritoneal carcinomatosis have positive cytology, in contrast to patients who develop malignancy-related ascites in association with primary or secondary tumours of the liver. Measurement of tumour markers in ascitic fluid rarely provides additional information over and above that which may be obtained

Table 1 **Serum-ascites albumin gradient**	
Wide (>11 g/L)	**Narrow (<11 g/L)**
Chronic liver disease (cirrhosis)	Peritoneal carcinomatosis
Veno-occlusive disease	Reduced plasma oncotic pressure (e.g. nephrotic syndrome)
Massive hepatic metastases	Secondary peritonitis
Congestive cardiac failure	Tuberculous peritonitis
Spontaneous bacterial peritonitis	

Table 2 **Spontaneous bacterial peritonitis compared with secondary infection**		
Ascitic fluid parameter	**Spontaneous bacterial peritonitis**	**Secondary**
Glucose (mmol/L)	>2.8	<2.8
Lactate dehydrogenase	<upper limit of reference interval	>upper limit of reference interval
Total protein (g/L)	<10	>10

Table 3 **Modified Light's criteria for identification of an exudate**
Pleural fluid is classified as an exudate if *any* of the following criteria are met:
■ Ratio of total protein measured in pleural fluid to total protein measured in serum is greater than 0.5
■ Pleural fluid lactate dehydrogenase (LDH) activity is greater than two-thirds of the upper limit of the serum reference interval
■ Ratio of LDH measured in pleural fluid to LDH measured in serum is greater than 0.6

by serum measurements of the same tumour markers.

Pleural fluid

Diagnosis

Pleural fluid is the fluid found in the pleural cavities between the visceral and parietal pleura (usually less than 10 mL). Pleural effusions can usually be detected by clinical examination of the chest (e.g. by dullness to percussion) or on chest X-ray. As with ascites, composition varies according to the cause.

Transudate or exudate?

Clinicians usually request pleural fluid analysis because they want to know what is causing an effusion. In some cases, a specific cause is suspected, but much more frequently the question is posed in more general terms, by asking if the effusion is a transudate or an exudate. The underlying assumption is that fluid formed by 'exudation' from inflamed or tumour-infiltrated pleura is likely to be high in protein, whereas fluid formed by 'transudation' from normal pleura due to an imbalance in hydrostatic and oncotic forces is likely to be low in protein; in general terms, exudates are more likely to reflect local pathology, and to warrant further investigation. The criteria established by Light and colleagues in 1972, and subsequently modified, continue to be applied widely in classifying pleural fluids as exudates or transudates. They are summarized in Table 3.

Application of Light's criteria in routine practice sometimes results in the misclassification of transudates as exudates. For this reason, alternative markers have been proposed e.g. pleural fluid cholesterol. However, there is no single test, or combination of tests, which is clearly better than modified Light's criteria. In addition, analysis of pleural fluid protein and LDH alone usually produces the same categorization of pleural effusions as modified Light's criteria; thus a blood sample may not always be necessary.

Is it empyema?

Infection of the pleural space usually occurs in association with bacterial pneumonia, and manifests initially as an exudative pleural effusion. If this does not resolve, it can become purulent (when it is referred to as empyema). Empyema is resistant to antibiotic therapy and often only amenable to surgical drainage. So when pleural fluid is frankly purulent or turbid on sampling, insertion of a chest tube is clearly indicated. If it is not clear that an empyema is developing, biochemical analysis may be helpful, in exactly the same way as it is in distinguishing between SBP and secondary infection – bacteria and neutrophils in the pleural fluid consume glucose, and anaerobic metabolism increases with heavier bacterial loads. This results in the production of lactate, which correlates inversely with pH. A pleural fluid pH of less than 7.2 is the most useful predictor of empyema.

Other questions

■ *Malignant pleural effusions.* As with ascites, finding malignant cells in pleural fluid indicates the presence of malignancy, although only 70% of patients with malignant effusions will have positive cytology. Again, measurement of tumour markers in pleural fluid is rarely indicated. This in part reflects the utility of other modalities of investigation in the diagnosis of malignancy, e.g. imaging.

■ *Is it chyle?* Chyle is the fluid found in intestinal lymphatics during absorption of food postprandially. Chylothorax is defined as lymphatic fluid (chyle or lymph) in the pleural space; it usually results from the leak or rupture of the thoracic duct or one of its major divisions. There is no unique marker for chyle, although chylomicrons are relatively specific, except postprandially. Triglycerides are more readily measured than chylomicrons and are widely used instead.

Pleural fluid glucose

For reasons that are not entirely clear, pleural effusions in patients with rheumatoid arthritis characteristically have very low concentrations of glucose; the explanations usually given – consumption of glucose by inflammatory and other cells, or altered pleural permeability to glucose – are not very convincing, since concentrations are relatively normal in other connective tissue disorders like systemic lupus erythematosus. Glucose concentrations are sometimes low in other conditions such as empyema, malignancy and tuberculosis, but are sufficiently variable that they are not diagnostically useful in these contexts.

Ascites and pleural fluid
■ The serum-ascites albumin gradient correlates directly with the portal pressure; a wide gradient indicates portal hypertension.
■ The neutrophil count in the ascitic fluid is the best single test for early detection of peritonitis.
■ Positive cytology (including the finding of malignant cells in the ascetic fluid) indicates the presence of malignancy but negative cytology does not exclude it.
■ Modified Light's criteria are widely used to classify pleural fluids as transudates or exudates.
■ A low pleural fluid pH may help predict the presence of empyema.

Cerebrospinal and other body fluids

Cerebrospinal fluid

Cerebrospinal fluid (CSF) is produced by the choroid plexuses, partly by ultrafiltration and partly by secretion, and fills and circulates through the ventricles and spinal cord. Compared with plasma, it has less protein, and the concentrations of protein-bound components like bilirubin are similarly reduced. Its electrolyte composition is similar to but distinct from plasma (more chloride, less potassium and calcium). Infection or the presence of blood in the CSF alters its composition. This provides the basis for biochemical analysis of CSF in the diagnosis of subarachnoid haemorrhage (SAH) and meningitis.

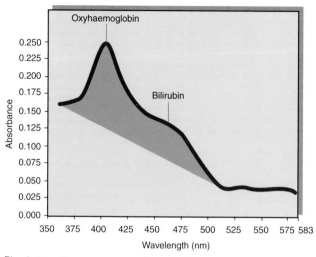

Fig. 1 **Absorbance spectrum of CSF in subarachnoid haemorrhage.**

Lumbar puncture

Lumbar puncture (LP) is the procedure performed in order to obtain a specimen of CSF. If signs of intracranial pressure such as hypertension, bradycardia and papilloedema are present then an LP should not be performed.

When collecting CSF in suspected infection, e.g. meningitis, microbiological examination takes priority. If subarachnoid haemorrhage is suspected, it may help to collect the CSF as several separate aliquots. These will be equally blood-stained in SAH, but progressively less so if the blood in the CSF results from damage to a blood vessel during the LP procedure (a so-called 'traumatic tap').

Subarachnoid haemorrhage

Bleeding into the subarachnoid space most frequently results from rupture of an aneurysm (swelling) in

one or more of the arteries located within the space. The patient typically complains of a severe headache of sudden onset ('thunderclap'), often associated with vomiting and a reduced level of consciousness. Where CT or MRI is readily available, it may be possible to diagnose SAH without doing an LP. However, the earliest changes in the composition of CSF precede the development of changes on imaging, and where SAH is suspected, LP should not be delayed unless there are signs of raised intracranial pressure.

Xanthochromia

Xanthochromia simply means yellow discoloration of the CSF. It results from the presence of blood pigments derived from red blood cells (RBCs) that have undergone lysis. It can be detected by visual inspection, but

this is unreliable, and where possible scanning spectrophotometry should be used instead. This involves measuring the absorbance of the CSF specimen across a range of wavelengths; the blood pigments have characteristic absorbance peaks (Fig. 1).

Meningitis

Meningitis refers to inflammation of the meninges which line the central nervous system (CNS). Bacterial meningitis presents acutely and is a medical emergency. CSF biochemistry tends to reflect the nature of the infective organism (Table 1) but is characteristic rather than diagnostic. Microbiological analysis should take priority. It is important when interpreting the relative concentrations of, for example, glucose in the CSF to take a blood sample for comparison.

Table 1 **CSF parameters in health and some common disorders**						
	Normal	**Subarachnoid haemorrhage**	**Acute bacterial meningitis**	**Viral meningitis**	**Tuberculous meningitis**	**Multiple sclerosis**
Pressure	50–180 mm of water	Increased	Normal/increased	Normal	Normal/increased	Normal
Colour	Clear	Blood-stained; xanthochromic	Cloudy	Clear	Clear/cloudy	Clear
Red cell count	0–4/mm³	Raised	Normal	Normal	Normal	Normal
White cell count	0–4/mm³	Normal/slightly raised	1000–5000 polymorphs	10–2000 lymphocytes	50–5000 lymphocytes	0–50 lymphocytes
Glucose	>60% of blood level	Normal	Decreased	Normal	Decreased	Normal
Protein	<0.45 g/L	Increased	Increased	Normal/increased	Increased	Normal/increased
Microbiology	Sterile	Sterile	Organisms on Gram stain and/or culture	Sterile/virus detected	Ziehl–Neelsen/ auramine stain or tuberculosis culture positive	Sterile
Oligoclonal bands	Negative	Negative	Can be positive	Can be positive	Can be positive	Often positive

From Haslett C et al, Davidson's Principles and Practice of Medicine. Churchill Livingstone, Edinburgh, 2002.

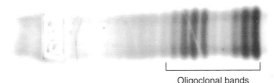

Fig. 2 **Oligoclonal CSF bands.**

Inherited metabolic disorders

CSF analysis may be helpful in the diagnosis of several inherited metabolic disorders. For example, high CSF lactate may be seen in inborn errors of metabolism affecting the respiratory chain, even when plasma lactate is normal or only slightly increased. This may reflect tissue specificity of electron transport chain proteins, or the high-energy demand (and lactate production) of the brain. CSF pyruvate concentrations are also high in these conditions. CSF amino acid analysis may similarly be helpful in diagnosing various inherited disorders of amino acid metabolism; these are sometimes considered in children with unexplained seizures but are very rare.

Other conditions

Analysis of CSF may be helpful in the evaluation of a variety of non-acute conditions, but as with meningitis the findings are rarely diagnostic. Very high CSF protein concentrations may be seen where there is interruption to the circulation of CSF, e.g. spinal tumours; the mechanisms include increased capillary permeability (to plasma proteins) and CSF fluid reabsorption due to stasis. Increased capillary permeability is best revealed by CSF electrophoresis; the high-molecular-weight plasma proteins, which are not normally found in CSF, can readily be identified. This non-specific pattern is found in many infective/inflammatory conditions involving the CNS.

CSF electrophoresis may also reveal the presence of oligoclonal bands (Fig. 2). If these are not seen also in the serum, they reflect local (i.e. CNS) synthesis of immunoglobulin. Ninety per cent of patients with multiple sclerosis (MS) have these bands, but they are not specific for this condition. Thus their absence in cases of suspected MS is more diagnostically useful than their presence.

Dementia

Currently, no biochemical markers meet the criteria that would allow reliable differentiation of Alzheimer's disease from other dementias (e.g. vascular), although there are various candidates. The most promising include the ratio of a phosphorylated form of tau protein (see below) to a protein known as beta-amyloid peptide 42. Recent research claims to have identified an 'Alzheimer's phenotype', based on plasma concentrations of proteins involved in intercellular communication. Though promising, these findings require to be replicated in larger studies.

Identification of body fluids

Cerebrospinal fluid

Not infrequently clinicians ask the laboratory to identify specimens of fluid collected from patients with rhinorrhoea or otorrhoea. The finding in the specimen of the so-called tau protein identifies it as CSF. This is an isoform of β-transferrin that is specific to the CSF.

Urine

Urine is often suspected as a contaminant of drain fluids. Contamination can usually be detected fairly easily by measuring urea and/or creatinine in serum, urine, and the fluid specimen under consideration; urinary concentrations of urea and creatinine greatly exceed serum concentrations.

Chyle

Chyle is the fluid found in the intestinal lymphatics during absorption of food postprandially. It appears milky due to the presence of fats. The intestinal lymphatics drain into the thoracic duct, and thence into the venous system. Occasionally the presence of chyle in the thoracic or abdominal cavities (known as chylothorax and chylous ascites respectively) is suspected, due for example to a leak from the thoracic duct. Although there is no unique marker of chyle, measurement of triglycerides may be helpful. Concentrations that are significantly greater in the suspected fluid than in fasting serum are suggestive.

Other fluids

Laboratory identification of other body fluids is not usually performed. In some cases, e.g. ascites and pleural fluid, there is no unique marker, and identification is rarely an issue. Other fluids, e.g. bile, are identifiable by visual inspection. Occasionally it may be helpful to distinguish amniotic fluid from maternal urine or vaginal fluid (in the context of suspected premature rupture of the fetal membranes). Although fetal fibronectin is relatively specific to amniotic fluid, it is not widely available, and diagnosis of labour can usually be made on other grounds.

🩺 *Clinical note*
The commonest side effect after the removal of CSF through lumbar puncture is headache, which occurs in up to 30% of adults and up to 40% of children.

Cerebrospinal and other body fluids

- CSF analysis may be helpful in a number of conditions but biochemical analysis alone is rarely diagnostic.
- When collecting CSF in suspected infection, e.g. meningitis, microbiological examination takes priority over biochemical examination.
- Xanthochromia may be due to blood pigments in the CSF from red cell lysis.
- CSF electrophoresis may reveal the presence of oligoclonal bands, which are commonly found in patients with MS.
- Biochemical analysis of other body fluids may be useful in identifying them.

Lipoprotein metabolism

The lipoprotein system evolved to solve the problem of transporting fats around the body in the aqueous environment of the plasma. A lipoprotein is a complex spherical structure that has a hydrophobic core wrapped in a hydrophilic coating (Fig. 1). The core contains triglyceride and cholesteryl esters, while the surface contains phospholipid, free cholesterol and proteins – the apolipoproteins (Table 1). Cholesterol is an essential component of all cell membranes and is a precursor for steroid hormone and bile acid biosynthesis. Triglyceride is central to the storage and transport of energy within the body.

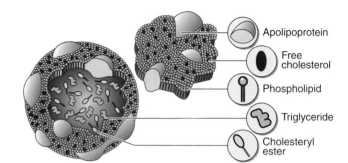

Fig. 1 **Structure of a lipoprotein.**

Nomenclature

Several different classes of lipoproteins exist whose structure and function are closely related. Apart from the largest species, the chylomicron, these are named according to their density, as they are most commonly isolated by ultracentrifugation. The four main lipoproteins and their functions are shown in Table 2.

Metabolism

Lipoprotein metabolism (Fig. 2) can be thought of as two cycles, one exogenous and one endogenous, both centred on the liver. These cycles are interconnected.

Two key enzyme systems are involved in lipoprotein metabolism, i.e.:

- Lipoprotein lipase (LPL) releases free fatty acids and glycerol from chylomicrons and VLDL into the tissues.
- Lecithin: cholesterol acyl transferase (LCAT) forms cholesteryl esters from free cholesterol and fatty acids.

The exogenous lipid cycle

Dietary lipid is absorbed in the small intestine and incorporated into chylomicrons that are secreted into the lymphatics and reach the bloodstream via the thoracic duct. In the circulation, triglyceride is gradually removed from these lipoproteins by the action of lipoprotein lipase. This enzyme is present in the capillaries of a number of tissues, predominantly adipose tissue and

Table 1 Properties of some human apolipoproteins

Apolipoprotein	Molecular weight	Site of synthesis	Function
A-I	28 000	Intestine, liver	Activates LCAT
A-II	17 000	Intestine, liver	–
B$_{100}$	549 000	Liver	Triglyceride and cholesterol transport Binds to LDL receptor
B$_{48}$	264 000	Intestine	Triglyceride transport
C-I	6600	Liver	Activates LCAT
C-II	8850	Liver	Activates LPL
C-III	8800	Liver	? Inhibits LPL
E	34 000	Liver, intestine, macrophage	Binds to LDL receptor and probably also to another specific liver receptor

LCAT = Lecithin; cholesterol acyl transferase.
LPL = Lipoprotein lipase.

Table 2 The four main lipoproteins and their functions

Lipoprotein	Main apolipoproteins	Function
Chylomicrons	B$_{48}$, A-I, C-II, E	Largest lipoprotein. Synthesized by gut after a meal. Not present in normal fasting plasma. Main carrier of dietary triglyceride
Very low density lipoprotein (VDL)	B$_{100}$, C-II, E	Synthesized in the liver. Main carrier of endogenously produced triglyceride
Low density lipoprotein (LDL)	B$_{100}$	Generated from VLDL in the circulation. Main carrier of cholesterol
High density lipoprotein (HDL)	A-I, A-II	Smallest lipoprotein. Protective function. Takes cholesterol from extrahepatic tissues to the liver for excretion

skeletal muscle. As it loses triglyceride, the chylomicron becomes smaller and deflated, with folds of redundant surface material. These remnants are removed by the liver. The cholesterol may be utilized by the liver to form cell membrane components or bile acids, or may be excreted in the bile. The liver provides the only route by which cholesterol leaves the body in significant amounts.

The endogenous lipid cycle

The liver synthesizes VLDL particles that undergo the same form of delipidation as chylomicrons by the action of lipoprotein lipase. This results in the formation of an intermediate density lipoprotein (IDL), which becomes low density lipoprotein (LDL) when further delipidated. LDL

may be removed from the circulation by the high affinity LDL receptor or by other scavenger routes that are thought to be important at high LDL levels and the main way in which cholesterol is incorported into atheromatous plaques.

HDL particles are derived from both liver and gut. They act as cholesteryl ester shuttles, removing the sterol from the peripheral tissues and returning it to the liver. The HDL is taken up either directly by the liver, or indirectly by being transferred to other circulating lipoproteins, which then return it to the liver. This process is thought to be anti-atherogenic, and an elevated HDL-cholesterol level has been shown to confer a decreased risk of coronary heart disease on an individual.

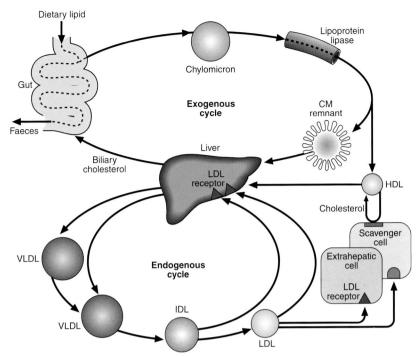

Fig. 2 **Lipoprotein metabolism.**

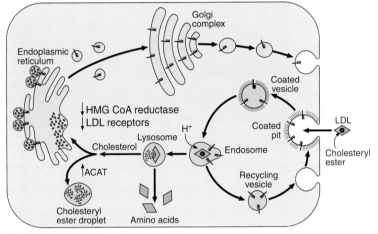

Fig. 3 **The LDL receptor pathway.**

Apolipoproteins

Apolipoproteins are the protein components of the lipoproteins (Table 1). They are important in:

- maintaining the structural integrity of the lipoproteins
- regulating certain enzymes that act on lipoproteins
- receptor recognition.

The LDL receptor

The LDL receptor (Fig. 3), a glycoprotein present on the surface of all cells, spans the cell membrane and is concentrated in special membrane recesses, called 'coated' pits. It binds to lipoproteins containing apolipoprotein B and E, and internalizes them for breakdown within the cell. Receptors are then recycled to the cell surface. The number and function of receptors dictate the level of circulating LDL. When the cell has sufficient cholesterol, the synthesis of receptors is down-regulated; when the cell is cholesterol depleted, the receptors increase in number. Inherited malfunction or absence of these receptors leads to familial hypercholesterolaemia (FH).

A specific mutation of apolipoprotein B results in defective binding of LDL to its receptor and produces an identical clinical picture to FH called familial defective apo B (FDB).

Clinical note
About 25% of the UK population have plasma cholesterol concentrations above the desirable level. In most cases this is the result of diet and lifestyle.

Case history 52

A 3-year-old boy with a history of chronic abdominal pain was admitted as an emergency. His blood was noted to be pink in the syringe, and the serum was milky.

Na⁺	K⁺	Cl⁻	HCO₃⁻	Urea	Glucose
			— mmol/L —		
103	3.8	70	20	3.1	5.2

Serum osmolality was measured as 282 mmol/kg and amylase 1780 U/L.
His triglyceride was reported to be >50 mmol/L.

- Why is there a discrepancy between the calculated and measured osmolality?
- What are the likely causes of the hypertriglyceridaemia?

Comment on page 167.

Lipoprotein metabolism

- Lipoproteins are complexes of lipid and proteins that facilitate lipid transport.

- Their metabolism can be thought of as two interconnected cycles centred on the liver.

- Lipoproteins are defined by their density and differ in composition, structure and function.

- Apolipoproteins have a functional as well as structural importance.

- Cholesterol can only be excreted from the body by way of the liver.

Clinical disorders of lipid metabolism

Lipoprotein disorders are some of the commonest metabolic diseases seen in clinical practice. They may present with their various sequelae which include:

- coronary heart disease (CHD)
- acute pancreatitis
- failure to thrive and weakness
- cataracts.

Classification

Currently there is no satisfactory comprehensive classification of lipoprotein disorders. Genetic classifications have been attempted but are becoming increasingly complex as different mutations are discovered (Table 1). *Familial hypercholesterolaemia* (FH), which may present with xanthelasma (Fig. 1), tendon xanthomas, severe hypercholesterolaemia and premature coronary heart disease, may be due to any of over 500 different mutations of the LDL receptor gene. Mutations of the apolipoprotein (apo) B gene can give an identical syndrome. *Familial hyperchylomicronaemia*, which presents with recurrent abdominal pain and pancreatitis, may result from genetic mutations of the lipoprotein lipase or apo C-II genes. Eruptive xanthomas (Fig. 2) are characteristic of hypertriglyceridaemia.

Until gene therapy and/or specific substitution therapy become more available, genetic classifications, while biologically very illuminating, are unlikely to prove very useful in practice. In practice, lipoprotein disorders are simplistically classified as being:

- *Primary* – when the disorder is not due to an identifiable underlying disease.
- *Secondary* – when the disorder is a manifestation of some other disease.

Table 1 Some genetic causes of dyslipidaemia

Disease	Genetic defect	Fredrickson	Risk
Familial hypercholesterolaemia	Reduced numbers of functional LDL receptors	IIa or IIb	CHD
Familial hypertriglyceridaemia	Possibly single gene defect	IV or V	
Familial combined hyperlipidaemia	Possibly single gene defect	IIa, IIb, IV or V	CHD
Lipoprotein lipase deficiency	Reduced levels of functional LPL	I	Pancreatitis
Apo C-II deficiency	Inability to synthesize apo C-II (cofactor for lipoprotein lipase)	I	Pancreatitis
Abetalipoproteinaemia	Inability to synthesize apo B	Normal	Fat soluble vitamin deficiencies, neurological deficit
Analphalipoproteinaemia (Tangier disease)	Inability to synthesize apo A	Normal	Neurological deficit. Cholesteryl ester storage in abnormal sites

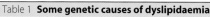

Fig. 1 **Xanthelasmas in younger individuals (age <40 years) usually indicate hypercholesterolaemia.** In the elderly they do not carry the same significance.

Primary

The Fredrickson or World Health Organization classification is the most widely accepted for the primary hyperlipidaemias (Fig. 3). It relies on the findings of plasma analysis, rather than genetics. As a result, patients with the same genetic defect may fall into different groups, or may change grouping as the disease progresses or is treated (Table 1).

The major advantage of this classification is that it is widely accepted and gives some guidance for treatment.

The six types of hyperlipoproteinaemia defined in the Fredrickson classification are not equally common. Types I and V are rare, while types IIa, IIb and IV are very common. Type III hyperlipoproteinaemia, also known as familial dysbetalipoproteinaemia, is intermediate in frequency, occurring in about 1/5000 of the population.

Secondary

Secondary hyperlipidaemia is a well-recognized feature of a number of diseases (Table 2) that divide broadly into two categories:

- Clinically obvious diseases such as renal failure, nephrotic syndrome and cirrhosis of the liver.

Table 2 Common causes of secondary hyperlipidaemia

Disease	Usual dominant lipid abnormality
Diabetes mellitus	Increased triglyceride
Alcohol excess	Increased triglyceride
Chronic renal failure	Increased triglyceride
Drugs, e.g. thiazide diuretics	Increased triglyceride
Hypothyroidism	Increased cholesterol
Nephrotic syndrome	Increased cholesterol

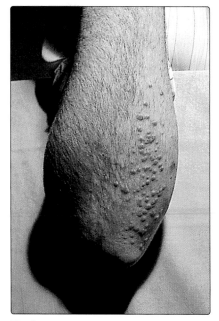

Fig. 2 **Eruptive xanthomas in a patient with hypertriglyceridaemia.**

- Covert conditions that may present as hyperlipidaemia. These include hypothyroidism, diabetes mellitus and alcohol abuse.

Atherogenic profiles

The causal association of certain forms of hyperlipidaemia and CHD is clearly the major stimulus for the measurement of plasma lipids and lipoproteins in clinical practice. The most common lipid disorder linked with atherogenesis and an increased risk of CHD is an elevated plasma LDL cholesterol level, but increasingly it is being recognized that individuals with low plasma HDL cholesterol and hypertriglyceridaemia are also at increased risk.

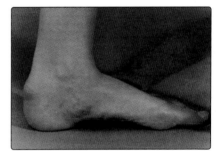

Type	Normal	Type I	Type IIa	Type IIb	Type III	Type IV	Type V
Sample							
Lipoprotein	N	↑ Chylomicrons	↑ LDL ↑ VLDL	↑ LDL	↑ IDL	↑ VLDL ↑ VLDL	↑ Chylomicrons
Total cholesterol	N	N or ↑	↑	↑	↑	N or ↑	N or ↑
Triglycerides	N	↑↑	N	↑	↑	↑	↑↑
LDL-CHOL	N	N or ↓	↑	↑	N or ↓	N	N
HDL-CHOL	N	N or ↓	N or ↓	N or ↓	N or ↓	N or ↓	N or ↓

Fig. 3 **Fredrickson (WHO) classification of dyslipidaemia.** This is based on the appearance of a fasting plasma sample after standing for 12 hours at 4°C and analysis of its cholesterol and triglyceride content.

Clinical note

The physical signs of the hyperlipidaemias are not specific for any particular disease and may sometimes be present in normolipidaemic patients, e.g. arcus senilis (Fig. 4). Their presence is, however, highly suggestive of raised lipids. Tendon xanthomas (Fig. 5) are particularly associated with familial hypercholesterolaemia.

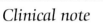

Fig. 4 **Arcus senilis.**

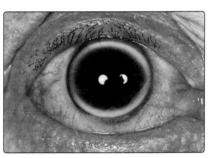

Fig. 5 **Tendon xanthomas.** These are pathognomic for familial hypercholesterolaemia and are often first seen on the Achilles tendon as in this patient.

Case history 53

A 53-year-old man was found to have the following results on a fasting blood sample:

Total cholesterol	Triglyceride	Glucose	γGT
mmol/L			U/L
8.4	6.8	9.8	138

A non-smoker, his blood pressure was 145/95 mmHg and he was obese with central fat distribution.

- What other information and investigations would be helpful in this man's management?
- What treatment options would you consider in this case?

Comment on page 168.

Clinical disorders of lipid metabolism

- The Fredrickson classification is still commonly used to classify hyperlipoproteinaemias by phenotype.

- The genetic and environmental nature of many causes of primary hyperlipidaemia are, as yet, unknown.

- Secondary causes of hyperlipidaemia are common and include hypothyroidism, diabetes mellitus, liver disease and alcohol abuse.

Hypertension

Hypertension is a common clinical problem. It is defined as chronically increased systemic arterial blood pressure. The definition of hypertension has changed over the years, as more effective treatments have become available. The WHO classification of hypertension is shown in Table 1. It is important not to base clinical decisions on a single blood pressure reading. Some patients have 'white coat' hypertension, where readings taken by doctors or other health professionals are misleadingly high. Ambulatory blood pressure measurement over a whole day provides the most detailed information (Fig. 1).

If hypertension is left untreated, patients are at risk of several complications. These include:

- stroke
- left ventricular hypertrophy leading eventually to heart failure
- chronic kidney disease
- retinopathy.

Occasionally patients present with severe hypertension associated with a severe form of retinopathy known as papilloedema, and progressive renal failure. This is known somewhat misleadingly as malignant hypertension and requires urgent treatment.

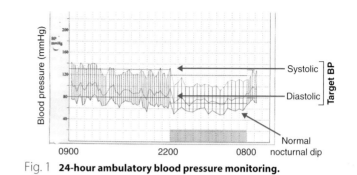

Fig. 1 **24-hour ambulatory blood pressure monitoring.**

identifiable causes (see below), some of which may be diagnosed or monitored biochemically. However, other modalities of investigation are at least as important in the investigation of hypertension. For example, imaging of renal arteries, or isotope renograms, may provide vital diagnostic information.

- *Renal parenchymal disease.* This can be confirmed by the finding of a reduced estimated glomerular filtration rate (eGFR) and/or proteinuria.
- *Renal artery stenosis.* This should be suspected in refractory hypertension, especially if creatinine rises on treatment with angiotensin-converting enzyme inhibitors (ACEIs) or angiotensin receptor blockers (ARBs). This is best diagnosed with magnetic resonance angiography.

It may be associated with grossly elevated renin concentrations.

- *Primary hyperaldosteronism.* This is dealt with in more detail on page 97. It should be suspected if hypokalaemia (often with associated alkalosis) is present, especially if there is a failure to respond to potassium supplementation. The ratio of aldosterone to renin is characteristically elevated, although imaging studies (CT or MRI) are required to make the diagnosis.
- *Phaeochromocytoma.* This is a relatively rare cause of secondary hypertension. It should be suspected if hypertension occurs in paroxysms, or if symptoms (like palpitations, headaches) are episodic. Urinary catecholamine is usually but not always raised, and there are often false positive results as well. In doubtful cases, normal isotope

Causes of hypertension
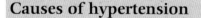

Hypertension is related to genetic and environmental factors. Often it runs in families, more than would be expected simply on the basis of a shared environment. Often it is associated with obesity or alcohol consumption (acquired). In many patients, the cause is not known, and in these patients it is referred to as 'primary' or 'essential' hypertension. So-called secondary hypertension is due to clearly

Table 1 **WHO classification of hypertension**	
Category	**BP (mmHg)**
Optimal blood pressure	<120/80
Normal blood pressure	<130/85
Mild hypertension	140/90–159/99
Moderate hypertension	160/100–179/109
Severe hypertension	≥180/110

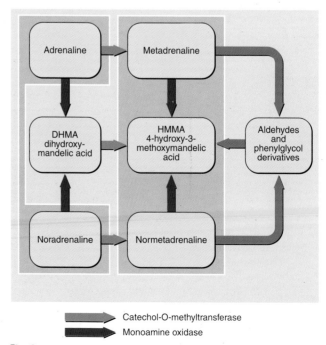

Fig. 2 **Pathway for production of catecholamine metabolites.**

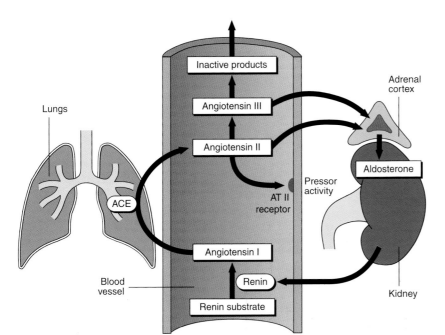

Fig. 3 **Mechanism of primary hyperaldosteronism**.

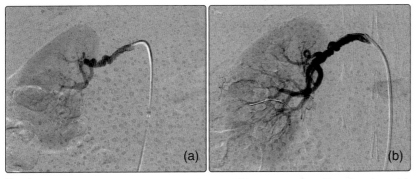

(a) (b)

Fig. 4 **Renal artery stenosis: (a)** pre-angioplasty and **(b)** post-angioplasty. Note the substantial increase in blood flow into the kidney post procedure. The functional impact of renal artery stenosis can be assessed clinically by the response to antihypertensive treatment, and biochemically by measurement of plasma renin activity.

(MIBG) scans are the best way of excluding the condition. The biochemical pathways involved in the production of catecholamines are illustrated in Figure 2.

- *Cushing's syndrome*. This is dealt with in more detail on pages 96–97. It is not usually a diagnostic dilemma, since the signs and symptoms of Cushing's syndrome, and the association with hypertension, are well recognized. However, if there is doubt, a dexamethasone suppression test (p. 81) may be useful.
- *Obesity/sleep apnoea*. Obesity is an increasingly common cause of secondary hypertension, especially if it is associated with sleep apnoea. The latter is likely in the presence of an increased neck circumference.
- *Other*. Less common causes of secondary hypertension include acromegaly, hyperthyroidism and hypothyroidism, and coarctation of the aorta.

Treatment of hypertension

Various groups of antihypertensive drugs are used in the management of hypertension. When patients fail to respond to one or more agents, many physicians add in other drugs, on the grounds that increasing the dose of existing treatments often increases side effects without enhancing the efficacy. Thus many patients end up on multiple drugs for their hypertension. Commonly used groups of drugs include the following:

- *ACEIs/ARBs*. ACEIs inhibit angiotensin-converting enzyme, and so reduce production of angiotensin II (a potent vasoconstrictor) and, ultimately, aldosterone (a potent mineralocorticoid). ARBs block angiotensin receptors (Fig. 3). Both groups of drugs may in some

patients reduce the renal damage induced by hypertension; this can be monitored by their effect on reducing proteinuria. In some patients with refractory hypertension, the introduction of ACEI/ARBs is associated with a rapid rise in creatinine. In this scenario, the drug should be stopped and renal artery stenosis suspected (see above).

- *Beta blockers*. Although these drugs now compete with more effective alternatives, they are still widely used. They act by blocking beta-adrenergic receptors in the heart, kidneys and brain, thereby reducing cardiac output, renin and noradrenaline release.
- *Calcium channel blockers*. These drugs are also widely used. They reduce entry of calcium into vascular smooth muscle, thereby reducing vascular tone and peripheral arterial resistance.
- *Diuretics*. These all induce natriuresis. Thiazide diuretics like bendroflumethiazide enhance the efficacy of other drugs, and are commonly used. Loop diuretics such as furosemide induce a more powerful natriuresis than thiazide diuretics. Spironolactone and other aldosterone antagonists (also known as potassium-sparing diuretics) are often associated with hyperkalaemia; potassium should be checked before and after their introduction.
- *Other drugs*. Doxazosin (an alpha blocker) and moxonidine (centrally acting) are also used. Other drugs are reserved for specialist care.
- Please insert two new figures (figures 4 a and 4b). Suggest move Figure 2 onto the previous page (p134) for balance. Figures are attached and will be sent electronically as well.

Hypertension

- In most patients with hypertension no specific cause can be found.
- Simple biochemical tests (e.g. U & Es) are useful for monitoring the biochemical effects of treatment, e.g. hypokalaemia.
- Biochemical tests are useful in monitoring renal damage, which can be a cause of hypertension or a manifestation of it.
- Less commonly, biochemistry may be helpful in the diagnosis of rarer causes of hypertension such as Conn's and Cushing's syndromes.

Cancer and its consequences

In Western societies one death in five is caused by cancer. The effects of tumour growth may be local or systemic (Fig. 1), e.g. obstruction of blood vessels, lymphatics or ducts, damage to nerves, effusions, bleeding, infection, necrosis of surrounding tissue and eventual death of the patient. The cancer cells may secrete toxins locally or into the general circulation. Both endocrine and non-endocrine tumours may secrete hormones or other regulatory molecules.

A tumour marker is any substance that can be related to the presence or progress of a tumour (see pp. 138–139).

Local effects of tumours

The local growth of a tumour can cause a wide range of abnormalities in commonly requested biochemical tests. This may be a consequence of obstruction of blood vessels or ducts, e.g. the blockage of bile ducts by carcinoma of head of pancreas causes elevated serum alkaline phosphatase and sometimes jaundice. The symptoms that result from such local effects may be the first sign to the patient that something is wrong, but there may be no initial suspicion that there is an underlying malignancy.

The liver is often the site of metastatic spread of a tumour. An isolated increase in the serum alkaline phosphatase or γGT is a common finding when this occurs. Even with significant liver involvement, there may be no biochemical abnormalities. Modest increases in the aminotransferases, ALT and AST, are observed if the rate of cell destruction is high.

Metastatic spread of a tumour to an important site may precipitate complete system failure. For example, destruction of the adrenal cortex by tumour causes impaired aldosterone and cortisol secretion, with potentially fatal consequences.

Rapid tumour growth gives rise to abnormal biochemistry. Leukaemia and lymphoma are often associated with elevated serum urate concentrations due to the rapid cell turnover. Serum lactate dehydrogenase is often elevated in these patients, reflecting the high concentration of the enzyme in the tumour and the cellular turnover. Large tumours may not have an extensive

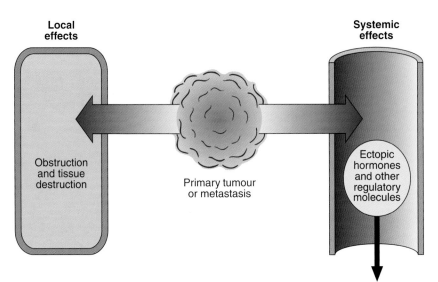

Fig. 1 **Biochemical effects of tumour growth.**

blood supply and the tumour cells meet their energy needs via anaerobic glycolysis. This may result in the generation of a lactic acidosis.

Renal failure may occur in patients with malignancy for the following reasons:

- obstruction of the urinary tract
- hypercalcaemia
- Bence Jones proteinuria
- hyperuricaemia
- nephrotoxicity of cytotoxic drugs.

Cancer cachexia

Cancer cachexia describes the characteristic wasting often seen in cancer patients. The features include anorexia, lethargy, weight loss, muscle weakness, anaemia and pyrexia. The development of cancer cachexia is due to many factors and is incompletely understood. Certainly, there is an imbalance between dietary calorie intake and body energy requirements. This results from a combination of factors:

- *Inadequate food intake.*
- *Impaired digestion and absorption.*
- *Competition between the host and tumour for nutrients.* The growing tumour has a high metabolic rate and may deprive the body of nutrients, especially if it is large. One consequence of this is a fall in the plasma cholesterol level in cancer patients.

- *Increased energy requirement of the cancer patient.* The host reaction to the tumour is similar to the metabolic response to injury, with increased metabolic rate and altered tissue metabolism.

Tumour spread may cause infection, dysphagia, persistent vomiting and diarrhoea, all of which may contribute to the overall picture seen in cancer cachexia. The observation that small tumours can have a profound effect on host metabolism suggests that cancer cells secrete or cause the release of humoral agents that mediate the metabolic changes of cancer cachexia. Some of these, such as tumour necrosis factor, have been identified. This cytokine is secreted by activated macrophages and acts on a variety of tissues including muscle, adipose tissue and liver.

Ectopic hormones

It is a characteristic feature of some cancers that they secrete hormones, even though the tumour has not arisen from an endocrine organ. Referred to as ectopic hormone production, hormone secretion by tumours has frequently been invoked but rarely proven (Fig. 2). Small cell carcinomas are the most aggressive of the lung cancers and are the most likely to be associated with ectopic hormone production. Ectopic ACTH secretion causing Cushing's syndrome is the most common. However, the classic clinical features of Cushing's syndrome are not usually apparent in the rapidly progressing ectopic ACTH disorder. Biochemical features include hypokalaemia and metabolic alkalosis and these may be the sole indicators of the problem.

Not infrequently, patients with malignancy develop the syndrome of inappropriate antidiuresis (SIAD). Water is retained and patients present with hyponatraemia. This is probably the commonest biochemical abnormality seen in patients with cancer and is almost invariably due to pituitary AVP secretion in response to non-osmotic stimuli. SIAD is often, incorrectly, attributed to ectopic AVP secretion, which is in fact very rare.

Some cancers may cause hypercalcaemia. In many cases this is due to the secretion of parathyroid hormone related protein, PTHrP, so called because of its relationship with PTH both in its structure and function.

Consequences of cancer treatment

Anti-tumour therapy can have serious effects. Gonadal failure arising from radiotherapy or chemotherapy is frequently encountered. Hypomagnesaemia and hypokalaemia may be a consequence of the use of the cytotoxic drug cisplatin. Patients treated with methotrexate may become folate deficient.

Hyperuricaemia is a consequence of the massive cell death that occurs in the treatment of some tumours with cytotoxic drugs, particularly lymphomas and some leukaemias, and is known as tumour lysis syndrome.

(a)

Condition resolves after surgical removal of tumour or irradiation. Good evidence, but may be due to tumour secretion of a releasing factor, e.g. secretion of growth hormone may be due to the production of growth hormone releasing hormone.

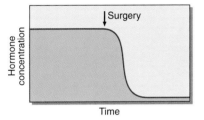

(b)

Demonstration that hormone level in arterial supply to tumour is less than in venous drainage. Good evidence, especially if combined with **(a)**.

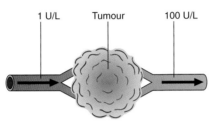

(c)

Hormone may be extracted from tumour. Good evidence, but may be due to absorption of hormone by tumour.

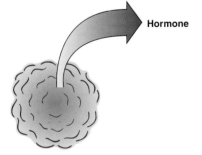

(d)

Histochemical demonstration of hormone in tumour cell secretory granules and mRNA for hormone in tumour. Definitive evidence.

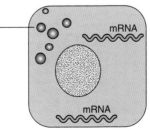

Fig. 2 **Evidence for ectopic hormone production.**

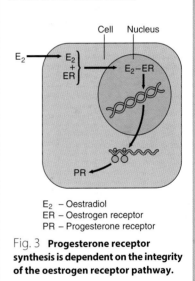
Case history 55

SI, a 37-year-old man, presented to this GP complaining of nocturia, frequency of micturition and polydipsia. On examination, he had mild truncal obesity, plethora, and ankle oedema. He had purpura of his arms but no striae. His blood pressure was 185/115 mmHg. Biochemistry results in a serum specimen showed:

Na+	K+	Cl−	HCO₃⁻	Urea	Creatinine	Glucose
		— *mmol/L* —			*µmol/L*	*mmol/L*
146	2.1	96	34	7.0	135	8.5

- What is the most likely diagnosis?
- What further biochemistry tests should be requested?

Comment on page 168.

Tumour markers

A tumour marker is any substance that can be related to the presence or progress of a tumour. In practice, the clinical biochemistry laboratory measures markers that are present in blood, although the term 'tumour markers' can also be applied to substances found on the surface of or within cells fixed in frozen or paraffin sections. A tumour marker in plasma has been secreted or released by the tumour cells. Such markers are not necessarily unique products of the malignant cells, but may simply be expressed by the tumour in a greater amount than by normal cells.

Tumour markers fall into one of several groups: they may be hormones, e.g. human chorionic gonadotrophin (HCG) secreted by choriocarcinoma; or enzymes, e.g. prostate specific antigen (PSA) in prostate carcinoma; or tumour antigens, e.g. carcinoembryonic antigen (CEA) in colorectal carcinoma.

The use of tumour markers

Tumour markers can be used in different ways. They are of most value in monitoring treatment and assessing follow-up (Fig. 1), but are also used in diagnosis, prognosis and screening for the presence of disease.

Monitoring treatment

Treatment monitoring is the area in which most tumour markers have found a useful role. The decline in concentration of the tumour marker is an indication of the success of the treatment, whether that be surgery, chemotherapy, radiotherapy, or a combination of these. However, the rate of decline of marker concentration should match that predicted from knowledge of the marker's half-life. A slower than expected fall may well indicate that not all the tumour has been eliminated.

Assessing follow-up

Even when a patient has had successful treatment, it is often valuable to continue to monitor the marker long after the levels have appeared to stabilize. An increase indicates recurrence of the malignancy. Detection of increasing marker concentration allows second-line therapy to be instituted promptly. The frequency of sampling, with the attendant cost implications, is much discussed.

Diagnosis

Markers alone are rarely used to establish a diagnosis. Their detection in blood when there is clinical evidence of the tumour as well as radiological and, perhaps, biopsy evidence, will often confirm the diagnosis.

Prognosis

To be of value in prognosis, the concentration of the tumour marker in plasma should correlate with tumour mass. For example, HCG correlates well with the tumour mass in choriocarcinoma, HCG and alpha-fetoprotein (AFP) correlate with the tumour mass in testicular teratoma, and paraproteins correlate with the tumour mass in multiple myeloma.

Screening for the presence of disease

In routine clinical practice tumour markers should not be used to screen for malignancy, however appealing this might be in theory.

The exception to this rule is the screening of specific high-risk populations. For example, the hormone calcitonin, which is increased in all patients with medullary carcinoma of thyroid, may be used to screen close relatives. Prophylactic thyroidectomy may then be advised if any are found to have elevated calcitonin concentrations.

A practical application of tumour markers

Some of the uses of tumour markers discussed above can be illustrated with reference to Figure 2. This shows how the tumour marker AFP was helpful in the management of a young man with a malignant teratoma. The presence of AFP together with the hormone HCG

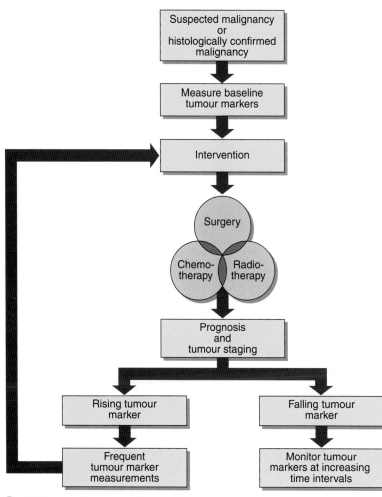

Fig. 1 **The use of tumour markers.**

confirmed the diagnosis. Between 75 and 95% of all patients presenting with testicular teratoma have abnormalities in one or both of these markers. The very high concentration of AFP (>10 000 kU/L) indicated that the prognosis was not good, and that it was likely there would be tumour recurrence after treatment. In fact, AFP concentrations fell in response to chemotherapy, but when the levels reached a plateau, surgery was carried out. Thereafter, chemotherapy was continued,

and AFP fell to very low levels. Continued monitoring of AFP levels in such a patient would provide early warning of tumour recurrence.

Tumour markers with established clinical value

Markers play a major role in the management of germ cell tumours and choriocarcinoma. Unfortunately, there are many cases in which markers are available but the tumours are resistant to chemotherapy, so their use is not mandatory. Table 1 shows which markers have gained an established place in the repertoire of tests commonly offered by the clinical biochemistry laboratory.

The future

Monoclonal antibodies raised against tumour cells and their membranes have led to the development of many new tumour marker assays, although few have as yet gained an established place in the management of patients with cancer. There is no doubt that tumour markers are an efficient and cheap way to monitor treatment. The search goes on for the 'perfect' marker that could be used in population screening, diagnosis, prognosis, monitoring treatment and for follow-up of tumour recurrence. However, the capacity for tumours to alter the expression of their surface antigens may make this goal unattainable.

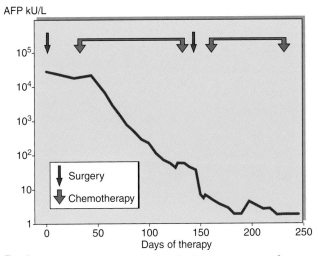

Fig. 2 **The use of AFP measurements in the management of a patient with a testicular teratoma.**

Marker	Tumour	Screening	Diagnosis	Prognosis	Monitoring	Follow-up
AFP	Germ cell		✓	✓	✓	✓
AFP	Hepatoma	✓	✓		✓	✓
HCG	Germ cell		✓	✓	✓	✓
HCG	Choriocarcinoma	✓	✓	✓	✓	✓
CA 125	Ovarian		✓		✓	✓
Acid phosphatase	Prostate		✓		✓	✓
Prostate specific antigen (PSA)	Prostate		✓		✓	✓
CEA	Colorectal				✓	✓
Calcitonin	Medullary carcinoma of thyroid	✓	✓		✓	✓
Hormones	Endocrine		✓		✓	✓
Paraprotein	Myeloma		✓		✓	✓

Table 1 **Clinical situations where tumour markers have been found to be useful**

Clinical note

Sometimes a man may act as a negative control when his partner uses a pregnancy test kit at home. Teratoma of the testis has a peak incidence in men in their twenties, and this tumour frequently secretes large amounts of HCG. This will give rise to a positive pregnancy test in the man! Such a finding should be taken very seriously and followed up immediately.

Case history 56

KS, a 72-year-old man, had complained of pains in his lower chest and abdomen for 2 months. His general practitioner detected dullness at both lung bases and referred him to a chest physician. On 23 June he was admitted to hospital. Examination revealed an enlarged liver. He had been a heavy drinker. Biochemistry results were:

Date	Bilirubin μmol/L	ALP	AST	ALT	LDH	γGT
				U/L		
23/6	24	1540	83	98		719
1/7	25	2170	80	107	430	1020

■ What is your differential diagnosis in the light of the liver function test results?
■ How might AFP be of help in this case?

Comment on page 168.

Tumour markers

■ The main use of tumour markers is in monitoring treatment, although they may also be of use in screening, diagnosis, prognosis, and in long-term follow-up.

■ Calcitonin is used to screen the relatives and family of a patient with medullary carcinoma of thyroid.

■ AFP, paraproteins, prostate specific antigen and a variety of hormones are helpful in establishing the diagnosis of certain tumours.

■ AFP and HCG are of value in predicting the outcome of non-seminomatous germ cell tumours.

Multiple endocrine neoplasia

Multiple endocrine neoplasias (MEN) are inherited tumour predisposition syndromes, characterized by tumours in two or more endocrine glands. Clinical manifestations of these syndromes result either from hormone overproduction by the tumours or from other adverse effects of tumour growth. Inheritance is autosomal dominant.

MEN 1

A clinical diagnosis of MEN 1 can be made if the patient has at least two of the following:

- parathyroid adenoma
- pancreatic endocrine tumour
- pituitary adenoma
- adrenal cortex adenoma
- carcinoid tumour.

The approximate frequencies of these tumours in MEN 1 are shown in Figure 1.

The inactivated gene in MEN 1 is a tumour suppressor gene, the protein product of which (menin) normally inhibits genes involved in cell proliferation. MEN 1 gene mutations invariably lead to endocrine tumours, but family members carrying the same MEN 1 gene mutation can have completely different clinical manifestations of the syndrome. Genetic testing for MEN 1 allows earlier recognition and surgical removal of tumours. In the past patients with MEN 1 died from,

e.g. peptic ulceration due to gastrinoma, or nephrolithiasis resulting from hyperparathyroidism.

Pituitary tumours in MEN 1 most often overproduce prolactin, but sometimes produce ACTH or growth hormone, resulting in Cushing's disease or acromegaly respectively. The pancreatic tumours can produce gastrin, insulin, vasoactive intestinal polypeptide (VIP), glucagon or somatostatin, resulting in characteristic clinical features. The adrenocortical tumours seen in MEN 1 are often non-functional.

MEN 2

In MEN 2 the RET (REarrranged during Transfection) encodes a tyrosine kinase receptor for a family of growth factors. Unlike MEN 1, different mutations of this gene are associated with specific tumours or tumour combinations. Clinically, MEN 2 presents as several distinct phenotypes.

MEN 2A

Medullary carcinoma of the thyroid (MCT) is present, often with phaeochromocytoma or hyperparathyroidism (Fig. 1). Phaeochromocytoma is bilateral in about 50% of affected cases.

MEN 2B

MCT is again present, along with phaeochromocytomas, but parathyroid adenomas are rare. Additional features

specific to MEN 2B include mucosal ganglioneuromas in the gastrointestinal tract and a Marfanoid habitus. MEN 2B presents at an earlier age than MEN 2A, and carries a worse prognosis.

Familial medullary carcinoma of the thyroid

This shares many of the genetic and clinical features of MEN 2, but phaeochromocytomas and parathyroid adenomas occur less frequently.

Screening and treatment

Some of the endocrine tumours associated with MEN, e.g. parathyroid and pituitary adenomas, are common, and only rarely part of a wider syndrome. MEN should be suspected where these tumours present early (<35 years), or where there is a family history of a MEN-associated tumour. By contrast, pancreatic endocrine tumours are rare and their diagnosis should prompt routine biochemical screening for, e.g. hyperparathyroidism or prolactinoma. In cases where MEN is diagnosed, all family members should be screened.

All carriers of MEN mutations will develop one or other of the associated endocrine tumours. Periodic biochemical screening has an important role to play in the follow-up of identified carriers. However, *definitive confirmation or exclusion of an individual's MEN predisposition requires genetic testing.* In some cases provocation tests may be necessary (Fig. 2).

Prophylactic surgical removal of the predisposed gland(s) may be indicated where the certainty of early cancer presentation is high. In particular, thyroidectomy is recommended for pre-school children who carry the RET mutations with the worst prognosis.

The APUD concept

Carcinoid and pancreatic islet cell tumours are seen in MEN syndromes but also occur sporadically. They arise from specialized neuroendocrine cells that have the capacity for amine precursor uptake and decarboxylation (APUD). Some of the peptides and amines secreted by these cells act like

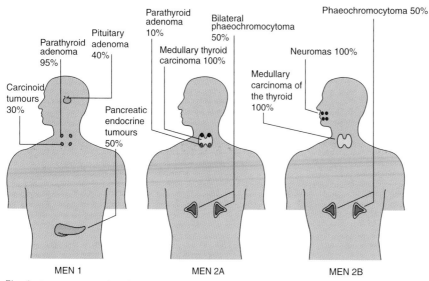

Fig. 1 **Tumours associated with MEN syndromes.** Percentages are approximate.

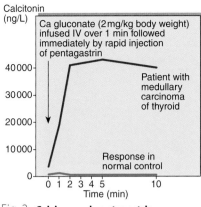

Fig. 2 **Calcium and pentagastrin provocation test of calcitonin secretion.** There is an exaggerated response to combined calcium and pentagastrin provocation in a patient with medullary carcinoma of the thyroid.

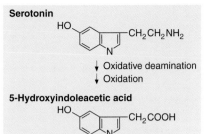

Fig. 3 **Serotonin and its urinary metabolite 5-hydroxyindoleacetic acid.** Certain foodstuffs such as bananas and tomatoes contain 5-hydroxyindoleacetic acid and may interfere with the urinary determination.

> **Clinical note**
> The H_2 receptor antagonists such as cimetidine are widely used to treat peptic ulcers. They may cause an increase in plasma gastrin concentrations to values that might suggest the presence of a gastrinoma. These drugs should be stopped before samples are taken for gastrin measurements.

classical hormones, being delivered through the bloodstream, while others are local paracrine regulators or neurotransmitters (Table 1). Overproduction of peptides or amines by tumours gives rise to associated tumour syndromes.

Carcinoid tumours

These most commonly arise in the appendix and ileocaecal region where the fore- and mid-gut meet. Carcinoid tumours may convert as much as half of the dietary intake of tryptophan into serotonin, secretion of which causes distinctive clinical effects, known as the carcinoid syndrome. This is characterized by flushing, diarrhoea and sometimes valvular heart disease. Intestinal carcinoid tumours only produce carcinoid syndrome if they have metastasized to the liver, whereas extra-intestinal carcinoids, e.g. bronchial, which do not drain into the portal circulation, may cause it even in the absence of metastasis. Serotonin may be measured directly in plasma or platelets, but the diagnosis is more often made by measurement in urine of its metabolite, 5-hydroxyindoleacetic acid (Fig. 3).

Insulinomas

These are the commonest pancreatic endocrine tumours.

Others

Gastrinomas, VIPomas, glucagonomas and somatostatinomas are all either rare or very rare.

Table 1 **Selected molecules which regulate gastrointestinal function**

Substance	Type of regulator	Major action
Gastrin	Hormone	Gastric acid and pepsin secretion
Cholecystokinin (CCK)	Hormone	Pancreatic enzyme secretion
Secretin	Hormone	Pancreatic bicarbonate secretion
Gastric inhibitory polypeptide (GIP)	Hormone	Enhances glucose mediated insulin release, inhibits gastric acid secretion
Vasoactive intestinal polypeptide (VIP)	Neurotransmitter	Smooth muscle relaxation. Stimulates pancreatic bicarbonate secretion
Motilin	Hormone	Initiates interdigestive intestinal motility
Somatostatin	Hormone Neurotransmitter Paracrine	Numerous inhibitory effects
Pancreatic polypeptide (PP)	Hormone Paracrine	Inhibits pancreatic bicarbonate and protein secretion
Enkephalins	Neurotransmitter	Opiate-like actions
Substance P	Neurotransmitter Paracrine	Contraction of smooth muscle

Case history 57

DC, a 50-year-old man, was referred to a neurologist after complaining of a 6-month history of severe headache. He was found to be slightly hypertensive. U & Es and LFTs were unremarkable. The only abnormality initially noted was a serum adjusted calcium concentration of 2.80 mmol/L.

■ What further investigations are required in this patient?

Comment on page 168.

> ### Multiple endocrine neoplasia
>
> ■ Multiple endocrine neoplasias are inherited cancer predisposition syndromes.
> ■ Diagnosis of MEN should prompt screening of family members.
> ■ Prophylactic surgical removal of endocrine glands may be appropriate.
> ■ The carcinoid syndrome is related to overproduction of serotonin.
> ■ Pancreatic islet cell tumours are rare.

Hyperuricaemia

Nucleic acids contain bases of two different types, pyrimidines and purines. The catabolism of the purines, adenine and guanine, produces uric acid. At physiological hydrogen ion concentration, uric acid is mostly ionized and present in plasma as sodium urate (Fig. 1). An elevated serum urate concentration is known as hyperuricaemia. Uric acid and urate are relatively insoluble molecules that readily precipitate out of aqueous solutions such as urine or synovial fluid (Fig. 2). The consequence of this is the medical condition gout.

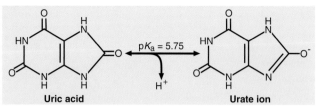

Fig. 1 **Uric acid and urate.**

Urate formation and excretion

Urate is formed in three ways. These are:

■ by de novo synthesis
■ by the metabolism of endogenous DNA, RNA and other purine-containing molecules such as ATP
■ by the breakdown of dietary nucleic acids.

Urate is excreted in two ways:

■ *Via the kidney.* The majority of urate is excreted via the kidney. Renal handling of urate is complex. It is freely filtered at the glomerulus, but 99% is reabsorbed in the proximal tubule. The distal tubules also secrete urate, but again much is reabsorbed. The amount of urate excreted in the urine is around 10% of that filtered at the glomerulus.
■ *Via the gut.* Smaller amounts of urate are excreted into the gut where it is broken down by bacteria. This process is called uricolysis.

Urate concentrations in serum are higher in men than women. Even within the reference interval, serum urate is near its aqueous solubility limit. The presence of protein helps to keep the molecule in solution. A high serum urate may arise from increased urate formation, or from decreased excretion. The common causes of hyperuricaemia are summarized in Figure 3. Genetic causes of hyperuricaemia are known as primary disorders, and there are also secondary causes. Most primary causes are due to decreased excretion of urate (90% of cases) rather than increased production (10%).

Lesch–Nyhan syndrome

One genetic disorder that should be singled out is Lesch–Nyhan syndrome, an X-linked disorder caused by a deficiency of hypoxanthine-guanine phosphoribosyltransferase, an enzyme that is involved in salvaging purine bases for resynthesis to purine nucleotides. The syndrome is characterized clinically by excessive uric acid production, hyperuricaemia and neurological problems that include self-mutilation and mental retardation.

Gout

Gout is a clinical syndrome that is characterized by hyperuricaemia and recurrent acute arthritis. Whereas all patients who develop gout will have had hyperuricaemia at some point in the development of the disease, only a minority of patients with hyperuricaemia develop gout. The reason for this is not known.

Acute gout is triggered by the tissue deposition of sodium urate crystals that cause an inflammatory response. In the chronic situation, tophaceous deposits of sodium urate may form in the tissues (Fig. 4). Gout is exacerbated by alcohol. The reason for this is twofold. Ethanol increases the turnover of ATP and urate production. Ethanol in excess may cause the accumulation of organic acids that compete with the tubular secretion of uric acid. Disorders such as ethanol intoxication, diabetic ketoacidosis and starvation lead to elevations of lactic acid, β-hydroxybutyric acid and acetoacetic acid, and will cause hyperuricaemia.

Treatment

The symptoms of acute gout respond to anti-inflammatory drugs such as indometacin, but it should be noted that these drugs have no direct effect on the serum urate level. Low-dose aspirin should be avoided as it inhibits renal urate excretion. Treatment must also be directed at the hyperuricaemia.

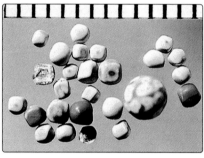

Fig. 2 **Urate stones from the urinary tract.**

Drugs such as probenecid, which promote urate excretion, can be used prophylactically. A diet that is low in purines and alcohol may be prescribed in an effort to reduce the plasma urate concentration. Allopurinol, a specific inhibitor of the enzyme xanthine oxidase that catalyses the oxidation of hypoxanthine to xanthine and uric acid, may also be effective in reducing urate concentrations.

A number of other crystalline arthropathies may present as gout but are not associated with hyperuricaemia. Most notably, pseudogout is due to the deposition of calcium pyrophosphate crystals.

Renal disease and hyperuricaemia

Renal disease is a common complication of hyperuricaemia. Several types of renal disease have been identified. The most common is urate nephropathy, which is caused by the deposition of urate crystals in renal tissue or the urinary tract to form urate stones. This may be associated with chronic hyperuricaemia. Acute renal failure can be caused by the rapid precipitation of uric acid crystals that commonly occurs during treatment of patients with leukaemias and lymphomas. In the 'acute tumour lysis syndrome' (p. 137), nucleic acids are released as a result of tumour cell breakdown and are rapidly metabolized to uric acid.

Urate in pregnancy

Serum urate is of value in the monitoring of maternal well-being in pregnancy-associated hypertension (pre-eclampsia), alongside other markers such as blood pressure, urine protein excretion and creatinine clearance (p. 153).

Comment on page 168.

Case history 58

A 50-year-old man was awakened by a severe pain in his left toe. He was shivering and feverish, and the pain became so intense that he could not bear the weight of the bedclothes.

- What biochemical tests would help make the diagnosis?

Clinical note

The definitive diagnosis of gout is by examination of synovial fluid from an acutely inflamed joint. Sodium urate crystals will be observed within polymorphonuclear leucocytes viewed under polarizing light.

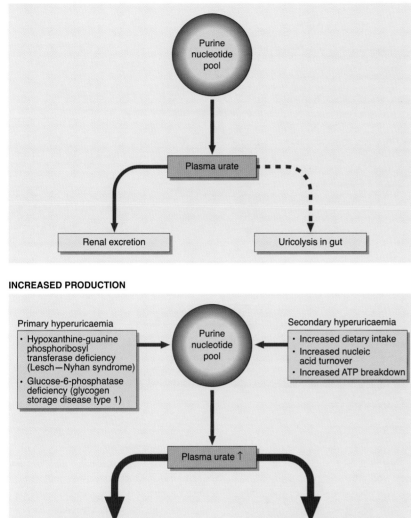

NORMAL

Purine nucleotide pool → Plasma urate → Renal excretion / Uricolysis in gut

INCREASED PRODUCTION

Primary hyperuricaemia
- Hypoxanthine-guanine phosphoribosyl transferase deficiency (Lesch–Nyhan syndrome)
- Glucose-6-phosphatase deficiency (glycogen storage disease type 1)

Secondary hyperuricaemia
- Increased dietary intake
- Increased nucleic acid turnover
- Increased ATP breakdown

Purine nucleotide pool → Plasma urate ↑ → Increased renal excretion / Uricolysis in gut

DECREASED EXCRETION

Primary hyperuricaemia
- Idiopathic

Secondary hyperuricaemia
- Renal insufficiency
- Elevated lactic acid or ketones, thiazide diuretics and low dose aspirin cause decreased tubular secretion
- Increased tubular reabsorption

Purine nucleotide pool → Plasma urate ↑ → Decreased renal excretion / Uricolysis in gut

Fig. 3 **The causes of hyperuricaemia.**

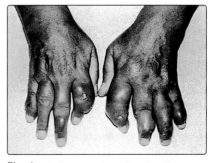

Fig. 4 **Tophaceous deposits of sodium urate in tissues.**

Hyperuricaemia

- Uric acid is formed from the breakdown of endogenous or exogenous purines.

- Hyperuricaemia may be caused by:
  – an increased rate of purine synthesis
  – an increased rate of turnover of nucleic acids, as in malignancies, tissue damage or starvation
  – a reduced renal excretion.

- Hyperuricaemia is a risk factor for gout that occurs when urate crystals are deposited in tissues.

- Hyperuricaemia is aggravated by a diet high in purines and alcohol.

Skeletal muscle disorders

Myopathies are conditions affecting the muscles that lead to weakness and/or atrophy. They may be caused by congenital factors (as in the muscular dystrophies), by viral infection or by acute damage due to anoxia, infections, toxins or drugs. Muscle denervation is a major cause of myopathy. Muscle weakness can occur due to a lack of energy-producing molecules or a failure in the balance of electrolytes within and surrounding the muscle cell necessary for neuromuscular function.

Normal muscle that is overused will end up weak or in spasm until rested. In severe cases of overuse, especially where movements are strong and erratic as might occur during convulsions, damage to muscle cells may result. Severely damaged muscle cells release their contents, e.g. myoglobin, a condition known as rhabdomyolysis.

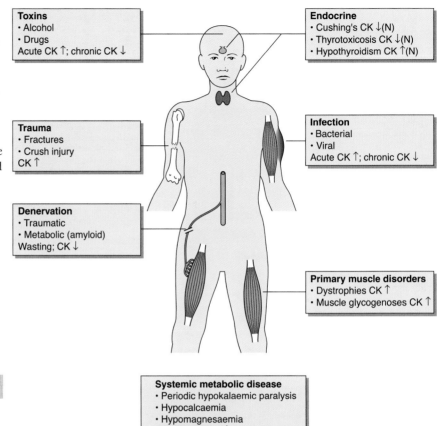

Fig. 1 **Causes of myopathy, with associated changes in serum creatine kinase (CK).**

Muscle weakness

Muscle weakness, which may or may not progress to rhabdomyolysis, has many causes (Fig. 1). Diagnosis of the condition will depend on the clinical picture and will include investigation of genetic disorders by enzymic or chromosomal analysis, endocrine investigations and the search for drug effects. Infective causes may be diagnosed by isolation of the relevant organism or its related antibody, but often no organism is detected. These cases, known as myalgic encephalitis (ME), post-viral syndrome or chronic fatigue syndrome, are relatively common and are now regarded as true diseases, whereas formally they were thought to be psychosomatic.

Investigation

In all cases of muscle weakness, serum electrolytes should be checked along with creatine kinase (CK). A full drug

history should be taken to exclude pharmacological and toxicological causes, and a history of alcohol abuse should be excluded. Neuromuscular electrophysiological studies should be performed to detect neuropathies. Where a genetic cause is suspected, a muscle biopsy should be taken for histopathological studies and measurement of muscle enzymes (Table 1). In contrast to rhabdomyolysis, serum CK and myoglobin are frequently normal in patients with myopathy.

Rhabdomyolysis

Muscle cells that are damaged will leak creatine kinase into the plasma. This enzyme exists in different isoforms. CK-MM or total CK is used as an index of skeletal muscle damage. Very high serum levels may be expected in patients who have been convulsing or have muscular damage due to electrical shock or crush injury. Creatine kinase concentrations may also be high in acute

spells in muscular dystrophy. For these reasons, when CK is used as an indicator of myocardial infarction, it is better to measure the MB isoenzyme, which is more specific for cardiac muscle damage (pp. 52–53).

The damaged muscle cells will also leak myoglobin. This compound stores oxygen in the muscle cells for release under conditions of hypoxia, as occurs during severe exercise. The dissociation curve of myoglobin is compared with haemoglobin in Figure 2. It delivers up its oxygen only when the PO_2 falls to around 3 kPa. When muscle cells become anoxic or are damaged by trauma, myoglobin is released into the plasma. It is filtered at the glomerulus. Urine containing myoglobin will be an orange or brown colour. The damaged muscle cells also release large amounts of potassium ions into the extracellular fluid, causing hyperkalaemia, and also tend to take up calcium ions, reducing serum calcium concentration.

Severe muscle damage is frequently accompanied by a reduction in the blood volume. This may occur directly

Table 1 **Cellular enzymes that may be measured in the investigation of muscle weakness**	
Type of myopathy	**Enzyme**
Glycogen storage disease	Myophosphorylase
	Glycerol kinase
	Lactate dehydrogenase
	Phosphofructokinase
	Phosphoglycerate kinase
	Myoadenylate deaminase
Lipid disease	Carnitine palmityl transferase

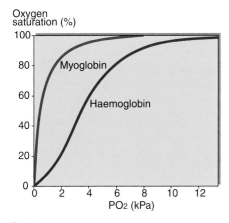

Fig. 2 **Comparison of oxygen saturation curves for haemoglobin and myoglobin.**

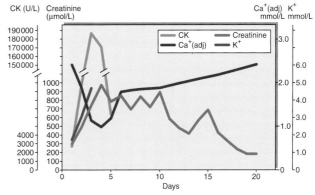

Fig. 3 **Biochemical results following rhabdomyolysis in a patient who had taken a drug overdose.**

as a result of haemorrhage in severe trauma, or indirectly because of fluid sequestration in the damaged tissue. The resultant shock frequently causes acute renal failure.

Myoglobin itself is not nephrotoxic. Children with muscular dystrophy do not develop renal failure despite having increased levels of myoglobin in urine for many years.

Investigation and treatment

The biochemistry laboratory has a major role to play in the diagnosis and investigation of rhabdomyolysis (Fig. 3). This includes:

- serum total creatine kinase, which allows the diagnosis to be made
- urea and electrolytes, to look for evidence of resulting renal impairment
- alcohol and drugs of abuse screen, to look for specific causes
- urine myoglobin, may also be useful in the diagnosis.

Treatment is directed towards maintaining tissue perfusion and the control of electrolyte imbalances. It includes

- cardiac monitoring
- control of hyperkalaemia and hypocalcaemia.

Haemodialysis may be necessary where renal function is severely compromised.

Other causes of myoglobinaemia and myoglobinuria

Myoglobin is not specific for skeletal muscle and is also released following myocardial infarction, where it may be used as an early marker of myocardial damage (see pp. 52–53).

Duchenne muscular dystrophy

This X-linked recessive disorder results from abnormalities in the dystrophin gene. Clinically, it is characterized by progressive muscle weakness, usually in boys, from the age of 5. Very high serum CK may precede the onset of symptoms but later in the disease the CK levels fall. Approximately 75% of female carriers also have raised CK levels.

> ### Clinical note
> Investigation of muscle weakness in an elderly patient should always include serum potassium, magnesium and calcium measurements. Hypokalaemia, hypocalcaemia and hypomagnesaemia may all develop insidiously. Correction can result in a dramatic improvement.

Case history 59

A 41-year-old labourer was admitted to hospital. He had collapsed and gave a 4-day history of flu-like illness, with shivering, myalgia, headaches, dyspnoea, vomiting and diarrhoea.

Serum enzymes (on admission)

AST	ALT	LDH	CK
		U/L	
149	88	1330	6000

- What tissues could have contributed to the high serum enzymes activities?
- What tests may help identify the source(s) of enzyme elevation?

Comment on page 168.

Skeletal muscle disorders

- Muscle weakness is a common complaint with a wide variety of causes.
- Biochemical investigation of muscle weakness can provide rapid diagnosis and effective treatment where ionic changes are the cause.
- Intracellular enzyme analysis from muscle biopsies can provide a diagnosis in some inherited disorders.
- Severely damaged muscle cells release potassium, creatine kinase, myoglobin and phosphate.
- Serum creatine kinase and myoglobin are frequently normal in patients with myopathy.
- Severe rhabdomyolysis, e.g. following injury, is an important cause of acute renal failure.

Biochemistry in the elderly

By the year 2050 more than 20% of the world's population will be over 65 years of age. As the population ages, more clinical biochemical resources will need to be directed towards the problems of the elderly population.

There is considerable variation in the onset of functional changes in body systems because of age. Many organs show a gradual decline in function even in the absence of diseases; but since there is often considerable functional reserve, there are no clinical consequences. The problem facing the clinical biochemist is how to differentiate between the biochemical and physiological changes that are the consequences of ageing, and those factors that indicate disease is present. Just because the result of a biochemistry test in an elderly patient is different from that in a young person does not mean some pathology is present. Serum creatinine is an example. Renal function deteriorates with age (Fig. 1) but finding a serum creatinine of 140 μmol/L in an 80-year-old woman should not be cause for alarm. Indeed, this creatinine result may represent a remarkably good glomerular filtration rate considering the age of the patient.

The interpretation of biochemical measurements in the elderly requires that laboratories establish age-related reference ranges for many of the tests undertaken.

Disease in old age

Some diseases are more commonly encountered in the elderly than in the young. In addition, common diseases may present in a different way to that in the young. Elderly patients may have more than one disease or may take several medications that mimic or mask the usual disease presentation.

The admission of a patient for geriatric assessment involves a degree of 'screening' biochemistry that may point towards the presence of disorders that may not be suspected (Table 1).

The metabolic diseases that occur most commonly in the elderly and may present in unusual ways include:

- thyroid disease
- diabetes mellitus
- renal disease
- pituitary disease
- impaired gonadal function
- bone disease.

Thyroid disease

Thyroid dysfunction is common in the elderly. Diagnosis may be overlooked since many of the clinical manifestations of thyroid disease may be misinterpreted as just the normal ageing process (Fig. 2). Unusual presentations are common, e.g. elderly patients with hyperthyroidism are more likely than younger patients to present with the cardiac-related effects of increased thyroid hormone.

The interpretation of TSH, T_4 and T_3 results may not be straightforward in the elderly population as these patients usually have more than one active disease process. A patient with a severe non-thyroidal illness may show low T_4, T_3 and TSH (p. 89). A patient's thyroid function can only be satisfactorily investigated in the absence of non-thyroidal illness. Elderly patients may also be taking drugs that affect thyroid function (Table 2).

Table 1 Biochemical assessment in a geriatric patient

Test	Associated conditions
Potassium	Hypokalaemia
Urea and creatinine	Renal disease
Calcium, phosphate and alkaline phosphatase	Bone disease
Total protein, albumin	Nutritional state
Glucose	Diabetes mellitus
Thyroid function tests	Hypothyroidism
Haematological investigation and faecal occult blood	Blood and bleeding disorders

Table 2 Some common drugs known to affect thyroid action

Effect	Drugs
Increase TBG	Oestrogens
Decrease TBG	Androgens, glucocorticoids
Inhibit TBG binding	Phenytoin, salicylates
Suppress TSH	L-DOPA, glucocorticoids
Inhibit T_4 secretion	Lithium
Inhibit T_4–T_3 conversion	Amiodarone, propranolol
Reduce oral T_4 absorption	Colestyramine, colestipol

Hypothermia is often encountered in an elderly patient. It is important to establish if there is an underlying endocrine disorder such as thyroid disease, or even adrenal or pituitary hypofunction (Fig. 3).

Diabetes mellitus

Diabetes mellitus is common in old age (Fig. 4). Genetic factors and obesity contribute to the insulin resistance that underlies the development of NIDDM (pp. 60–61).

Glucose tolerance declines with age even in the absence of diabetes mellitus, and the renal threshold for glucose rises. These observations can make the diagnosis of diabetes mellitus difficult in an elderly patient.

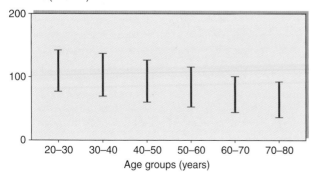

Fig. 1 **Age-related fall in the creatinine clearance reference interval.**

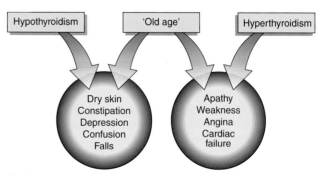

Fig. 2 **The clinical manifestations of thyroid disease may be misinterpreted as characteristics of 'normal' ageing.**

the long term. The benefits of postmenopausal hormone replacement therapy (HRT) are well established in relation to menopausal symptoms, and maintenance of bone structure, although its impact on the risk of coronary heart disease remains controversial.

Bone disease

Bone disease in general is more common in elderly patients than in the young. Osteoporosis is the most common bone disease that occurs in the elderly (p. 76). The risk of hip fracture increases dramatically with increasing age because of a reduction in bone mass per unit volume. Bone loss accelerates when oestrogen production falls after the menopause in women, but both sexes show a gradual bone loss throughout life. The common biochemical indices of calcium metabolism are normal in patients even with severe primary osteoporosis, and currently are of little help in diagnosis and treatment, except to ensure that other complicating conditions are not present.

Vitamin D deficiency remains a cause of osteomalacia in the elderly, housebound or institutionalized patients. Vitamin D status can be assessed by measurement of the main circulating metabolite, 25-hydroxycholecalciferol. In severe osteomalacia due to vitamin D deficiency, serum calcium will fall, and there will be an appropriate increase in PTH secretion. Alkaline phosphatase will be elevated.

Paget's disease is characterized by increased osteoclastic activity that leads to increased bone resorption. Bone pain can be particularly severe. Serum alkaline phosphatase is very high, and urinary hydroxyproline excretion is elevated.

Myeloma is frequently encountered in older patients. However, although a sizeable proportion of the elderly population will have a paraprotein band on electrophoresis, only a minority will have overt myeloma.

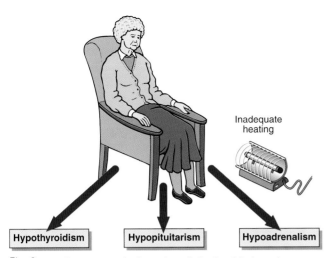

Fig. 3 **Possible reasons for hypothermia in the elderly patient.**

Renal disease

Renal function gradually deteriorates throughout life as shown by the increases in the upper limit of the age-related reference intervals for both urea and creatinine. Creatinine clearance falls even though the amount of creatinine produced decreases as a consequence of reduced muscle mass. A degree of cardiac insufficiency may enforce this fall. The ability of the kidneys to concentrate urine and to excrete a dilute urine both decline with age.

Pituitary disease

With increasing age the pituitary gland decreases in size, and the incidence of microadenomas and focal necrosis increases. Gonadotrophin and AVP secretion increase, and growth hormone secretion decreases. The significance of the latter is the subject of much current investigation.

Gonadal function

Both ovarian and testicular hormone secretion decline with age. The menopause in women may cause distressing symptoms in the short term, and serious bone disease in

Nutrition in elderly patients

Nutritional deficiencies are more common in the elderly, especially those who are neglected or who fail to eat a balanced diet. Recent evidence suggests that this is a factor in the reduced immune response found in all malnourished patients, which renders them more susceptible to infection.

> ### Clinical note
> When faced with a biochemical problem in an elderly patient it is important to remember that it is highly likely (in contrast to a young person) that more than one pathology is present.

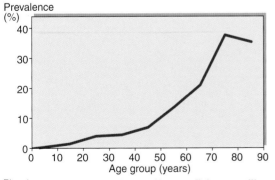

Fig. 4 **Age specific prevalence of known diabetes mellitus.**

Case history 60

A 72-year-old man presented to his GP in a confused state. On examination he was emaciated and had motor and sensory polyneuropathy. Alcohol could be smelt on his breath.

■ What further tests should be undertaken?

Comment on page 169.

Biochemistry in the elderly

■ The clinical biochemist must be aware of whether a change in a biochemical parameter is a normal occurrence of old age or indicates the presence of disease.

■ Common diseases in elderly patients may present in a different way to that in younger patients.

■ Elderly patients may be prescribed a number of medications that will complicate the interpretation of results.

DNA diagnosis

Molecular genetics is a tool used by many disciplines and is the study of the expression and inheritance of genes at the molecular level. In clinical biochemistry this involves studying base pair sequence differences in the DNA. Analysis of a patient's DNA and the genes that it contains can provide diagnostic information. Mutations in single genes may cause inherited diseases such as cystic fibrosis, sickle cell anaemia, familial hypercholesterolaemia and Duchenne muscular dystrophy. Compound disorders involving several genes are thought to be important in common diseases such as coronary heart disease, diabetes mellitus and cancer.

The human genome

Most of the human genome does not code for functional proteins; there are long untranslated regions between and even within genes. The genome is not identical from one person to the next, as on average every two hundredth base pair will be different. When a change occurs in the coding region, it may lead to the synthesis of an altered protein, defective in its function. Changes in the non-coding region are often neutral, but may be useful markers for the molecular geneticist. Recently, changes in non-coding DNA have been identified as the cause of such diseases as fragile X syndrome and myotonic dystrophy.

Restriction fragment length polymorphisms

In the laboratory, DNA can be cut into small pieces by enzymes called restriction endonucleases. These enzymes are restricted to cutting the DNA at specific base pair sequences. The presence of polymorphic sites, where there are differences in the base pair sequence of the DNA, may create or abolish a cutting site for a particular restriction endonuclease. In these instances, the polymorphisms are known as *restriction fragment length polymorphisms* (RFLPs) as they lead to the production of DNA fragments of different lengths after enzyme action detectable by Southern blot analysis (Fig. 1).

Linkage

In very few diseases, e.g. sickle cell anaemia, the mutation causing the disease occurs at a site that is recognized by a restriction enzyme. RFLP analysis is therefore immediately diagnostic. More commonly, however, the restriction site is close to the clinically important mutation site so that the two sites will remain linked during meiotic recombination. If the polymorphic restriction site and the mutation sought are closely linked then RFLP analysis will be highly informative, but as the distance between them increases the reliability of diagnosis decreases (Fig. 2).

VNTR polymorphism

RFLPs have the limitation that every individual has two copies of the relevant section of the DNA (one inherited from each parent) and is either +/+ or +/– or –/– for the polymorphic site.

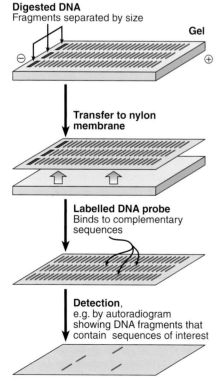

Digested DNA
Fragments separated by size

Gel

⊖   ⊕

Transfer to nylon membrane

Labelled DNA probe
Binds to complementary sequences

Detection,
e.g. by autoradiogram showing DNA fragments that contain sequences of interest

Fig. 1 **Southern blot analysis of human DNA.**

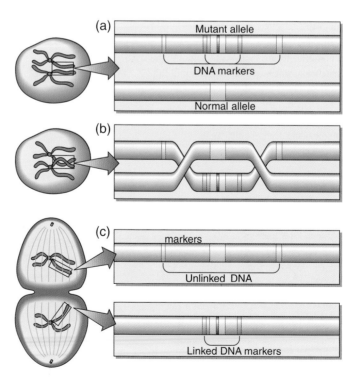

(a) Mutant allele
DNA markers
Normal allele

(b)

(c) markers
Unlinked DNA
Linked DNA markers

(a) Polymorphic DNA sequences may be regarded as DNA markers.

(b) During meiosis, chromatid crossover occurs and the DNA sequences are shuffled.

(c) Those markers that are physically close to the gene of interest remain linked, while those that are distant or on separate chromosomes are unlinked.

Fig. 2 **Linked and unlinked markers during meiotic recombination.**

Another type of polymorphism is called a variable number tandem repeat (VNTR). Here the restriction sites flank a region of the genome whose length varies between individuals due to different numbers of copies of a specific sequence (a 'tandem repeat'). The restriction fragment pattern obtained using probes that identify different sequences is almost completely unique to an individual and can be used as a 'genetic fingerprint'.

Polymerase chain reaction

The polymerase chain reaction (PCR) (Fig. 3) has revolutionized the study of genes. PCR allows a small section of human genomic DNA to be amplified many times in the test tube. The technique is simple, fast, and requires as little as a single cell. DNA for analysis may be obtained from any nucleated cell; most commonly used are white blood cells, but hair roots, mouth scrapings or sperm can also be used. Such small samples have obvious advantages for prenatal and forensic diagnoses, but great care must be taken to avoid contamination with cells or DNA from the laboratory.

The primers chosen to amplify the DNA are identical to short lengths of the sequence of the genomic DNA that flank the area of interest. The double stranded DNA is first denatured by heating. Primers anneal to their complementary sequences and, by the action of DNA polymerase, extension occurs completing the first cycle. This newly synthesized DNA is also used as a template for the 2nd cycle and so on. By the 30th cycle, the region flanked by the two primers will have been amplified more than a million fold.

Applications of DNA diagnosis: cystic fibrosis

Cystic fibrosis is relatively common, being encountered in 1/1600 Caucasian births. It is an autosomal recessive condition. Around one in twenty-two of the population are carriers, making the disease one of the most common serious genetic abnormalities. The disease affects exocrine secretions, and the onset of the disease may be at birth or later in childhood. Newborn screening has been largely unsuccessful, and traditional confirmation of the disease depended on the demonstration of an increased chloride concentration in a sample of sweat.

It is now possible to identify children who will be affected and also those who will be carriers so that genetic diagnoses and counselling can be given. The gene is on chromosome 7, and codes for a protein called cystic fibrosis transmembrane conductance regulator (CFTR). This regulates the function of a bicarbonate/chloride exchanger. DNA diagnosis of cystic fibrosis can be used in prenatal diagnosis. Furthermore,

cystic fibrosis is now regarded as a target for gene therapy. This procedure in which missing or defective parts of the human genome are replaced or repaired heralds the beginning of a new era in medicine.

Case history 61

A male infant has cystic fibrosis. He has two sisters and a brother. His mother and father are unrelated and appear well although his maternal uncle died as a child with the disease.

■ Draw his family tree.
■ How would this child have been diagnosed and how would you investigate his siblings?

Comment on page 169.

DNA diagnosis

■ Analysis of a patient's DNA can provide the clinician with diagnostic information.

■ The technology for studying DNA involves looking for the differences in the fragments formed when the DNA is digested by specific enzymes known as restriction endonucleases, or amplification of selected regions of the DNA by a technique called the polymerase chain reaction.

■ Genetic analysis can now help diagnose children with cystic fibrosis and identify carriers of the disease.

Clinical note
In the investigation of inherited diseases, it is often useful to sketch a patient's family tree to illustrate at a glance his or her family history. The simple rules and conventions for constructing these diagrams are shown in Figure 4.

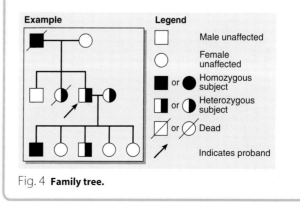

Fig. 4 **Family tree.**

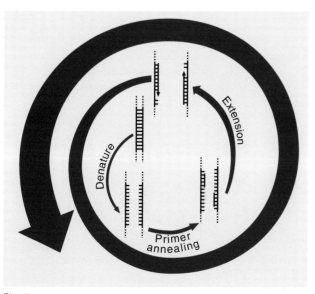

Fig. 3 **The polymerase chain reaction.**

Fetal monitoring and prenatal diagnosis

Biochemical tests have limited value in monitoring fetal development, but some components of maternal blood and urine and amniotic fluid may be measured to give evidence of pathology.

HCG

Human chorionic gonadotrophin (HCG) is a glycoprotein produced by the chorionic cells of the developing embryo that is detectable by sensitive assays within days of conception. Measurement of HCG is used to confirm pregnancy, and forms the basis of pregnancy tests (p. 9). The protein's rapid rate of synthesis in early pregnancy provides systemic evidence of the blastocyst 24 hours after implantation. HCG continues to be secreted by the developing placenta, and serum and urine concentrations increase during the first 9 weeks of pregnancy, then decline gradually until the third trimester (Fig. 1). The function of HCG is to maintain the activity of the corpus luteum sustaining progesterone synthesis. Measurement of HCG is also of value in:

- Assessing fetal viability in threatened abortion.
- Detecting ectopic pregnancy. HCG fails to rise at the expected rate.
- Detecting and monitoring hydatidiform mole and choriocarcinoma. HCG may be used as a tumour marker for diagnosis and monitoring of these trophoblastic malignancies (pp. 138–139).

Fetoplacental function

Human placental lactogen (HPL) is synthesized by the placenta. The HPL concentration in maternal blood increases during pregnancy until term.

It can be used to monitor placental function.

Oestriol is a steroid synthesized by the combined action of enzymes in the fetus and placenta. Its concentration in maternal blood increases throughout pregnancy, and it can be assayed in maternal urine or blood. Oestriol was at one time commonly used to monitor fetoplacental function.

These two biochemical tests have been superseded by physical investigations such as ultrasound and cardiotocography.

Prenatal diagnosis

Prenatal diagnostic techniques fall into two groups: invasive and non-invasive (Table 1). Prenatal diagnosis may be required because of increased risk of inherited disease. Neural tube defects cannot usually be predicted by family history, and pregnant women may be offered a screening test to detect these disorders.

Table 1 Techniques for prenatal diagnosis	
Invasive	Amniocentesis
	Chorionic villus sampling
	Cordocentesis
	Fetoscopy
	Fetal skin biopsy
	Fetal liver biopsy
Non-invasive	Ultrasound
	Radiography

Alpha-fetoprotein

Alpha-fetoprotein (AFP) is a small glycoprotein synthesized by the yolk sac and fetal liver and is a major fetal plasma protein. Because of its size it appears in fetal urine, and hence it is present in amniotic fluid and maternal blood. AFP concentrations increase in

maternal blood until 32 weeks of gestation in a normal pregnancy (Fig. 2).

Detection of higher than normal AFP concentrations can suggest CNS defects such as anencephaly or spina bifida early in pregnancy, because such malformations of the neural tube are associated with leakage of plasma or CSF proteins into amniotic fluid and consequently maternal serum AFP concentrations increase. In some countries all pregnant women in antenatal care are given the opportunity to have their serum AFP measured between 16 and 18 weeks of gestation, with appropriate counselling. When a high result is obtained, the test must be repeated on a fresh sample. Once other possibilities for an elevated AFP, such as wrong dates or multiple pregnancies, have been excluded, an amniocentesis is performed and the AFP determined in amniotic fluid. High levels suggest the presence of a neural tube defect.

Amniotic fluid acetylcholinesterase (an enzyme found in high concentrations in neural tissue) is also used in some centres to detect fetal malformations.

Serum AFP and HCG concentrations and maternal age may be considered together to assess the risk that chromosomal disorders such as Down's syndrome are likely to be present. If the risk is high then amniocentesis may be performed to obtain cells for karyotyping.

Cells for study of inborn errors may be obtained either by biopsy of the chorionic villus, which is genetically identical to the fetus, or by culture of cells from amniotic fluid. The latter process takes 3–4 weeks. Both enzyme studies and DNA analysis may be carried out on these tissue samples.

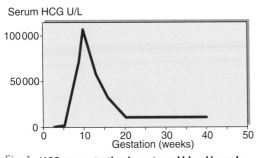

Fig. 1 **HCG concentration in maternal blood in early pregnancy.**

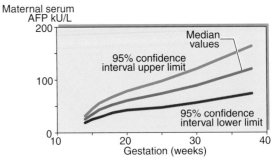
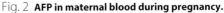

Fig. 2 **AFP in maternal blood during pregnancy.**

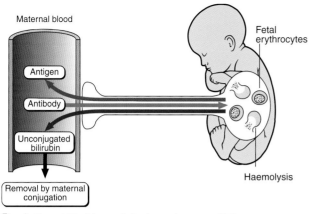

Fig. 3 **Hyperbilirubinaemia in rhesus incompatibility.**

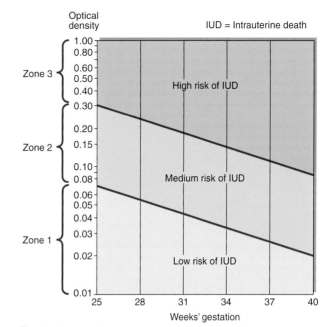

Fig. 4 **Liley graph.** Bilirubin absorbs light at 450 nm. The absorbance is directly related to its concentration and this enables the risk of intrauterine death (IUD) to be estimated.

Bilirubin

Bilirubin is measured in amniotic fluid to aid in the assessment of fetal risk in rhesus incompatibility. Incompatible red cell antigens can enter the maternal circulation either from the fetus at the time of delivery or, rarely, because of incompatible blood transfusion; specific red cell antibodies are stimulated in the mother. If a Rh–ve mother has a Rh+ve child these antibodies may cross the placenta and react with specific antigens to the fetal red cell membrane causing haemolysis (Fig. 3). This is unusual in a first pregnancy but may be a feature of subsequent pregnancies. Excess breakdown of red cells leads to anaemia, overproduction of bilirubin and, eventually, oedema.

During fetal life, unconjugated bilirubin crosses the placenta and is removed by the mother, so the baby may not be born with obvious jaundice. However, the baby will rapidly become jaundiced in the days immediately after birth. In utero, the level of bilirubin in the amniotic fluid can be used to predict the severity of the fetal condition. Amniocentesis is performed on women who have previously had an affected fetus and on women who show a high and rising Rh titre. The severity of the problem can be assessed by reference to a nomogram that relates bilirubin levels to gestational age, such as that in Figure 4. Fetal exchange blood transfusion or early delivery may be considered.

Rhesus incompatibility is much less common nowadays since susceptible women are given an intravenous injection of anti-rhesus antibody at the time of delivery to eliminate fetal red blood cells that may have entered the maternal circulation. As a consequence they do not survive long enough to be recognized as foreign antigens in the mother. However, haemolytic disease of the newborn cannot be completely eliminated, because it may be caused by other blood group incompatibilities.

Fetal blood gases

Hydrogen ion concentration, blood gases and serum lactate concentration can be measured in fetal blood. Such measurements are only requested when non-invasive investigations have indicated that the fetus is at risk. Fetal blood can be obtained by the technique of cordocentesis, where the blood is sampled from the umbilical cord through a fine needle inserted through the abdomen under ultrasound guidance.

Hydrogen ion concentration can also be measured in fetal blood to assess fetal distress during labour. Capillary blood samples can be obtained directly from the baby's scalp once the cervix is sufficiently dilated. Fetal hypoxia causes a lactic acidosis and elevated hydrogen ion concentration. Measurement of fetal PO_2 can be obtained directly using a transcutaneous oxygen electrode.

> ### Clinical note
> Fetal ultrasound scanning, related to time of conception and/or sequential measurements, has become the most widely used way of monitoring fetal growth. This technique has superseded many biochemical tests of fetal well-being that were once commonly performed.

> ### Case history 62
>
> A 30-year-old woman who had previously delivered one live child and had one miscarriage attended for antenatal care. She was known to be rhesus negative. At 30 weeks' gestation she was found to have a high titre of anti-D antibodies.
>
> ■ What investigations are needed now?
>
> *Comment on page 169.*

> ## Fetal monitoring and prenatal diagnosis
>
> ■ Confirmation of pregnancy is by detection of human chorionic gonadotrophin in maternal urine.
>
> ■ Elevated concentrations of alpha-fetoprotein in maternal blood and amniotic fluid may indicate the presence of a fetus with a neural tube defect or Down's syndrome.
>
> ■ Amniotic fluid bilirubin measurements are of value in the detection of risk of rhesus incompatibility.

Pregnancy

Maternal physiology

Maternal physiology changes so dramatically during pregnancy that reference intervals for biochemical tests in non-pregnant women are often not applicable. The main differences in the commonly requested tests are shown in Table 1. These differences should not be misinterpreted as indicating that some pathology is present.

Weight gain

The mean weight gain in pregnancy is 12.5 kg, but there is a very large standard deviation (about 4 kg). The gain in weight is made up of several components:

- *The products of conception.* These include the fetus, placenta and amniotic fluid.
- *Maternal fat stores.* These may account for up to 25% of the weight increase.
- *Maternal water retention.* Total body water increases by about 5 L, mostly in the extracellular fluid. The volume of the intravascular compartment increases by more than 1 L.

Respiratory function

Mild hyperventilation occurs from early pregnancy, probably due to a centrally mediated effect of progesterone, and PCO_2 falls. However, blood hydrogen ion concentration is maintained within non-pregnant limits, since the plasma bicarbonate falls due to an increased renal excretion of bicarbonate. Oxygen consumption increases by about 20%, but PO_2 is relatively unchanged.

Renal function

Because of increases in plasma volume and cardiac output, renal blood flow increases. The GFR rises early in pregnancy, and creatinine clearance may be 150 mL/minute or more by 30 weeks. Serum urea and creatinine concentrations fall. Tubular function alters and, in particular, there is a reduction in the renal threshold for glucose. Intermittent glycosuria may be present in up to 70% of pregnancies. Tubular reabsorption of uric acid and amino acids alters, and their excretion in urine increases.

Carbohydrate metabolism

The fasting blood glucose falls early in pregnancy, probably because of substrate utilization. The response to a standard carbohydrate challenge is altered in late pregnancy.

Protein metabolism

Serum albumin concentration falls gradually from early pregnancy and this is related to ECF expansion. The concentrations of many other proteins increase, particularly placental proteins such as alkaline phosphatase of placental origin, transport proteins such as transferrin, and hormone-binding glycoproteins such as thyroxine-binding globulin, and fibrinogen.

Hormonal changes

Oestrogens and progesterone are secreted in greater amounts early in pregnancy, and protein hormones such as HCG and HPL are produced by the placenta. These hormonal changes form the biochemical basis of the diagnosis of pregnancy. For example, HCG should be undetectable in the non-pregnant state.

Table 1 **Reference intervals in the third trimester of pregnancy, and how they compare with non-pregnant controls**		
Serum/blood measurement	Pregnant	Non-pregnant
Sodium (mmol/L)	132–140	135–145
Potassium (mmol/L)	3.2–4.6	3.4–4.9
Chloride (mmol/L)	97–107	95–105
Bicarbonate (mmol/L)	18–28	21–28
Urea (mmol/L)	1.0–3.8	2.5–8.0
Glucose (fasting) (mmol/L)	3.0–5.0	4.0–5.5
Calcium (mmol/L)	2.2–2.8	2.2–2.6
Magnesium (mmol/L)	0.6–0.8	0.7–1.0
Albumin (g/L)	32–42	40–52
Bilirubin (µmol/L)	3–14	3–22
Alanine aminotransferase (U/L)	3–28	3–55
Aspartate aminotransferase (U/L)	3–31	12–48
Alkaline phosphatase (U/L)	174–400	80–280
Blood H+ (nmol/L)	34–50	35–45
Blood PCO_2 (kPa)	3.0–5.0	4.4–5.6

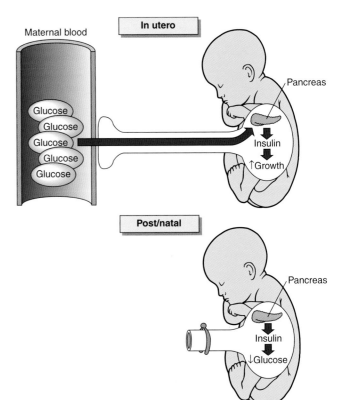

Fig. 1 **Diabetes mellitus in pregnancy is associated with fetal hyperinsulinaemia.** In utero this leads to increased growth, while post-natally the persisting hyperinsulinaemia causes neonatal hypoglycaemia.

Pregnancy-associated pathology

Morbidity during pregnancy may be due to pre-existing medical conditions in the mother such as diabetes mellitus, hypertension, renal disease, thyrotoxicosis, or due to pregnancy-associated conditions.

Diabetic pregnancy

Pregnancy in a diabetic patient, whether she is known to be diabetic before pregnancy or when diabetes mellitus manifests itself during pregnancy, is associated with increased fetal mortality and morbidity. Maternal hyperglycaemia promotes hyperinsulinism in the fetus (Fig. 1). Insulin is a growth factor, and babies of poorly controlled diabetic patients are large and bloated. Tight control of diabetes mellitus during pregnancy decreases complications.

Hypertension

The patient who develops hypertension in pregnancy – a condition described variously as pre-eclampsia or pregnancy-induced hypertension – is at increased risk of placental insufficiency and consequent fetal intrauterine growth retardation. The hypertension is thought to be the causative factor of eclampsia, a severe illness that usually occurs in the second half of pregnancy and is characterized by generalized convulsions, extreme hypertension and impaired renal function including proteinuria. This disease is a significant cause of maternal death, which occurs most commonly as a result of cerebral haemorrhage. The features of pre-eclampsia are shown in Figure 2. There are similarities between pre-eclampsia and two other conditions seen in pregnancy – namely the HELLP syndrome (haemolysis, elevated liver enzymes and low platelets) and acute fatty liver of pregnancy. Blood-borne factors from a poorly perfused placenta may activate the maternal endothelium, causing endothelial dysfunction and vascular damage. Altered liver metabolism may also contribute, especially to acute fatty liver of pregnancy, by contributing to triglyceride accumulation in the liver. All of these conditions place the mother and baby at risk. The only effective management is delivery of the baby, although magnesium sulphate may be used to treat hypertension in eclampsia. Frequently it is difficult to decide on the optimum time for delivery. Laboratory investigations may help to inform this decision. These include transaminases (AST and ALT), LDH, platelet count, triglyceride and urine protein estimation.

Obstetric cholestasis

This condition has become increasingly widely recognized recently. It is characterized by severe maternal itch

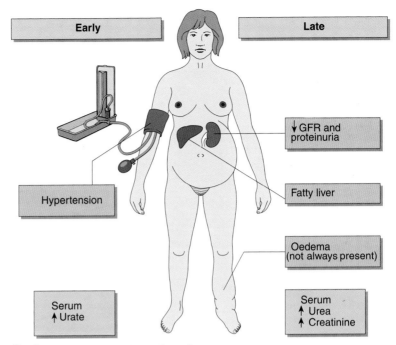

Fig. 2 **Clinical features of pre-eclampsia.**

- Early
- Late
- ↓GFR and proteinuria
- Hypertension
- Fatty liver
- Oedema (not always present)
- Serum ↑Urate
- Serum ↑Urea ↑Creatinine

(in the absence of a skin rash) and is important particularly because it places the baby at risk of intrauterine death. Deaths usually occur after 36 weeks, with little or no warning. Elevation of serum bile acids is the most sensitive indicator of obstetric cholestasis, the aetiology and pathogenesis of which remain obscure.

Drugs in pregnancy

Many women have, of necessity, to continue to take drugs during pregnancy. No drugs are without risk to the developing fetus, and drug levels should be kept as low as possible during gestation and thereafter if the mother is breast feeding, since many drugs are secreted in breast milk. Of particular concern are anticonvulsant drugs. Careful monitoring of levels is necessary to steer between the dangers of maternal seizures and potential fetal damage from the drug.

> **Clinical note**
> Pregnancy is the commonest cause of amenorrhoea in a woman of reproductive age. A pregnancy test should always be performed before other endocrine investigations of the cause of absent menstrual bleeding.

Case history 63

A 20-year-old woman in her first pregnancy was referred to hospital by her GP when she was 31 weeks pregnant. At 12 weeks pregnant she appeared well, had no oedema and her blood pressure was 110/70 mmHg. Now, she complained that she was unable to remove her wedding ring and that her vision was blurred. On examination ankle oedema was also observed and her blood pressure was found to be 180/110 mmHg.

- What is the most likely diagnosis?
- What sideroom test(s) should be performed?
- What biochemical investigations should be performed immediately?

Comment on page 169.

Pregnancy

- Physiological changes occur in pregnancy, altering many biochemical reference intervals. Do not be misled into believing that they indicate pathology.

- Diabetes in pregnancy is associated with increased fetal mortality and morbidity. Good diabetic control during pregnancy decreases complications. The baby of a diabetic mother has an increased probability of developing respiratory distress syndrome.

- Hypertension and a rising serum urate concentration are early features in the development of pre-eclampsia, a rapidly progressing condition that carries considerable risk to mother and fetus.

Screening the newborn for disease

Neonatal screening programmes

Many countries have screening programmes for diseases at birth. A blood sample is collected from every baby around the seventh day of life. Capillary blood sampling in the neonate is best performed on the plantar aspect of the foot, especially on the medial aspect of the posterior third, as shown in Figure 1. A 'blood spot' is collected on to a thick filter paper card (Fig. 2). The specimen can be conveniently sent by mail to a central screening laboratory. The following questions are usually considered when discussing the cost-effectiveness of a screening programme.

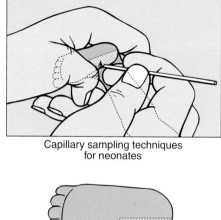

Capillary sampling techniques for neonates

Posterior medial third of foot (plantar aspect)

Fig. 1 **Capillary blood sampling in neonates.**

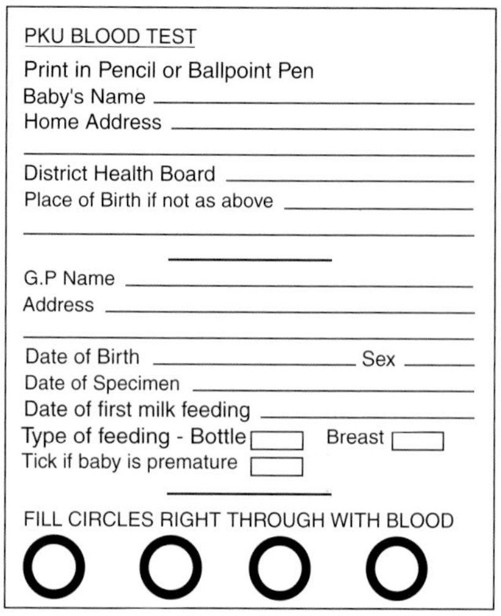

PKU BLOOD TEST

Print in Pencil or Ballpoint Pen
Baby's Name _____
Home Address _____
_____

District Health Board _____
Place of Birth if not as above _____

_____

G.P Name _____
Address _____

Date of Birth _____ Sex _____
Date of Specimen _____
Date of first milk feeding _____
Type of feeding - Bottle [ ] Breast [ ]
Tick if baby is premature [ ]

FILL CIRCLES RIGHT THROUGH WITH BLOOD
○ ○ ○ ○

Fig. 2 **Filter paper card ('Guthrie card') for the collection of 'blood spots.'**

- Does the disease have a relatively high incidence?
- Can the disease be detected within days of birth?
- Can the disease be identified by a biochemical marker which can be easily measured?
- Will the disease be missed clinically, and would this cause irreversible damage to the baby?
- Is the disease treatable, and will the result of the screening test be available before any irreversible damage to the baby has occurred?

Neonatal screening programmes for hypothyroidism and phenylketonuria have been established in many countries. Both these disorders carry the risk of impaired mental development, which can be prevented by prompt recognition of the disease. Local factors, such as population mix, lead to the setting up of specific screening programmes. For example, the high incidence of congenital adrenal hyperplasia (1:500 live births) among the Yupik Eskimo is the stimulus for a screening programme for this disease in Alaska. In Finland, the incidence of phenylketonuria is low and neonatal screening is not carried out.

Disagreement on the benefits and risks of tests, the presence of public pressure and availability of funding are factors that continue to determine whether neonatal screening programmes are established.

Congenital hypothyroidism

Primary hypothyroidism is present in one in every 3500 births in the UK. There is often no clinical evidence at birth that the baby is abnormal, yet if congenital hypothyroidism is unrecognized and untreated, affected children develop irreversible mental retardation and the characteristic features of cretinism (Fig. 3). Most cases of congenital hypothyroidism are due to thyroid gland dysgenesis, the failure of the thyroid gland to develop properly during early embryonic growth. The presence of a high blood TSH concentration is the basis of the screening test (Fig. 4).

A positive result of a screening test should be confirmed by demonstration of an elevated TSH in a serum specimen obtained from the infant. When necessary, thyroxine treatment should be initiated as soon as possible after diagnosis. The initial dosage is 10 µg/kg and this can be gradually increased during childhood to the adult dosage of 100–200 µg per day by 12 years of age. The absence of clinical signs of hypothyroidism or hyperthyroidism, together with normal serum T_4 and TSH concentrations, provides evidence of the adequacy of treatment.

If a positive screening test is obtained, the mother's thyroid function is usually also assessed. Maternal autoantibodies can cross the placenta and block receptor sites on the fetal thyroid. In this rare situation, after an initial transient hypothyroidism just after birth, the baby's own thyroid function will usually develop normally.

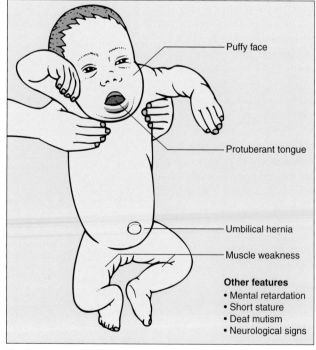

Puffy face

Protuberant tongue

Umbilical hernia

Muscle weakness

Other features
• Mental retardation
• Short stature
• Deaf mutism
• Neurological signs

Fig. 3 **Features of cretinism.**

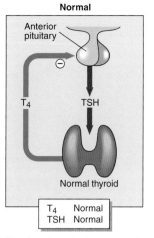

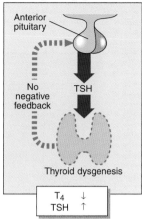

Fig. 4 **Control of TSH secretion.**

TSH screening does not detect secondary hypothyroidism due to pituitary disease. This is a much rarer disorder than primary hypothyroidism, occurring in one in every 100 000 births.

Phenylketonuria

The incidence of phenylketonuria is around one in every 10 000 births in the UK. Phenylketonuria arises from impaired conversion of phenylalanine to tyrosine, usually because of a deficiency of phenylalanine hydroxylase. Figure 5 shows how phenylalanine, an essential amino acid, is metabolized. In phenylketonuria, phenylalanine cannot be converted to tyrosine, accumulates in blood and

is excreted in the urine. The main urinary metabolite is phenylpyruvic acid (a 'phenylketone'), which gives the disease its name. The clinical features include:

- irritability, poor feeding, vomiting and fitting in the first weeks of life
- mental retardation
- eczema
- reduced melanin formation in the skin, resulting in the classical fair haired, blue eyed appearance.

Phenylalanine hydroxylase uses tetrahydrobiopterin (BH4) as a cofactor. Defective BH4 supply or regeneration, due to deficiency of dihydropteridine reductase, have been

identified as rare causes of 'hyperphenylalaninaemia', a term that better describes the group of disorders.

The detection of phenylketonuria was the first screening programme to be established. The screening test is based on the detection of increased phenylalanine concentration in the blood spot.

The mainstay of the management of phenylketonuria is to reduce the plasma phenylalanine concentration by dietary control. Mental retardation is not present at birth, and can be prevented from occurring if plasma phenylalanine concentrations are kept low in the early years of life. It was thought that dietary control need only be followed for 10 years or so but current views are that lifelong therapy is necessary.

Follow-up of screening tests

A positive or equivocal result in a screening test should be followed up rapidly and efficiently. A clearly positive result will require immediate referral to a paediatrician. Requests for a repeat specimen because the result was borderline, or there was insufficient sample, or the analysis was unsatisfactory, must be handled tactfully. Parents frequently find it distressing if their child is suspected of a serious disorder even if subsequently the baby is found to be normal.

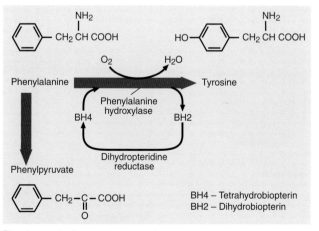

Fig. 5 **Metabolism of phenylalanine.**

> *Clinical note*
>
> *N*-aspartylphenylalanine methyl ester (aspartame) is a commonly used artificial sweetener. It is broken down in the gut to phenylalanine. Patients with phenylketonuria must avoid any food containing this additive. It is particularly important that foodstuffs, including soft drinks, should be clearly labelled with a warning that they contain this artificial sweetener.

Case history 64

The 'blood spot' analysis on a 6-day-old baby girl indicated a high TSH, 28 mU/L. A second blood sample was quickly obtained for a repeat TSH estimation. The laboratory reported a TSH concentration of 6 mU/L.

- What further investigations should be carried out?

Comment on page 169.

Screening the newborn for disease

- In some countries screening programmes have been established to detect specific diseases in babies.

- Analyses are performed on blood spots obtained around 1 week after birth.

- Common diseases tested for in this way are congenital hypothyroidism and phenylketonuria.

- For it to be worthwhile to screen for a disorder the disease should have a relatively high incidence, be detectable within days of birth, result in serious consequences if missed clinically, and be treatable.

Paediatric biochemistry

Paediatric biochemistry differs from adult biochemistry in several respects. Firstly, profound changes in physiological maturity occur from birth through to adulthood – and these are reflected in paediatric biochemistry. Secondly, the diseases of childhood are not the same as those of adulthood. Genetic and developmental disorders feature much more prominently, whereas disease processes that take many years to become clinically evident, e.g. atherosclerosis, do not. Finally, the practicalities of sample collection and processing differ significantly.

Immaturity

Children are by definition physiologically immature and in a state of development. After birth, immaturity of organ systems may persist for weeks, months or even years, and accounts for several common clinical presentations (see below).

Jaundice

The liver of a newborn baby may not be capable of conjugating all of the bilirubin presented to it. The consequence is neonatal jaundice, and many babies become jaundiced during the first week of life. In full-term babies this usually resolves rapidly, but in premature babies it may persist. As a general rule, jaundice during the first 24 hours after birth is always pathological, and often indicates increased unconjugated bilirubin resulting from red blood cell destruction (haemolysis) due to blood group incompatibility or infection. Similarly, jaundice that lasts more than 10 days after birth should always be investigated. It may indicate galactosaemia, congenital hypothyroidism, cystic fibrosis or glucose-6-phosphate dehydrogenase deficiency.

Persistent jaundice due to unconjugated hyperbilirubinaemia should not be ignored. Unconjugated bilirubin is lipophilic and can cross the blood–brain barrier and bind to proteins in the brain where it is neurotoxic. This happens when albumin (the normal carrier of unconjugated bilirubin) becomes saturated. The clinical syndrome of bilirubin-encephalopathy is called kernicterus (Fig. 1) and may result in death or severe mental handicap. Where the excess bilirubin is found to be conjugated, the pathology is different, and kernicterus is not a feature, since conjugated bilirubin is water-soluble rather than lipophilic. Causes include neonatal hepatitis, possibly contracted from the mother at birth; biliary atresia, resulting in severely impaired biliary drainage; and inherited deficiency of alpha-1-antitrypsin, a powerful protease, the absence of which is associated with liver and lung damage.

Hypoglycaemia

Before birth, the chief source of energy for the fetus is glucose obtained from the mother via the placenta. Any excess glucose is stored as liver glycogen. Free fatty acids cross the placenta and are stored in fat tissue. At birth the baby suddenly has to switch to its own homeostatic mechanisms in order to maintain its blood glucose concentration in between feeds. These include gluconeogenesis and glycogenolysis. However, glycogen stores are often insufficient to prevent neonatal hypoglycaemia. Lipolysis provides another energy source in the form of free fatty acids until feeding is established. Hypoglycaemia including neonatal hypoglycaemia is dealt with on pp. 66–67.

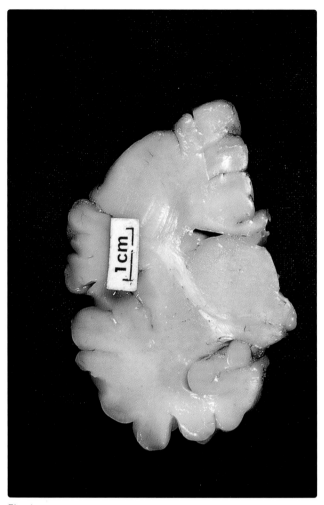

Fig. 1 **Kernicterus.** Reproduced with permission from Ellison D, et al, Neuropathology. A Reference Text of CNS Pathology, 2nd edn. Mosby, 2004.

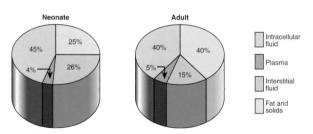

Fig. 2 **Body composition (% of body weight) in the neonate and adult.**

Dehydration

The total body water of a newborn baby is around 75% of body weight, compared with 60% in the adult (Fig. 2). In the first week after birth, the ECF contracts and this explains why most babies initially lose some weight before gaining it back subsequently. Infants are very vulnerable to fluid loss because their renal tubular function is not fully mature. Their ability to concentrate urine (and hence retain water) is poor – the maximum urine osmolality that can be produced is about 600 mmol/kg, compared with in excess of 1200 mmol/kg in a healthy adult. In addition, reabsorption of bicarbonate and glucose is reduced, leading to a low serum bicarbonate and glycosuria respectively.

In general, the dehydrated infant is relatively more water depleted than sodium depleted, partly because of the immature tubular function described above, but also because their larger ratio of body surface area to body weight renders them more susceptible to insensible water loss. Monitoring of fluid balance requires regular assessment of hydration status. Short of bladder catheterization, urine output is virtually impossible to assess with any degree of accuracy in infants and serial body weight measurement is often used instead as a good simple index of trends in hydration.

Prematurity

Prematurity presents an even more extreme challenge to organ function. A good example of organ failure resulting from prematurity is respiratory distress syndrome. Babies born before 32 weeks' gestation are unlikely to be able to make their own pulmonary surfactant, resulting in respiratory distress syndrome due to failure of alveolar expansion. Measurement of the lecithin/sphingomyelin ratio was used in the past in the assessment of fetal lung maturity, but has largely been superseded by the advent of surfactant therapy. Figure 3 illustrates the role of surfactant.

Practical considerations

- *Sampling.* Although venepuncture is preferred in older children, heelprick sampling is less traumatic for very young children. Heel puncture can, however, be complicated by calcaneal osteomyelitis, and there are preferred sites of collection (see p. 154).
- *Sample volume.* This is a major issue for paediatric biochemistry laboratories. A premature baby weighing less than 1000 g may have as little as 75 mL total blood volume. The sample volume must, therefore, be kept to an absolute minimum. At low sample volumes, e.g. 100 μL, evaporation from uncovered specimens can alter results of analyses by as much as 10% in 1 hour.
- *Plasma or serum.* In most laboratories that process paediatric specimens, plasma is preferred. In principle the

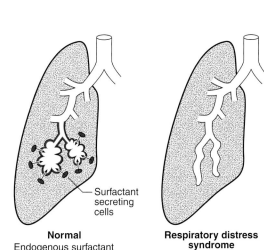

Normal
Endogenous surfactant supply, normal expansion of alveoli

Respiratory distress syndrome
No surfactant, failure of alveoli to expand

Surfactant therapy
Surfactant supplied exogenously

Fig. 3 **Surfactant and respiratory distress syndrome.**

turnaround time is reduced because one does not have to wait for clotting to occur before centrifuging the sample. Also there is generally less haemolysis.
- *Interferences.* Haemolysis increases plasma concentrations of potassium and some other analytes that are present in higher concentrations in red blood cells than in extracellular fluid. Hyperbilirubinaemia can interfere with creatinine measurement.
- *Instrumentation.* Automated analysers must be chosen with sample size in mind, as well as the 'dead volume' (the amount of sample that must remain in the sample cup after the sample has been aspirated for analysis); both of these should be kept to a minimum. Common interferences should, ideally, not affect results. Some analysers make use of slide technology to prevent interferences.

Case history 65

The baby of a diabetic mother weighed 1.64 kg (below 10th centile for weight) when born at gestational age of 32 weeks. The baby was well at birth, but her condition deteriorated within hours and she had respiratory problems.

- What biochemical determinations should be requested on this baby?
- Why is it important to consider each request carefully?

Comment on page 169.

Clinical note

Newborn babies have low levels of vitamin K, which is involved in the synthesis of blood coagulation factors. To minimize the risk of intracerebral haemorrhage, it has been recommended that all newborn babies, particularly those who are breast fed, be given this vitamin.

Paediatric biochemistry

- Jaundice is common in babies in the first week of life. In term babies, this usually resolves rapidly. Jaundice during the first 24 hours of life is always pathological.

- Neonatal hypoglycaemia may be encountered in the premature infant, the 'light-for-dates' baby or the infant of a diabetic mother.

- Relative to adults, babies have increased total body water and extracellular water. Renal function changes with age. Guidelines for fluid and electrolyte replacement therapy in babies are quite different from those in adults.

- Respiratory distress syndrome is the consequence of lack of surfactant, which prevents expansion and aeration of pulmonary alveoli.

Inborn errors of metabolism

The spectrum of genetic disorders is wide and encompasses chromosomal disorders as well as many common diseases in which multiple genes confer susceptibility to the effects of environmental influences. 'Classical' genetic diseases result from single gene mutations that result either in reduced synthesis of a particular protein, or the synthesis of a defective protein. In 1909 Garrod first defined the concept of *inborn errors of metabolism*, where blocks in specific metabolic pathways result from defects in particular enzymes. Certainly, in most inborn errors, the defective or absent protein is an enzyme; exceptions include familial hypercholesterolaemia, cystinuria and Hartnup disease, where the affected proteins are either receptors or are otherwise involved in transport processes.

Patterns of inheritance

Inborn errors can be autosomal (involving a chromosome other than X or Y) or X-linked, and the genetic defect can be either dominant or recessive. In dominant disorders, everyone who carries the gene is affected by the disease, so every affected individual has at least one affected parent. If the defective gene is recessive, it will be silent unless both copies (maternal and paternal) of the gene carry the mutation, i.e. affected individuals must be homozygous; parents carrying only one copy of the affected gene (heterozygotes) are carriers and are not clinically affected. These patterns of inheritance are illustrated in Figure 1.

Establishing pedigrees may not be straightforward. One reason for this is that the severity of the disease can vary widely between individuals even within the same family. Sometimes the clinical manifestations may be so mild that the disease cannot be detected, even though the defective gene is present. When this occurs the disease is said to be *non-penetrant*. Thus, dominant diseases may clinically appear to 'skip' generations.

Mechanisms of disease

Inborn errors of metabolism can manifest clinically in various ways:

- accumulation of substrate
- reduced product
- diversion of intermediates
- failure of negative feedback
- failure of transport mechanisms.

These are shown in Figure 2.

Clinical diagnosis

Several problems confront the clinician suspecting an inborn error of metabolism. Firstly, the clinical presentation is often non-specific. In an infant, the symptoms may include poor feeding, lethargy and vomiting, which are seen with any significant illness; in older children, failure to thrive or developmental delay may be the only presentation. Secondly, the range of specialist tests used to diagnose inborn errors is extensive and, for many, bewildering. Useful clues that should increase the index of suspicion include:

- parents are cousins (so-called consanguinous mating)
- history of unexplained premature death in an older sibling

Autosomal dominant

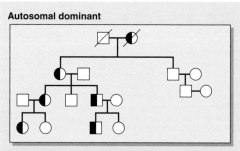

The second copy of the gene on the homologous chromosome cannot compensate for the mutated copy:
- Consecutive generations affected
- Half of offspring affected, male = female
- Unaffected individual cannot transmit disease

Autosomal recessive

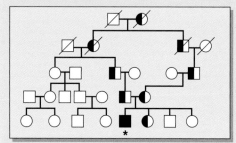

The second copy of the gene on the homologous chromosome compensates for the mutated copy:
- Unaffected carrier individuals transmit disease
- If both parents are carriers, then one-quarter of their offspring are affected, and one-half are carriers
- Usually only one generation is affected – denoted by *
Affected individuals may have two identical mutant copies arising from a common ancestor as shown, or different in 'compound heterozygotes'

X-linked recessive

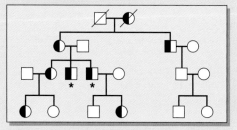

A second copy of the gene is only present in females. In X-linked recessive disease:
- Males only affected - denoted by *
- Unaffected female carriers transmit the disease
- All of carrier female's offspring inherit mutation – males are affected, and females are carriers
- Affected males cannot transmit the disease to their sons, but all of their daughters are carriers

Fig. 1 **Patterns of inheritance.**

- onset of symptoms following change in feeding regimen
- dysmorphic features
- unusual smell (see Table 1).

One useful classification of inborn errors includes both clinical and laboratory features (Table 2).

Laboratory diagnosis

Clearly if there is a clinical basis for suspecting a particular inborn error of metabolism, specific investigations should be requested. For example, the presence of cataracts should

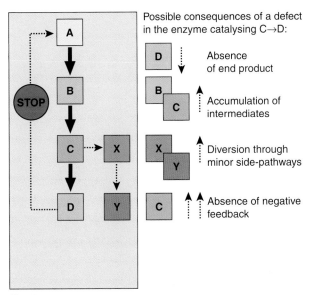

Possible consequences of a defect in the enzyme catalysing C→D:

Absence of end product

Accumulation of intermediates

Diversion through minor side-pathways

Absence of negative feedback

Fig. 2 **Pathogenic mechanisms resulting from enzyme deficiency.**

 Clinical note
Making the diagnosis of an inborn error post mortem is not pointless: it may permit genetic counselling and may save the life of a future sibling. Where possible blood and urine samples should be collected after discussion with a specialist laboratory. Inborn errors are also diagnosed sometimes using samples of skin, liver or vitreous humour.

Table 1 **Inborn errors of metabolism associated with characteristic smells due to volatile organic intermediates**

Inborn error of metabolism	Smell
Maple syrup urine disease	Maple syrup
Phenylketonuria	Musty
Isovaleric acidaemia	Sweaty feet or cheese
Trimethylaminuria	Fish
Hypermethioninaemia	Cabbage

make one suspect galactosaemia, for which the appropriate investigation is measurement of galactose-1-phosphate uridyl transferase in red blood cells. More often, however, there are no specific features. Routine laboratory investigations may help point the direction of further investigations by suggesting particular groups of metabolic disorders (see Table 3). In the acute situation, in the absence of clues, the following investigations should always be considered, and performed urgently if indicated:

- *Plasma ammonia.* Indicated particularly when there is neurological distress/intoxication; grossly elevated levels are most frequently due to urea cycle disorders.
- *Organic acids (urine)* and *amino acids (urine and plasma).* Organic and amino acid disorders collectively comprise a large group of inborn errors of metabolism.
- *Plasma lactate.* Should be measured especially if there is acidosis, hypoglycaemia or neurological distress. This test is readily available in most laboratories.
- *Galactose-1-phosphate uridyl transferase.* Unusual in this list in being specific to one disorder (galactosaemia). However, this is easily treated by excluding galactose from the diet, is frequently fatal if unrecognized (especially in neonates), and is sufficiently common that it is included in some population screening programmes.

Table 2 **Classification of inborn errors of metabolism on basis of clinical and laboratory features**

Presentation	Most likely diagnoses
'Intoxication', ketoacidosis (blood H+ not ↑↑)	Maple syrup urine disease (amino acid disorder)
'Intoxication', ketoacidosis	Organic acid disorders
'Energy deficiency', lactic acidosis	Congenital lactic acidoses
'Intoxication', high ammonia, no ketoacidosis	Urea cycle defects
'Energy deficiency', no metabolic disturbance	Peroxisomal disorders Non-ketotic hyperglycinaemia
Storage disorders, no metabolic disturbance	Lysosomal storage diseases
Hypoglycaemia, hepatomegaly, abnormal LFTs	Glycogen storage diseases

'Intoxication' and 'energy deficiency' are contrasting clinical manifestations of neurological distress in the neonatal period. 'Intoxication' is characterized by a symptom-free interval, then onset of lethargy or coma. 'Energy deficiency' is often associated with hypotonia, dysmorphic features. Lethargy and coma are rarely the initial signs, and often there is no symptom-free interval.

Table 3 **Biochemical investigations that may help to direct further investigations**

Test	Comment
Urinalysis	
■ reducing substances	■ Positive for reducing substances but not for glucose: suspect galactosaemia
■ ketones	■ Strongly positive: suspect hypoglycaemia (see below)
	■ Negative despite hypoglycaemia or fasting: suspect a disorder of fatty acid oxidation
■ pH	■ pH <5.5 excludes renal tubular acidosis as cause of metabolic acidosis and points to an organic acid disorder
Blood	
■ Anion gap ([Na+] + [K+] − ([Cl−] + [HCO3−]))	■ High anion gap metabolic acidosis (>20 mmol/L): suspect an organic acid disorder
■ Metabolic acidosis (low [HCO3−])	
■ Hypoglycaemia	■ Relatively non-specific – found in normal neonates, and compatible with many inborn errors of metabolism: – organic acid disorders – amino acid disorders – glycogen storage disorders – galactosaemia – fatty acid oxidation defects
■ Hyponatraemia	■ If found with ambiguous genitalia: suspect congenital adrenal hyperplasia
■ Respiratory alkalosis	■ If found with neurological distress: suspect urea cycle disorder
■ Abnormal liver function tests (LFTs)	■ Relatively non-specific – consistent with – glycogen storage disorders – tyrosinaemia – alpha-1-antitrypsin deficiency
■ Hyperammonaemia	■ Plasma [NH4+] >800 μmol/L: strongly suspect urea cycle disorder

Selected inherited disorders

Disorder	Main feature
Acute intermittent porphyria	The porphyrias are disorders of haem biosynthesis. The acute porphyrias which present with abdominal pain and neurological features all have increased urinary porphobilinogen during an attack, and this is diagnostic
Adrenoleucodystrophy	This rare neurodegenerative disease is characterized by the impaired metabolism and subsequent accumulation of long chain fatty acids in plasma and tissues
Agammaglobulinaemia	There is a complete absence of immunoglobulin production. Selective IgA deficiency is more common with affected children presenting with recurrent respiratory infections
Alpha-1-antitrypsin deficiency	Patients with deficiency of the protease inhibitor, alpha-1-antitrypsin, may present with liver disease in childhood or with pulmonary emphysema in adults. All patients with genotypes associated with low alpha-1-antitrypsin in the serum are likely to develop emphysema if they smoke or are exposed to environmental pollutants
Biotinidase deficiency	A failure of biotin recycling results in an organic aciduria, developmental delay, seizures, alopecia, hypotonia and hearing loss
Congenital adrenal hyperplasia	This name is given to disorders of the enzymes involved in steroid hormone biosynthesis. The most common is lack of the 21-hydroxylase on the pathways which lead to cortisol and aldosterone (pp. 92–93)
Cystic fibrosis	See pages 148–149
Cystinuria	An increased excretion of the amino acids cystine, lysine, arginine and ornithine leads to an increased incidence of renal calculi. A defective carrier protein causes impaired renal tubular reabsorption of these amino acids from the glomerular filtrate
Cystinosis	This is a lysosomal storage disorder where there is a defect in the membrane transport of cystine. Cystine crystals are deposited in kidney, liver, spleen, bone marrow and cornea
Familial hypercholesterolaemia	See pages 132–133
Galactosaemia	This defect is present in approximately 1:100 000 babies in the UK. A deficiency of galactose 1-phosphate uridyl transferase means that the baby cannot utilize the galactose component of the lactose which is present in milk. Such infants may present with failure to thrive, vomiting and diarrhoea and if untreated may die in the neonatal period or go on to develop liver disease, mental retardation, cataracts and renal tubular damage.
Glucose-6-phosphate dehydrogenase deficiency	This is an X-linked disorder associated with neonatal jaundice on the 2nd or 3rd day of life and drug-induced haemolytic crises
Glycogen storage disease (type I: von Gierke's)	Deficiency of glucose-6-phosphatase makes the glycogen stores of the body inaccessible. Children with this disorder have hepatomegaly and hypoglycaemia accompanied by hyperlipidaemia and lactic acidosis
Haemochromatosis	See pages 112–113
Homocystinuria	A deficiency of the enzyme cystathionine synthase leads to the accumulation of sulphur-containing amino acids. Affected children are normal at birth but develop eye problems, osteoporosis and mental retardation
Lesch–Nyhan syndrome	This is a severe form of hypoxanthine–guanine phosphoribosyltransferase deficiency, an enzyme involved in the metabolism of the purine bases (pp. 142–143)
Maple syrup urine disease	This defect in the decarboxylation of branched chain amino acids such as leucine, isoleucine and valine leads to severe brain damage and death during the first year of life
Mucopolysaccharidoses	This group of disorders is characterized by tissue accumulation of glycosaminoglycans such as heparin sulphate and dermatan sulphate. This results in skeletal deformities, mental retardation and premature death
Multiple endocrine neoplasias	See pages 140–141
Muscular dystrophy	See pages 144–145
Phenylketonuria	See pages 154–155
Propionic acidaemia	This is caused by deficiency of enzymes involved in the metabolism of propionyl coenzyme A
Urea cycle defects	Deficiency of enzymes of the urea cycle results in a build-up of ammonia in the blood. Severe cases are often fatal in the first few days after birth.
Vitamin D dependent rickets	See pages 74–75
Wilson's disease	This causes variable neurological and hepatic symptoms as a consequence of copper toxicity (pp. 114–115).

Case History Comments

Case history comments

Case history 1
The delay in transporting the specimen to the laboratory was not known and the pattern of results obtained (serum urea = 11.8 mmol/L, sodium = 130 mmol/L and potassium = 6.7 mmol/L) suggest that the patient may be sodium depleted with pre-renal uraemia and hyperkalaemia. This pattern, if correct, is typical of Addison's disease, an endocrine emergency. However, a delay in separating the serum from the clot makes the potassium and sodium concentrations unreliable as these ions move out of and into the erythrocytes along their concentration gradients. Thus another specimen is required to establish the patient's true electrolyte status.

Case history 2
As is common in these circumstances, the boy had consumed a large amount of refined carbohydrate – two cans of soft drinks, a jam doughnut and in excess of 200 g of assorted sweets over the preceding 2 hours. Thus, it is to be expected that the blood glucose would be high and a diagnosis of diabetes mellitus should not be made. A follow-up fasting glucose would, however, be appropriate if there were persisting worries about the diagnosis in this case.

Case history 3
After 2 days or so the kidneys adapt to the decreased input and would conserve sodium, potassium and water. However, he will continue to lose water insensibly and as a result the ICF and ECF will contract in equal proportion. After 3–4 days the contraction will become critical when the ECF may be insufficient to maintain the circulation and, if not corrected, will lead to death.

Many individuals in this situation will also be severely injured with significant blood loss. This would obviously further compromise the ECF volume and would make survival unlikely.

Case history 4
These urea and electrolytes are typical of dilutional hyponatraemia. Her normal blood pressure and serum urea and creatinine concentrations make sodium depletion unlikely as the mechanism of her hyponatraemia. The absence of oedema excludes

a significant increase in her total body sodium. These results are characteristic of the so-called syndrome of inappropriate antidiuresis (SIAD) and are due to secretion of AVP in response to non-osmotic stimuli. The ectopic production of AVP is extremely rare even in patients with malignant disease. The urine osmolality signifies less than maximally dilute urine, i.e. impaired water excretion, which is in keeping with SIAD. However, it is equally consistent with sodium depletion (the hypovolaemia resulting from sodium and water loss is a powerful non-osmotic stimulus to AVP secretion). In any case, maximally dilute urine (50 mmol/kg or less) is clinically obvious – it is associated with urine flow rates in excess of 500 mL/hour. Thus, measurement of urine osmolality usually adds little to the diagnosis of hyponatraemia.

Case history 5
This is a classic presentation of severe sodium and water depletion with clinical evidence (hypotension, tachycardia, weakness) and biochemical evidence (pre-renal uraemia with a significant increase in the serum urea and a modest increase in the serum creatinine), which indicate severe contraction of the ECF volume. It is worth noting that a serum sodium concentration is a very poor guide to the presence, or absence, of sodium depletion. This patient requires both sodium and water as a matter of urgency. In view of his gastrointestinal symptoms this will need to be given intravenously as a 0.9% sodium chloride solution.

Case history 6
The biochemical results strongly suggest pre-renal uraemia, as there is a marked increase in the serum urea with a very modest increase in the serum creatinine. He has severe hypernatraemia and these two observations would indicate that the patient is primarily suffering from water depletion. The serum potassium is normal as is his anion gap. These results would, therefore, indicate the presence of profound uncomplicated water depletion.

In cases such as this it is essential to exclude non-ketotic, diabetic, precoma.

His blood glucose was 9.2 mmol/L, which excludes this diagnosis. Ketones were not detected, nor did he have an acidosis. It was rapidly established from the clinical history that the man had not eaten or drunk for more than 3 days. A diagnosis of pure water depletion was therefore established on the basis of the history, clinical findings and biochemical features.

Case history 7
It would be unusual for her blood pressure to be this high if she was taking her prescribed medication. The first thing that should be done is to check compliance. Assuming she is compliant, renal artery stenosis should be considered, particularly given the history of vascular disease. This is best detected using imaging (e.g. MR angiography), although grossly elevated renin may be helpful in the diagnosis. In this case the hypokalaemia results from the increased mineralocorticoid activity. Other causes of increased mineralocorticoid activity, e.g. Conn's and Cushing's syndromes, might also explain these findings.

Case history 8
This woman displays features of sodium depletion; she is also likely to have a mild degree of water depletion. The evidence for sodium depletion is her progressive weakness, her pre-renal uraemia and her hyponatraemia. While her glomerular filtration rate has decreased her tubular function appears satisfactory as demonstrated by her ability to produce a concentrated urine and to conserve her urine sodium. This woman received inadequate intravenous fluid therapy postoperatively. Her treatment regimen was especially deficient in sodium, which led to a contraction of her ECF and this caused her to develop pre-renal uraemia. The contraction in her ECF will also have stimulated AVP secretion and thus she conserved water and became hyponatraemic. The contraction in her ECF also stimulated aldosterone secretion, which caused her renal tubules to conserve sodium.

Ideally, in order to prescribe appropriate fluid therapy for this woman, one needs to estimate her sodium, potassium and water deficits from her fluid balance charts. Particular note must be taken of losses that are relatively rich in sodium, such as drainage fluid, losses from fistulae, stomas or by nasogastric aspiration. Insensible water loss and urinary losses must also be taken into account.

Case history 9

The creatinine clearance is calculated using the formula below where U is the urine creatinine concentration, V is the urine flow-rate and P is the plasma or serum creatinine concentration. As there are 1440 minutes in a day this man's urine flow-rate, $V = 2160/1440 = 1.5$ mL/minute. His urinary creatinine must be in the same units as his serum creatinine. His urinary creatinine concentration:

$U = 7.5$ mmol/L $= 7500$ µmol/L. His serum creatinine: $P = 150$ µmol/L. Thus,

$$\frac{UV}{P} = \frac{7500 \times 1.5}{150} = 75 \, \text{mL/minute}$$

This is low for a young male.

When it was discovered that the urine collection was for 17 hours and not 24 hours his urine flow-rate was recalculated (2160/1020):

$V = 2.1$ mL/minute.

Recalculating his creatinine clearance:

$$\frac{UV}{P} = \frac{7500 \times 2.1}{150} = 105 \, \text{mL/minute}$$

This is in the range one would expect in a young male. One can see, therefore, how errors in the timing and collection of urine significantly influence the calculation of the creatinine clearance. Errors in collection are by far the most common and serious errors encountered when estimating the creatinine clearance.

Case history 10

One can make a confident diagnosis of central diabetes insipidus from the history of head trauma and the observation that she was producing large volumes of urine and complaining of thirst. Her blood glucose level excludes diabetes mellitus as a cause of her polyuria and her hypernatraemia accounts for her thirst. In normal circumstances a serum sodium concentration of 150 mmol/L will stimulate AVP production and cause the urine to be maximally concentrated. This patient's urine is, therefore, inappropriately dilute. It would be unnecessary and even dangerous to

attempt to perform a water deprivation test on this patient. Note that her serum urea is not increased. This reflects her high urine flow-rate despite her significant water depletion.

Case history 11

The most useful piece of information here is the finding of pitting oedema, because it considerably narrows the differential diagnosis of proteinuria, which would otherwise be extensive. The combination of proteinuria and pitting oedema could be explained by the nephrotic syndrome, in which protein loss in the urine results in hypoalbuminaemia. However, congestive cardiac failure is the most likely explanation. It is much commoner than nephrotic syndrome, and is frequently associated with proteinuria.

Case history 12

The marked increase in the serum urea with the modest increase in the serum creatinine would indicate the presence of pre-renal uraemia. Pyrexial patients are frequently hypercatabolic, which will contribute to his high serum urea. His low serum bicarbonate and high anion gap indicates that he has a metabolic acidosis. This acidosis will cause the potassium to move from the intracellular to the extracellular compartment. The reduction in his glomerular filtration rate results in his inability to maintain a normal serum potassium in the face of this efflux as both these factors contribute to his hyperkalaemia.

Case history 13

The serum urea in this case, though high, is relatively low in comparison to the serum creatinine. This would be consistent with a low protein intake. The serum bicarbonate is low, indicating the presence of a metabolic acidosis. However, the anion gap is normal and, hence, it is unlikely that this patient's [H$^+$] will be grossly abnormal. The hyperkalaemia, therefore, is likely to be entirely due to the low glomerular filtration rate with the efflux of potassium from the intracellular to the extracellular compartment being of minor importance. The hyponatraemia in this case reflects impaired water excretion resulting from the inability of the renal tubules to respond to AVP. These results clearly indicate that the patient needs to continue with dialysis. This woman's serum calcium status

should also be assessed. Hypocalcaemia should be excluded and a high serum alkaline phosphatase would indicate the presence of metabolic bone disease. A raised serum PTH concentration is another very sensitive marker of metabolic bone disease in patients with renal failure.

Treatment of metabolic bone disease in renal failure is aimed at correcting hypocalcaemia and hyper-phosphataemia, e.g. oral calcium salts and calcitriol (active form of vitamin D).

Case history 14

The low [H$^+$] and high bicarbonate concentration confirm that this patient has a metabolic alkalosis. The raised PCO$_2$ indicates partial respiratory compensation for this. The loss of H$^+$ will have been caused by his severe vomiting which, in view of the history, is likely to be due to pyloric stenosis. Ingestion of bicarbonate would not lead to this degree of metabolic alkalosis though it will have aggravated the situation. The severe vomiting has led to dehydration and this is manifested by the presence of pre-renal uraemia. The hypokalaemia is due to a combination of potassium loss in the vomitus and the metabolic alkalosis causing the influx of potassium from the ECF to the ICF.

The urine results are typical of a patient with dehydration and metabolic alkalosis due to vomiting. Aldosterone is being secreted in an attempt to expand his ECF and the patient is conserving sodium despite his hypernatraemia. The hyperaldosteronism is promoting potassium loss despite hypokalaemia, and hydrogen ion loss, resulting in the classical paradoxical acid urine.

Case history 15

The high [H$^+$] and PCO$_2$ confirm the presence of a respiratory acidosis which, from the history, will have been expected. Note that the bicarbonate is not abnormally increased, which indicates that this is an acute development, and renal compensation for the respiratory acidosis has not had time to have a significant impact on the respiratory acidosis.

Case history 16

The [H$^+$] is at the upper end of the reference interval. The PCO$_2$ is markedly elevated which would indicate the presence of a respiratory acidosis but the bicarbonate concentration is also markedly increased as the compensatory response for the respiratory acidosis. This man has type 2 respiratory failure.

Case history 17

The dominant feature in this patient's acid–base disorder is an alkalosis as the [H$^+$] is low. The bicarbonate concentration is increased, indicating a metabolic alkalosis. The PCO$_2$ is increased (respiratory acidosis) and this could be due to partial compensation for the metabolic alkalosis. However, the increase in PCO$_2$ is too high for this to be the only explanation. The background history of respiratory disease is the other reason for this patient's respiratory acidosis.

The PO$_2$ indicates that the patient is satisfactorily oxygenating her blood.

This patient's hypokalaemia and metabolic alkalosis can be explained by profound potassium depletion due to the use of a diuretic with an inadequate intake of potassium. The principles of therapy are potassium supplementation and alteration of her drug regimen to one that will ameliorate potassium loss, e.g. use of an ACE inhibitor.

Case history 18

By far the most likely diagnosis based on the information given is the nephrotic syndrome. In the nephrotic syndrome you would expect the serum albumin to be low and the urinary albumin to be high. The serum urea and electrolytes are frequently normal. Although the glomerular basement membrane may be damaged, the glomerular filtration rate is usually normal in the early stages of the nephrotic syndrome. Hypercholesterolaemia is a feature of the nephrotic syndrome. The history of recurrent infections suggests a degree of immune deficiency. This patient is likely to be losing immunoglobulin and some of the components of the complement system in her urine and this could lead to a relative immune deficiency.

Case history 19

This man is suffering from multiple myeloma. He is one of the approximately 20% of patients with myeloma that do not have a paraprotein in the serum but have Bence Jones proteinuria. His renal function should be tested and hypercalcaemia should be excluded.

Case history 20

This man's presentation is typical of an acute coronary syndrome which may be the manifestation of a full blown myocardial infarction in this case. He should have an ECG recorded as soon as possible which may, in combination with the history, confirm the diagnosis of an MI. His plasma troponin should be measured, though this may not be increased in patients with an acute coronory syndrome until 12 hours after the onset of pain.

Case history 21

Metastatic breast carcinoma is the most likely diagnosis in this case. The liver function tests indicate that there is little hepatocellular damage present and that bilirubin excretion is normal. These findings, however, do not exclude the possibility of hepatic metastasis, giving rise to localized areas of intrahepatic obstruction. If this were so, then the γGT should also be increased. A normal serum calcium does not exclude the possibility of bone metastasis, which is another source of the high alkaline phosphatase activity. This could be confirmed by studying alkaline phosphatase isoenzymes. A third possibility is that there may be a local recurrence with the tumour itself producing alkaline phosphatase, though this would be very unlikely. A bone scan would be very helpful in this case.

Case history 22

In this case, the most likely diagnosis is carcinoma of the head of the pancreas obstructing the common bile duct. The other major differential would be enlarged lymph nodes at the porta hepatis obstructing the common bile duct, which would explain the clinical picture as well as pancreatic cancer. This could result from any abdominal or haematological malignancy, e.g. hepatoma (he was a moderate drinker) or lymphoma. Other differentials include cholangiocarcinoma and gall stones, although these are unlikely. Carcinoma of the head of the pancreas classically gives rise to severe, painless, deep jaundice, which is in keeping with a bilirubin of 250 μmol/L. This is uncomplicated obstructive jaundice, which is characterized by an alkaline phosphatase activity that is more than three times the upper limit of the reference interval. The aspartate and alanine aminotransferase activities do not indicate severe hepatocellular damage. By far the most important

further investigations to be performed on this patient would be to image the structures in the vicinity of the head of the pancreas and the common bile duct looking for the cause of the obstruction. This could be done by ultrasound or radiology.

Case history 23

The most striking features of these results are the marked increase in the aspartate and alanine aminotransferase activities. These indicate the presence of acute hepatocellular damage. There is a degree of cholestasis as indicated by the increase in bilirubin associated with an increase in the serum alkaline phosphatase activity. As the increase in alkaline phosphatase is less than twice the upper limit of the reference interval, cholestasis is unlikely to be the dominant cause of the jaundice. The increase in the γGT is to be expected as this enzyme is increased in many forms of liver disease.

The differential diagnosis here includes viral hepatitis or alcoholic hepatitis. An idiosyncratic drug reaction is also possible.

Case history 24

(i) Diabetes mellitus could be diagnosed unequivocally here, on the basis either of the fasting glucose or the 2-hour glucose.

(ii) The 2-hour result is diagnostic of diabetes mellitus despite the normal fasting glucose result.

(iii) This man's 2-hour glucose result puts him in the impaired glucose tolerance category and his fasting glucose puts him in the impaired fasting glycaemia category.

(iv) This woman has impaired glucose tolerance, notwithstanding her normal fasting glucose result.

Case history 25

By far the most likely diagnosis in this case is diabetic ketoacidosis. This may be precipitated by a number of conditions, such as infection. This may have caused anorexia and, thus, the patient may have omitted to take her insulin. Trauma can increase a patient's requirement for insulin but there is nothing to suggest that in this case. The blood glucose can be checked at the bedside as can a specimen of urine for the presence of ketones. The laboratory tests that may be requested are urea and electrolytes to assess renal function, the presence or absence of hyperkalaemia and the serum sodium concentration. The patient's acid–base status should be assessed to quantitate the severity of the acidosis present, and the blood glucose should be accurately measured. These results will influence the patient's treatment. It is essential in cases such as this that samples of blood and urine and, if appropriate, sputum are sent to the microbiological laboratory to look for the presence of infection.

Case history 26

Nocturnal hypoglycaemia is the most likely cause of this woman's symptoms. The diagnosis can be made by measuring her blood glucose while she is symptomatic. However, this can be distressing to patients and is not always feasible. Indirect evidence of nocturnal hypoglycaemia may be obtained by measuring her urinary catecholamine excretion or urinary cortisol excretion overnight. A further clue may be obtained if the woman's glycated haemoglobin level indicates good diabetic control in the face of hyperglycaemia during the day. In many such cases a diagnosis of nocturnal hypoglycaemia is inferred if the symptoms are relieved by changing the insulin regimen or getting the patient to eat more food before she retires at night.

Case history 27

As renal failure is the most common cause of hypocalcaemia, her serum urea and electrolytes should be measured. However, unsuspected renal failure is unlikely as her serum phosphate is normal. Her plasma PTH should be measured and if high (appropriate to the low calcium) then vitamin D deficiency is the most likely diagnosis, and the cause should be sought. In particular, a detailed dietary history should be taken. An increased serum alkaline phosphatase would be compatible with vitamin D deficiency. The bone pain is due to the underlying osteomalacia.

A low PTH would indicate hypoparathyroidism. Other causes of hypocalcaemia would be unlikely in this case.

Case history 28

The two most likely diagnoses in this case are primary hyperparathyroidism and hypercalaemia of malignancy. The most important biochemical investigation to be performed at this stage would be plasma PTH measurement, which will be high in primary hyperparathyroidism

and suppressed in hypercalcaemia of malignancy. In patients with hypercalcaemia of malignancy, the underlying disease is usually detectable by a careful clinical history and examination. There are, however, notable exceptions, multiple myeloma being one, and therefore a sample of serum and urine should be sent for protein electrophoresis to see if a paraprotein band can be identified. A blanket request for tumour markers such as CEA or AFP should not be requested unless there is a clear clinical indication for doing so. The patient's alkaline phosphatase activity should be measured and alkaline phosphatase isoenzyme studies may be indicated, especially if the plasma PTH concentration is suppressed.

The patient shows evidence of dehydration and has severe hypercalcaemia, which should be treated by rehydration in the first instance.

Case history 29

Though this patient is hypocalcaemic, the expected compensatory rise in PTH may not occur in view of the severe hypomagnesaemia. Thus, the PTH may be low.

This patient needs magnesium supplements. As magnesium salts cause diarrhoea they need to be given parenterally, especially in this case where there is established diarrhoea and malabsorption. It is likely that once the patient is magnesium replete, her original vitamin D and calcium supplements will be sufficient to maintain her in a normocalcaemic state. However, she may require regular 'top-ups' of intravenous magnesium in the future.

Case history 30

As Paget's disease can be considered a disorder of bone remodelling, the serum alkaline phosphatase, which is a good marker of osteoblastic activity, can be used to monitor the disease activity. It cannot, however, be used to demonstrate the involvement of a specific bone or deformity; this has to be done radiologically. If a patient is being given a bisphosphonate it is important to monitor the serum calcium, as hypocalcaemia is a well-recognized side effect of these drugs.

Case history 31

If panhypopituitarism is suspected, a lower dose of insulin should be used. This is because the relative deficiency of

glucocorticoids and growth hormone is associated with an increase in insulin sensitivity.

The basal prolactin was so high in this case that prolactinoma was the diagnosis until proven otherwise. Imaging of his pituitary confirmed the diagnosis.

The hypoglycaemic stress induced in this patient did not cause the expected rise in serum cortisol. It is essential, therefore, that he is commenced on steroid replacement before surgery. His low free T_4 combined with the abnormal response in his TSH (i.e. the 60 minute level being greater than the 30 minute level) would support a diagnosis of secondary hypothyroidism. He should, therefore, also be commenced on thyroxine replacement. As prolactinomas frequently shrink dramatically in response to dopamine agonists, he should be commenced preoperatively on either bromocriptine or cabergoline to reduce the size of the tumour.

Case history 32

Growth hormone deficiency should be suspected particularly in view of the documented fall-off in the patient's growth rate over the previous year. Random GH measurement is potentially misleading – false-positive and false-negative results are frequent. Many endocrinologists measure exercise-stimulated GH; a result >20 mU/L excludes GH deficiency.

Case history 33

This patient has a high serum T_4 because the oestrogen component of hormone replacement therapy stimulates the synthesis of thyroxine-binding globulin. Thus, to maintain a normal level of the physiologically active Free T_4 the total serum T_4 needs to be increased.

By far the most important investigation for this woman is a fine-needle aspiration biopsy of the thyroid nodule. Frequently, cystic lesions will be drained by this procedure and may not recur. It is important, however, that adequate thyroid epithelium be obtained to enable the diagnosis of thyroid cancer to be excluded or confirmed.

Case history 34

The low free T_4 and markedly elevated TSH results suggest primary hypothyroidism. Skeletal and cardiac muscles are affected in hypothyroidism, causing the release of creatine kinase into the circulation. This, combined with a decrease in the catabolic rate of creatine kinase, will be sufficient to cause the creatine kinase to increase to the levels observed in this case. The aspartate aminotransferase is at the upper end of the reference interval and this will fall along with the creatine kinase and cholesterol after a few weeks' treatment with thyroxine. In view of the evidence of myocardial ischaemia it is prudent to introduce thyroxine replacement cautiously (a low dose would be no more than 50 μg daily). High initial doses can precipitate myocardial ischaemia, and where the hypothyroidism is severe, as in this case, pericardial effusions and impaired ventricular function.

Case history 35

It is likely that this patient has suffered a relapse of her thyrotoxicosis. The severity of the derangement in her thyroid biochemistry (free T_4 66 pmol/L) makes it likely that she will be clinically thyrotoxic and symptomatic.

Repeated failure of medical therapy may warrant consideration of alternative treatment options, namely radioactive iodine and surgery. The former ablates the production of thyroid hormones irreversibly, and the patient would need to take replacement thyroxine therapy permanently thereafter.

Case history 36

Whenever one encounters the combination of hyponatraemia with hyperkalaemia, adrenocortical failure must be suspected. There is a modest increase in the serum creatinine with a normal serum urea that is not typical of Addison's disease. In adrenal failure the patient usually has pre-renal uraemia, which causes the serum urea to rise more than the creatinine. The low serum bicarbonate is a feature of adrenal insufficiency, and may reflect both the lack of mineralocorticoid activity and lactic acidosis, the latter resulting from hypovolaemia and associated reduced tissue perfusion.

It is essential that, at the very least, a timed random cortisol is requested on this patient. Unless the result is grossly elevated, thus excluding adrenal insufficiency, a Synacthen test is warranted. As the patient has severe skeletal muscle pain the creatine kinase should be measured as the hyperkalaemia may be due to

potassium released from damaged muscle. If rhabdomyolysis were detected, it would be important to monitor renal function and calcium status carefully.

Case history 37

This presentation is classical of acute adrenal failure with characteristic symptoms, physical findings and electrolyte pattern. The diagnosis is confirmed by the Synacthen test.

On presentation, this woman was sodium depleted with pre-renal uraemia. As her ECF was expanded with 0.9% sodium chloride, this improved her glomerular filtration rate, which is sufficient, even in the absence of aldosterone, to correct the hyperkalaemia by increasing her urinary potassium excretion. The reduction in this patient's blood volume will stimulate vasopressin secretion, giving rise to the hyponatraemia. The sodium chloride infusion by restoring her blood volume will inhibit AVP secretion, enabling her to correct the hyponatraemia.

Case history 38

Cushing's syndrome is the most likely diagnosis in this case. One can be confident of the diagnosis in view of the increased urinary cortisol:creatinine ratio, and the failure to suppress with low-dose dexamethasone.

Establishing a diagnosis of Cushing's syndrome is insufficient as it is essential to discover the underlying cause to enable the correct treatment to be given. This patient should have a high-dose dexamethasone suppression test with measurement of serum cortisol and ACTH. Suppression of the cortisol would point to the pituitary-dependent Cushing's syndrome as would an abnormally increased ACTH concentration. An adenoma should be actively sought in her pituitary and adrenal glands by CT or MRI scanning. If her ACTH is abnormally increased she may undergo selective venous catheterization to locate the source, which may be due to a carcinoid tumour of the lung.

Case history 39

This clinical presentation combined with biochemical findings of increased testosterone, reduced SHBG and increased LH/FSH ratio are characteristic of the polycystic ovarian syndrome. Ultrasound examination of her ovaries would confirm the diagnosis. Patients

with obesity and/or PCOS are insulin resistant. This stimulates compensatory hyperinsulinaemia. In many insulin-resistant women, the ovaries remain relatively more insulin sensitive than other tissues, and the hyperinsulinaemia stimulates ovarian androgen production.

Case history 40

An accurate measurement of height and serial measurements of weight are the most important means of monitoring the nutritional progress of such a patient. Patients are at risk of developing micronutrient deficiency if they experience difficulty in swallowing and, as a consequence, alter their diet to one that may be deficient in one or more components. For example, fresh fruit and vegetables may be sacrificed in favour of highly processed foods, thus causing vitamin C deficiency. Another alternative that has to be considered in these patients is that because of the relentless, incurable, nature of their disease they may ingest excessive amounts of vitamin and trace element supplements in the vain attempt to halt the progression of their disease. A careful dietary assessment should be made in this man and, if suspected, vitamin or trace element deficiencies or excesses tested for biochemically.

Case history 41

Measuring the serum vitamin B_{12} concentration is inappropriate in patients on parenteral treatment. A routine blood count is much more valuable. In a patient with pernicious anaemia feeling 'run down', other autoimmune diseases should be suspected. It would be reasonable to request thyroid function tests and glucose. The incidence of carcinoma of the stomach is increased among patients with pernicious anaemia and this diagnosis should also be borne in mind.

Case history 42

This patient has insufficient small bowel to enable him to be fed enterally. He will, therefore, require long-term parenteral nutrition. It is important that he is encouraged to take some oral fluids and nutrients to maintain the integrity of his remaining bowel.

The caloric and nitrogen requirements for restoration and maintenance of his skeletal muscle and body mass should be assessed. It is important to assess his baseline micronutrient status so that any deficiencies can be corrected. As he will receive the bulk of his nutrition parenterally in the future, his micronutrient status will need to be monitored. Once he is stable this should be formally checked at 6-monthly intervals along with his weight, skin-fold thickness and skeletal muscle mass.

Case history 43

In a patient such as this in ITU the biochemical measurements that are most frequently helpful are:

- *Serum urea and electrolytes* to monitor renal function and *serum potassium* as he may become hyperkalaemic as a result of tissue damage.
- *Pulse oximetry* to assess tissue oxygenation.
- *Blood gas analysis and plasma lactate,* to detect and quantify acid–base disorders that may arise.
- *Serum muscle enzymes,* such as CK may help detect a compartment syndrome or monitor rhabdomyolysis.

Case history 44

Recurrence or metastatic spread of the breast cancer would need to be excluded in this woman by imaging her liver and skeleton. Measurement of γGT and alkaline phosphatase isoenzyme studies may help to localize the source of the alkaline phosphatase. However, increased bone alkaline phosphatase does not necessarily signify bony metastases. In view of the history and symptoms, osteomalacia due to malnutrition or malabsorption may be the reason. If the patient has malabsorption or malnutrition she may have a macrocytic anaemia due to folate or B_{12} deficiency and may be deficient in other vitamins or other micronutrients such as zinc. Malabsorption is often difficult to detect clinically and she should undergo tests for malabsorption such as faecal fat measurement.

Case history 45

This patient has the classic symptoms and signs of iron deficiency anaemia. The finding of a low serum ferritin with a low serum iron and per cent transferrin saturation are typical of this condition. However, if iron deficiency anaemia is suspected, the most important and usually the only investigation required is to demonstrate the presence of a hypochromic

microcytic anaemia by examining the blood film.

Case history 46

The finding of a high liver copper concentration would indicate that the patient died from Wilson's disease, which is an autosomal recessive disorder. The patient's sister (and brothers, if any) should be screened for Wilson's disease. Serum copper, caeruloplasmin and urinary copper excretion may indicate if she also has the disease. A liver biopsy may be indicated to confirm the diagnosis and allow treatment to be initiated. DNA analysis is becoming available to assist in the diagnosis. Due to the very large number of mutations DNA testing is only of value within families to detect affected members and identify carriers.

Case history 47

Erythromycin inhibits the metabolism of theophylline. Since the erythromycin treatment was still required, her theophylline was stopped for 2 days and restarted at a lower dose. Once the infection was clear she was restarted on her original dose of theophylline.

Case history 48

These results would indicate that the man has taken an overdose of salicylate. The plasma salicylate of 4.6 mmol/L will contribute to his relatively high anion gap of 18 mmol/L. Salicylate poisoning is associated with a metabolic acidosis due to uncoupling of oxidative phosphorylation, and a respiratory alkalosis, due to direct stimulation by salicylate of the respiratory centre. The $[H^+]$ and PCO_2 indicate that the respiratory alkalosis is dominant at this stage.

In all cases of salicylate overdose the plasma paracetamol should also be measured as many proprietary analgesics contain aspirin and paracetamol. In the early stages of paracetamol poisoning, and when treatment is effective, patients will not display any specific signs or symptoms.

Case history 49

Many imported cosmetic agents contain lead. Not infrequently children will ingest these agents accidentally and may develop lead poisoning. It is, therefore, appropriate to measure the whole blood lead and erythrocyte protoporphyrin levels.

Case history 50

A high serum γGT is not diagnostic of alcohol abuse. γGT is induced by a number of enzyme-inducing agents such as phenytoin and phenobarbital, which this boy was taking. Currently, there is no definitive biochemical test to confirm alcohol abuse. However, the combination of an increased serum γGT and urate with a macrocytosis is strongly suggestive of alcohol abuse.

The alkaline phosphatase of 520 U/L is entirely appropriate for a teenager during his pubertal growth spurt. It should not be taken as indicative of liver disease.

Case history 51

Hypoglycaemia and diabetic ketoacidosis must be excluded. Blood glucose should be measured and blood or urine checked for ketones. Hypoglycaemia is more likely and should be treated with intravenous glucose. It is possible that the combination of hypoglycaemia, with or without alcohol intoxication, may have caused him to have an accident that could have resulted in a head injury causing his coma. Thus, in addition to monitoring his vital signs and grading his coma, it is essential to look for any superficial or neurological signs suggestive of head injury. It is essential that this be done even if he is demonstrated to be hypoglycaemic and rapidly recovers when given glucose, as the complications of a head injury such as subdural haematoma may not be immediately apparent.

Case history 52

This boy's calculated osmolality is approximately 206 mmol/kg. Thus, the osmolal gap is approximately 76 mmol/kg. This has arisen because of his severe hyperlipidaemia, which causes pseudohyponatraemia. In severe hyperlipidaemia the increased lipids occupy a larger fraction of the plasma volume than usual, and the water a smaller fraction. Sodium is distributed in the water fraction only, and, in reality, these patients have a normal plasma sodium concentration. However, many of the instruments used to measure sodium take no account of this, and thus produce artefactually low sodium results.

Severe hypertriglyceridaemia in a child may be caused by a decrease in lipoprotein lipase activity. This may result from genetic defects in the enzyme itself or in the enzyme's cofactor, apolipoprotein CII. Lipoprotein lipase is essential for the normal catabolism of chylomicrons and VLDL.

Case history 53

This man has diabetes mellitus, which is the most likely cause of his hyperlipidaemia. His γGT is high, which may be due to the presence of a fatty liver, a common finding in non-insulin-dependent diabetics on presentation. The high γGT may also be due a high alcohol intake, which may contribute to his hypertension. However, the combination of diabetes mellitus with central obesity and hypertension would suggest insulin resistance or the so-called metabolic syndrome.

Details of his family history with respect to coronary heart disease should be obtained. Palmar or tuberous xanthomas should be looked for and, if present, would suggest type III hyperlipidaemia. His Apo E genotype should then be established.

This patient should be treated with dietary measures. Particular attention should be paid to his alcohol intake. Liver disease should be excluded as its presence would preclude the use of metformin, which would be an appropriate drug to treat his diabetes, or the use of statins or fibric acid derivatives to treat his hyperlipidaemia.

Case history 54

This man is most likely to have essential hypertension, but it is important to consider other secondary causes especially in a relatively young patient. Acromegaly and phaeochromocytoma may present with the combination of hypertension, excessive sweating and glycosuria. Once considered, the signs and symptoms of acromegaly are usually readily recognized. However, phaeochromocytoma may not give rise to any symptoms or signs suggestive of the diagnosis apart from the episodic nature of the sweating. The patient's fundi should be checked for any evidence of malignant hypertension.

In suspected phaechromocytoma, urinary catecholamines or their metabolites should be measured. If the patient does not experience symptoms during the period of collection these tests may be normal. Hyperglycaemia and hypercalcaemia are other recognized consequences of excessive catecholamine secretion in patients

with phaeochromocytomas. If a phaeochromocytoma is diagnosed then the possibility of familial disease should be considered and family members screened.

Case history 55

The concern would be that this patient has Cushing's syndrome due to ectopic (malignant) production of ACTH. This is most frequently seen with carcinoma of the lung. As this disease is usually very aggressive, patients tend to develop florid metabolic features of the disease compared with the physical signs, which may be minimal. His serum urea and electrolytes indicate that he has developed profound hypokalaemic alkalosis and glucose intolerance. These can all be attributed to hypercortisolism. Cortisol will also cause muscle wasting that, combined with hypokalaemia, will lead to weakness. The nocturia and polyuria can cause profound potassium depletion.

Cushing's syndrome should be confirmed by performing a dexamethasone suppression test. If the suspicion of malignant ectopic ACTH production is high, the low and high-dose suppression tests should be performed back to back. Measurement of urinary cortisol output will confirm cortisol over-production. His plasma ACTH concentration should be grossly elevated. In such cases, if carcinoma of the lung is demonstrated radiologically and/or by bronchoscopy, the diagnosis of ectopic ACTH production is made without necessarily confirming it biochemically. Conn's syndrome and other conditions that may give rise to hypokalaemia with hypernatraemia are much rarer.

Case history 56

Though he is not clinically jaundiced the high alkaline phosphatase and γGT with modest increases in the AST and ALT would suggest cholestasis. This may be due to liver cirrhosis or malignant disease affecting the liver, both of which would be likely diagnoses in this case. Liver congestion resulting from cardiac failure would explain the clinical findings, but the biochemistry of congestion is classically dominated by raised transaminases; cholestasis is usually only a minor feature. This is the opposite of the picture here.

An AFP level may be helpful as it is a good tumour marker for hepatocellular carcinoma, which is

also a likely diagnosis in this case. The most common predisposing factors to the development of hepatocellular carcinoma are alcoholic cirrhosis in Western countries and hepatitis B in the developing world.

Case history 57

The patient's plasma PTH should be measured and, if increased, a diagnosis of primary hyperparathyroidism can be made. However, hyperparathyroidism with a serum calcium of 2.8 mmol/L is usually asymptomatic and thus another cause for his hypertension, headaches and anxiety should be sought. If the symptoms were episodic this would suggest the possibility of a phaeochromocytoma, which is associated with hyperparathyroidism in families with MEN. The patient should have his urinary catecholamines measured and, if the diagnosis is made, it is important that other members of his family be screened for hyperparathyroidism and phaeochromocytoma.

Case history 58

Acute severe pain in the metatarsophalangeal joint is the classic presentation of gout. The serum urate level is usually high in gout, but only a minority of patients with hyperuricaemia develop gout and frequently patients with acute gout may have a normal serum urate level. The presence of fever would be compatible with septic arthritis. The joint should be aspirated and, in addition to looking for urate crystals that would confirm a diagnosis of gout, some of the aspirate should be sent for microbiological studies to exclude the possibility of infection.

Case history 59

The large increase in the CK and LDH relative to the AST and ALT would indicate that muscle is the major tissue contributing to the increase in serum enzyme activities. However, muscle cells do not contain ALT, while AST and LDH are found in muscle, liver and erythrocytes. Thus, the tissues that could have contributed to the serum enzyme activities include muscle (either skeletal or cardiac), the liver or erythrocytes.

Muscle is the only source of CK and by measuring troponin T or I one can determine whether or not cardiac muscle is involved. If the liver is involved then the serum γGT should be increased as this is one of the most sensitive indicators of liver disease. Although LDH isoenzyme studies may help to identify erythrocyte damage as a possible source of LDH and AST, it may be more useful to look for other evidence of haemolysis, e.g reticulocytosis and absent or low haptoglobin.

Case history 60
Elderly people living on their own frequently have an inadequate diet. This is particularly true of men if they are unused to cooking for themselves. This patient may have a number of micronutrient deficiencies but, acutely, the most important would be possible thiamine deficiency. This can be detected by demonstrating an increase in the percentage activation of erythrocyte transketolase in vitro by the addition of thiamine or the measurement of thiamine pyrophosphate in erythrocytes. These investigations are often unavailable in the acute situation and patients are usually treated empirically with multivitamin preparations. When micronutrient deficiency is suspected, the diagnosis can only be confirmed if the appropriate samples are collected before the patient is given supplements.

Case history 61
Family tree
This child may have been picked up from neonatal screening. In the UK, this is routinely performed at 5 days and, along with other tests, immunoreactive trypsin (IRT) is measured. If elevated, DNA analysis is performed. If the child had symptoms, the primary screening test is the sweat test for chloride levels, which can be performed from around 2 weeks of age. The concentration of chloride in sweat is high in cases of CF. It would be appropriate to perform the same test on his siblings though the test cannot be used to detect heterozygote carriers. DNA diagnosis of both those with CF and heterozygous carriers is possible, and such tests may be

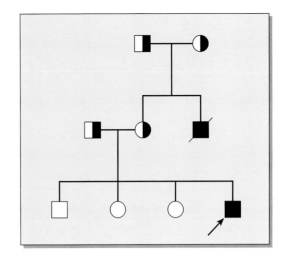

used if the sweat test is equivocal in the proband. It can also be used to test the carrier status of his siblings or for prenatal diagnosis in future pregnancies.

Case history 62
This woman should have an amniocentesis performed with bilirubin being measured in her amniotic fluid. In Rhesus incompatibility the amniotic fluid bilirubin concentration will rise because of the destruction of fetal red cells by maternal antibodies.

Case history 63
Pre-eclampsia is the most likely diagnosis. The most appropriate side room test to perform would be to test for albuminuria. Biochemical investigations that should be performed on this woman are:

- *Serum urate*, as this is a sensitive indicator for pre-eclampsia.
- *Serum urea and electrolytes* should be measured as she may be developing renal failure.
- *Serum albumin and liver function* tests should be performed to detect liver disease.
- *Glomerular filtration rate* should be measured as should urinary protein excretion to monitor her condition.

Case history 64
No other investigations should be performed, but the parents should be reassured that their daughter does not have congenital hypothyroidism.

Over 99% of all 6-day-old children will have a TSH of <10 mU/L while the majority of patients with congenital hypothyroidism will have a TSH >100 mU/L. Babies with a blood TSH between 15 and 40 mU/L on their first test are considered to have an equivocal result. If in a second sample a normal result is obtained, as is usually the case, no further investigation need be made.

Case history 65
This baby's blood gas status should be assessed as she is at risk of developing the respiratory distress syndrome. In view of her maternal history, weight and gestational age, she may be hypoglycaemic and her blood glucose should be measured. Hypocalcaemia is another possibility that should be considered, so her serum calcium should be measured.

The total blood volume in neonates is small and could be less than 100 mL in this baby. It is, therefore, very important to collect the minimum blood from neonates as they can become anaemic if a large number of investigations are performed.

Web Resources

Web resources

The internet is a remarkable resource and its value as an educational tool cannot be overestimated. However, it is also a highly dynamic affair with a distinct air of 'here today and gone tomorrow'. In selecting useful websites for these pages we have concentrated on well-established sites that in all probability will still be accessible for the lifetime of this edition. There are many other sites that can support and extend what is contained in this book and the reader is urged to access these through normal searches. One word of caution though – remember our subject has a number of pseudonyms – Clinical Biochemistry, Clinical Chemistry, Chemical Pathology, or just plain Pathology. If you are conducting general searches you may have to use more than one of these terms to get the return you are hoping for. As Clinical Chemistry is the term used most frequently in the United States you will find that this term yields the most hits (4.6 million versus 1.9 million for Clinical Biochemistry). Many university departments throughout the world have specific pages devoted to clinical cases and tutorial work related to Clinical Biochemistry which readers of this book may find useful. Occasionally complete slide sets and lecture notes are also available, but these are best searched for afresh as they are particularly prone to deactivation. Happy hunting.

Key journals

http://www.clinchem.org/
Clinical Chemistry is the most cited journal in the field of clinical chemistry, clinical (or anatomic) pathology, analytical chemistry, and the subspecialties, such as transfusion medicine, clinical microbiology. The journal, issued monthly, publishes contributions, either experimental or theoretical, that concern basic materials or principles, analytical and molecular diagnostic techniques, instrumentation, data processing, statistical analyses of data, clinical investigations in which chemistry has played a major role, or laboratory animal studies of chemically oriented problems of human disease.

http://www.elsevier.com/locate/ clinbiochem
Clinical Biochemistry publishes articles relating to the applications of molecular biology, biochemistry, chemistry and immunology to clinical investigation and to the diagnosis, therapy, and monitoring of human disease.

http://www.rsmpress.co.uk/acb. htm
Annals of Clinical Biochemistry is the official journal of the Association for Clinical Biochemistry, edited in collaboration with de Nederlandse Vereniging voor Klinische Chemie and Japan Society of Clinical Chemistry. One of the world's foremost in its field, it publishes fully refereed papers of international authorship that contribute to existing knowledge in all fields of clinical biochemistry, especially that pertaining to the understanding, diagnosis and treatment of human disease.

Key professional bodies

http://www.aacc.org/AACC/
The American Association for Clinical Chemistry (AACC) is an international scientific/medical society of clinical laboratory professionals, physicians, research scientists and other individuals involved with clinical chemistry and related disciplines. Founded in 1948, the society has 10 000 members and is headquartered in Washington, DC.

http://www.acb.org.uk/
The Association of Clinical Biochemistry (ACB) was founded in 1953, and is one of the oldest such associations in the world. Based in the United Kingdom, it is a professional body dedicated to the practice and promotion of clinical science. The ACB has medical and non-medical members in all major UK healthcare laboratories, in many university departments and in industry. The links with its corporate members lead to a fruitful relationship with the clinical diagnostics industry. The ACB liaises with and is consulted by many national and international organizations on issues relating to Clinical Biochemistry.

http://www.ifcc.org/
The mission statement of the International Federation of Clinical Chemistry and Laboratory Medicine (IFCC) is to be the leading organization in the field of Clinical Chemistry and Laboratory Medicine worldwide. This site has numerous useful links.

General sites

http://www.labtestsonline.org/
Lab Tests Online has been designed to help patients or carers understand the many clinical lab tests that are part of routine care as well as diagnosis and treatment of a broad range of conditions and diseases. If you are a medical professional, this site can also serve as a quick reference tool or as a resource for keeping up with advances in laboratory science. The content of the site is available in English, Spanish and German.

http://www.nlm.nih.gov/ medlineplus/laboratorytests. html
This site from the National Institutes of Health in the United States is directed at patients and contains a number of links to other patient-oriented sites for the explanation of the use and interpretation of laboratory tests.

http://www.geocities.com/ HotSprings/2255/endocrine.html
This portal provides access to a range of secondary sites that contain a variety of useful clinical case material in endocrinology and metabolic medicine.

http://www.merck.com/mmpe/ sec12.html
This is a convenient source of basic and more advanced information on a variety of fluid and electrolyte, acid–base and endocrine disorders. It is well arranged and easy to navigate.

http://www.lipidsonline.org
This site provides an up-to-date resource for clinicians and academics dealing with atherosclerosis and its consequences. Complete slide sets are available on many topics in this area, which was developed by Baylor College of Medicine in Houston, Texas.

http://www.nobelprize.org/ nobel_prizes/medicine/ laureates/1985

This site tells the story of the discovery of receptor mediated endocytosis and of the molecular defect in familial hypercholesterolaemia, and describes the scientific chase which led to the award of the Nobel Prize in Medicine/ Physiology in 1985.

http://ghr.nlm.nih.gov/

The Genetics Home Reference of the National Library of Medicine in the United States is a useful website that gives a lot of information about human genetic diseases. Although designed for the public it is also a useful resource for the professional.

http://Genomics.energy.gov/

This provides access to a range of resources relating to current genetic research including the Human Genome Project information site which has a host of useful educational links.

http://www.hoslink.com/plhome. htm

This Australian site describes itself as a resource portal for medical and biomedical professionals. It has well illustrated sections of laboratory

findings in different disease states arranged by systems.

http://www.pathmax.com/main. html

This is a useful American portal that covers all aspects of pathology and serves as a link to numerous other relevant sites. By clicking on the Chemistry/Lab Mgmt tab you will be directed to a list of potentially useful sites.

History

http://www.clinchem.org/cgi/ collection/Hist?page=1

These pages established by the journal Clinical Chemistry provide access to a range of interesting papers that deal with different aspects of the history of this subject. It is worth noting that from the same site there is a link to a related case study site which was still under construction at the time of writing.

http://www.ifcc.org/ejifcc/ vol13no4/130304003.pdf

This site provides access to an interesting review paper on the birth of Clinical Chemistry.

Careers in clinical biochemistry

http://www.acb.org.uk/site/ clinscicareers.asp

This section of the Association of Clinical Biochemists website contains some useful pointers for those considering a career in clinical science. The website contains several useful links for an insight into the career path of a clinical biochemist.

http://www.rcpath.org/index. asp?PageID=411

This page from the Royal College of Pathologists website contains a very useful description of a career in Chemical Pathology written by Dr William Marshall. There is also a number of links to training programmes for medical and science graduates interested in a career in Clinical Biochemistry.

Index